Molecular and Translational Medicine

Series Editors
William B. Coleman
Gregory J. Tsongalis

For further volumes:
http://www.springer.com/series/8176

W. Edward Highsmith, Jr.
Editor

Molecular Diagnostics

12 Tests That Changed Everything

Humana Press

Editor
W. Edward Highsmith, Jr.
Department of Laboratory Medicine and Pathology
Mayo Clinic College of Medicine
Rochester, MN, USA

ISBN 978-1-4939-4265-7 ISBN 978-1-4614-8127-0 (eBook)
DOI 10.1007/978-1-4614-8127-0
Springer New York Heidelberg Dordrecht London

Softcover reprint of the hardcover 1st edition 2014

Printed on acid-free paper

Humana Press is a brand of Springer
Springer is part of Springer Science+Business Media (www.springer.com)

Foreword: From Molecular Pathology to Genomic Pathology

Since the first report of PCR in 1985, a new discipline has evolved within laboratory medicine based on detecting nucleotide sequences in clinical samples. This discipline was first designated "molecular pathology" in David Weatherall's book "The New Genetics and Clinical Practice" where he wrote "(D)uring the last few years there have been remarkable advances in molecular biology…(that) have been applied to the study of human genes, both in health and disease. It is now possible to define many diseases in terms of their *molecular pathology*, a level of diagnostic precision that would have been undreamed of 10 years ago."

Molecular diagnostic testing has changed the practice of laboratory medicine and, thus, affected the practice of many of the medical specialties that utilize these test results. In each of the categories in this book—Infectious Disease, Oncology, Genetics—the authors describe how the advent of molecular testing protocols has changed medical practice, giving credence to the title "12 Tests that Changed Everything." But probably the most significant area of change is discussed in the final section—Future Directions—because the very nature of technology is forward thinking. And thinking forward in molecular diagnostics must include Next Generation (NextGen) Sequencing.

While the term *Molecular Pathology* is used in the context of applying molecular tools to existing disciplines, such as infectious disease, hematopathology, or genetics, *Genomic Pathology* truly represents the essence of "personalized medicine," where specific alterations in an individual's human genome, transcriptome, or proteome lead to alterations in therapeutics and improved outcomes. For example, recently new interventions were described for cystic fibrosis and Duchenne muscular dystrophy in which patients with specific mutations were treated with individualized therapeutics.

In the succeeding chapters, we will see how CMA (chromosomal microarrays, which replaces aCGH, or array comparative genomic hybridization) and FISH have transformed conventional cytogenetics into cytogenomics. Newer SNP microarrays detect homozygosity in addition to CNV's (copy number variants), parameters which are leading to expanded understanding of heritable disorders. Perhaps the most dramatic case for "personalized medicine" is in the area of oncology, both hematological and solid organ malignancies. In the chapters on Cancer PGx, EGFR, and Her2, sequence-specific analyses are tied to individualized therapeutics, similar to the examples described above for cystic fibrosis and Duchenne muscular dystrophy. Using various techniques, Her2 amplification is intimately tied to Herceptin treatment. Monitoring therapy in leukemias by assessing the level of novel fusion proteins via their respective transcripts has become the standard of practice in CML. Reports of recent success in AML, ALL, and APML are tied to NextGen sequencing of individual translocation breakpoints followed by quantitative assessment of fusion proteins (or their transcripts). We have had a longer time to evaluate the heritable breast/ovarian cancer genes, BRCA 1 and 2, and the effect that genetic counseling has had in providing options for mutation positive patients and their families. Other solid tumor susceptibility genes provide similar scenarios. But the majority of malignancies are not heritable; for these, the ability to use targeted NextGen sequencing panels that encompass multiple genes provides an attractive approach for *Genomic Pathology*.

The management of patients with infectious diseases has been an area where significant changes have been seen in detection, identification, epidemiological surveillance, and treatment as exemplified in the chapter on HSV in CSF. The exquisite sensitivity of PCR allows molecular methods to replace many conventional culture-based identification methods, for both bacterial and viral organisms. Of course, viral loads in hepatitis and HIV have improved monitoring while viral genotyping allows matching of specific subtypes with more efficacious drugs.

There are some obvious dramatic improvements directly related to molecular techniques. Blood bank screening using molecular techniques, or NAT (nucleic acid testing), is now standard practice and represents a major success story in making the blood supply safe from infectious agents. Furthermore, molecular techniques are being used for genotyping as an alternative or adjunct to conventional antibody-based blood group typing.

In the NBS (newborn screening) arena, tandem mass spectrometry, with molecular confirmation, is performed in many, if not most, states today. Tomorrow, the potential for NBS DNA sequencing (either whole exome or whole genome) begs the (ELSI) questions of ethical, legal, and societal issues—not only what we test for but how we handle the information. Added to this paradigm is the bioinformatics issue which needs to be addressed, not only for NBS but also for NextGen sequencing in general. But as molecular techniques have been adopted into clinical practice, this has been a recurring story. We haven't always had answers at the time, but the speed of technological advances hasn't slowed.

Charlottesville, VA, USA Lawrence M. Silverman

Preface

When I was asked by my friends and colleagues, Drs. Greg J. Tsongalis and Bill Coleman, to edit a book in their series on Molecular Medicine, I was, of course, quite flattered. But that feeling changed fairly quickly to one of disquiet—because I did not know what subject to try and explore in a book format. Most of the things that I have spent the past 20 or so years doing—technology development, genotype–phenotype correlations in genetic disease, and laboratory management—had all been covered by a number of books and reviews, and I was not sure that the world needed more on these topics.

The advent of next generation sequencing (NGS), and the surrounding excitement and predictions that it will "change everything," made me think of the last time a new technology was introduced into clinical laboratories with the breathless predictions that it would "change everything." That technology, of course, was the polymerase chain reaction or PCR. Just as we are seeing with NGS, whole scientific meetings were almost completely devoted to symposium after symposium about PCR and what had been and could be accomplished with its use. Indeed, new organizations were created to provide forums for physicians and scientists to share knowledge about this new application of molecular biology and molecular pathology.

I thought that the book that I would like to read would be one that looked at the question of whether the introduction of PCR did indeed "change everything." One could call it a quality control step, assessing how well we are able to predict which technologies will be transformative in laboratory medicine. With respect to PCR, I think we hit the bull's-eye with the majority of the predictions. It did "change everything." The fields of infectious disease, genetics, and oncology have all been transformed over the past years by the introduction of molecular testing methods in the clinical laboratory. And, I have no doubt that the next decade will see further transformations as new methods such as chromosome arrays and massively parallel sequencing begin to be used for patient care.

Although superficially, there may appear to be little in common between HIV testing, cystic fibrosis carrier screening, EGFR genotyping, and many of the other topics of this volume, I believe that they all follow a common theme—they were all developed in response to a clinical need, and developed from the same toolkit. The majority of molecular pathology laboratories in the USA offer tests in all of the three primary areas of molecular pathology: infectious disease, oncology, and genetics. This is not a volume about the history of molecular testing. Indeed, all of the clinical laboratory tests addressed in this volume are the cornerstones of the modern molecular diagnostics laboratory, and their use is transforming and improving the lives of countless patients in the USA and around the world. Thus, I hope that this volume will be useful to molecular pathologists, clinical laboratory directors, genetics/pathology residents/fellows, and clinical laboratory science students.

In order to focus on the similarities rather than the differences with these tests, I asked the chapter authors to follow the same format for each of the topics. I asked that the following subheadings be used:

Background on the Test
Clinical Applications
Methodology
Standard Reagents
Regulatory Issues
Interpretation
How the Test(s) Have Changed Medical Practice
Future Directions

Although there is some variability, the authors have all followed this plan. It is our hope that a similar format will be advantageous for the reader.

The topics selected for this book may seem somewhat arbitrary and subjective, since there are many areas besides these that have had molecular tests that truly changed how medicine is practiced. The selections were mine alone—and I take responsibility for the many omissions. A quick count of the number of chapters reveals 13 chapters in a book entitled "12 Tests that Changed Everything." The last chapter addresses a technology that has not yet, but almost undoubtedly will, change everything—again. As there are many unanswered questions in the field of clinical NGS regarding many of the topics that the first 12 authors were asked to address as subheadings, the final chapter does not adhere to this organization.

In selecting authors for the various topics that I wanted to cover, I followed the advice of Chef Duff, star of The Ace of Cakes on the Food Network. He said that after finishing school, he wanted to open a bakery that would do innovative things that had not been done before, so "…I hired the most creative bunch of people I know. My friends." Although I knew several of the chapter authors in this volume only by reputation (and now by e-mail), a large number are indeed my friends, from either professional organizations or institutions where we were employed together. To all of the chapter authors—a heartfelt thank you. I think we have put together something here to be proud of.

Rochester, MN, USA W. Edward Highsmith, Jr.

Contents

Contributors

Karim M. Abdel-Hady, B.Sc. Yousef Jameel Science & Technology Research Center, The American University in Cairo, AUC Avenue, New Cairo, Egypt

Swaroop Aradhya, Ph.D. Neurogenetics, Array Services, Genedx, Gaithersburg, MD, USA

Umut Aypar, Ph.D. Department of Laboratory Medicine and Pathology, Mayo Clinic, Rochester, MN, USA

Hassan M.E. Azzazy, Ph.D. Department of Chemistry, The American University in Cairo, New Cairo, Egypt

Yousef Jameel Science & Technology Research Center, The American University in Cairo, New Cairo, Egypt

Matthew J. Binnicker, Ph.D. Division of Clinical Microbiology, Department of Laboratory Medicine and Pathology, Mayo Clinic, Rochester, MN, USA

John Logan Black III, M.D. Nucleotide Polymorphism Laboratory, Division of Clinical Biochemistry and Immunology, Department of Laboratory Medicine and Pathology, Mayo Clinic, Rochester, MN, USA

Karla R. Bowles, Ph.D. Myriad Genetic Laboratories, Inc., Salt Lake City, UT, USA

Niel T. Constantine, Ph.D., M.T. (A.S.C.P.) Department of Pathology, University of Maryland School of Medicine, Baltimore, MD, USA

Anna DeMarinis, M.A., M.T.(A.S.C.P.)S.B.B., C.Q.A.(A.S.Q.) The DeMarinis Group, LLC, North Attleborough, MA, USA

Mark J. Espy, M.S. Division of Clinical Microbiology, Department of Laboratory Medicine and Pathology, Mayo Clinic, Rochester, MN, USA

Matthew J. Ferber, Ph.D. Molecular Genetics Laboratory, Department of Laboratory Medicine and Pathology, Mayo Clinic, College of Medicine, Rochester, MN, USA

Kevin C. Halling, M.D., Ph.D. Department of Laboratory Medicine and Pathology, Molecular Anatomic Pathology and Molecular Genetics Laboratories, Mayo Clinic, Rochester, MN, USA

W. Edward Highsmith Jr., Ph.D. Molecular Genetics Laboratory, Department of Laboratory Medicine and Pathology, Mayo Clinic College of Medicine, Rochester, MN, USA

Sean Hofherr, Ph.D. Laboratory Medicine, Children's National Medical Center, Washington, DC, USA

Nicole Hoppman, Ph.D. Clinical Cytogenetics Laboratory, Department of Laboratory Medicine and Pathology, Mayo Clinic College of Medicine, Rochester, MN, USA

Hutton Kearney, Ph.D., F.A.C.M.G. Cytogenetics, Mission Health Hospital, Asheville, NC, USA

Benjamin R. Kipp, Ph.D. Department of Laboratory Medicine and Pathology, Molecular Anatomic Pathology and Molecular Genetics Laboratories, Mayo Clinic, Rochester, MN, USA

Eric W. Klee, Ph.D. Division of Biomedical Informatics, Department of Health Sciences Research, Mayo Clinic, College of Medicine, Rochester, MN, USA

Neal I. Lindeman, M.D. Molecular Diagnostics Laboratory, Harvard Medical School, Brigham and Women's Hospital, Boston, MA, USA

Christa Martin, Ph.D. Emory Genetics Laboratory, Emory University, Atlanta, GA, USA

Joseph Ntumbong Nkeze, M.S. Department of Pathology, University of Maryland School of Medicine, Baltimore, MD, USA

Devin Oglesbee, Ph.D. Laboratory Genetics, Mayo Clinic, Rochester, MN, USA

Department of Laboratory Medicine and Pathology, Mayo Clinic, Rochester, MN, USA

Department of Medical Genetics, Mayo Clinic, Rochester, MN, USA

Eric Rosenthal, Ph.D., Sc.M. Myriad Genetic Laboratories, Inc., Salt Lake City, UT, USA

Ahmed Saleh, Ph.D. Department of Pathology and Institute of Human Virology, University of Maryland School of Medicine, Baltimore, MD, USA

Faculty of Science, Zoology Department, Cairo University, Cairo, Egypt

Lawrence M. Silverman, Ph.D. Department of Pathology, University of Virginia, Charlottesville, VA, USA

David I. Smith, Ph.D. Division of Experimental Pathology, Department of Laboratory Medicine and Pathology, Mayo Clinic, College of Medicine, Rochester, MN, USA

Thomas F. Smith, Ph.D. Division of Clinical Microbiology, Department of Laboratory Medicine and Pathology, Mayo Clinic, Rochester, MN, USA

Sarah South, Ph.D. ARUP Laboratories, Department of Pediatrics, University of Utah, Salt Lake City, UT, USA

Laura J. Tafe, M.D. Department of Pathology and the Geisel School of Medicine at Dartmouth, Dartmouth-Hitchcock Medical Center, Lebanon, NH, USA

Eric C. Thorland, Ph.D. Clinical Cytogenetics Laboratory, Department of Laboratory Medicine and Pathology, Mayo Clinic, Rochester, MN, USA

Gregory J. Tsongalis, Ph.D., F.A.C.B, H.C.L.D., C.C. Department of Pathology, Geisel School of Medicine at Dartmouth, Dartmouth Hitchcock Medical Center and Norris Cotton Cancer Center, Lebanon, NH, USA

Patricia A. Wright, B.A., M.T.(A.S.C.P.)S.B.B. Signature Healthcare-Brockton Hospital, Brockton, MA, USA

Richard Y. Zhao, Ph.D. Department of Pathology, University of Maryland School of Medicine, Baltimore, MD, USA

Department of Microbiology and Immunology, University of Maryland School of Medicine, Baltimore, MD, USA

Part I

Oncology

Clinical FISH Testing for the Diagnosis of Solid Tumors

1

Benjamin R. Kipp and Kevin C. Halling

Background

Cancer genomes contain numerical and structural somatic alterations, including single base substitutions, structural rearrangements, small insertions, small deletions, and copy number variation [1, 2]. Theodor Boveri, a German zoologist, is credited for first describing the association between numerical chromosome anomalies and cancer in his 1914 monograph *Concerning the Origin of Malignant Tumours* [3]. Nearly a century has passed since this sentinel paper and cancer biologists are still trying to better understand aneuploidy and its role in carcinogenesis. Recent large-scale DNA copy number analyses of tumors highlight how common aneuploidy is in malignant tumors. Beroukhim and colleagues [1] evaluated 3,131 tumors comprising 26 different tumor types and identified, on average, 24 gains (median = 12) and 18 losses (median = 12) for each tumor. In addition, approximately 17 % of the genome was amplified and 16 % was deleted in a typical cancer specimen.

B.R. Kipp, Ph.D. (✉) • K.C. Halling, M.D., Ph.D.
Department of Laboratory Medicine and Pathology, Molecular Anatomic Pathology and Molecular Genetics Laboratories, Mayo Clinic, Rochester, MN, USA
e-mail: kipp.benjamin@mayo.edu

Fluorescence in situ hybridization (FISH) is a technique that uses fluorescently labeled DNA probes to detect chromosomal abnormalities in peripheral blood, paraffin-embedded tissue, or cytology specimens. Since tumor cells generally contain chromosomal alterations, FISH is able to detect cells that have chromosomal abnormalities consistent with neoplasia. Different types of DNA probes can be designed to target different chromosomal alterations including aneuploidy, deletions, amplifications, and translocations. Centromere enumeration probes (CEP) are designed to target highly repetitive human α-satellite DNA sequences (171 base pair repeats) located near the centromeres of individual chromosomes. These probes are used to enumerate the number of copies of a given chromosome in an individual cell. Locus-specific identifier (LSI) probes are designed to hybridize to specific chromosomal regions and can detect chromosomal loss (e.g., *CDKN2A*, *TP53*), gains/amplifications (e.g., *EGFR*, *HER2*), or translocations (e.g., *EML4-ALK*, *BCR-ABL*). LSI probes are becoming more popular because in addition to diagnosing cancer, alterations in specific genes (e.g., HER2 amplification) help predict whether a patient will respond to a targeted therapy (e.g., Herceptin). This chapter will focus on the diagnosis of solid tumors by FISH and discuss how this technique has changed clinical practice over the past decade.

W.E. Highsmith Jr. (ed.), *Molecular Diagnostics: 12 Tests That Changed Everything*, Molecular and Translational Medicine, DOI 10.1007/978-1-4614-8127-0_1,

Clinical Applications

FISH for Bladder Cancer Detection

Bladder cancer is estimated to account for 73,510 new cases and 14,880 deaths in 2012 [4]. Most patients with bladder cancer present with painless and intermittent hematuria. However, only 10–20 % of patients with gross hematuria and 2–5 % with microscopic hematuria will actually have bladder cancer [5]. The diagnostic work-up for patients with bladder cancer includes initial cystoscopy followed by biopsy or resection of suspicious lesions, urine cytology, and upper urinary tract evaluation. Urine cytology complements cystoscopy in that it can detect tumors that are not visible by cystoscopy. However, urine cytology has relatively poor sensitivity for detecting bladder cancer, especially low-grade tumors. The reported combined sensitivity of cytology for grade 1, 2, and 3 tumors has been shown to be 21, 53, and 78 %, respectively [6]. Because urine cytology suffers from low sensitivity, numerous tumors markers have been investigated to help increase the diagnostic sensitivity [5].

FISH testing has become an excellent tool for overcoming some of the limitations of cytology. Much of the success of FISH testing for the diagnosis of solid tumors can be attributed to the FISH UroVysion assay™ (Abbott Molecular, Abbott Park, IL), which was the first commercially available FISH probe set for the detection of bladder cancer. In 2000, Sokolova et al. published the first manuscript describing UroVysion, a four-target, multicolor FISH probe set containing CEP probes targeting chromosomes 3, 7, and 17 and an LSI probe targeting 9p21 [7]. Halling et al. published a study later that year, which was the first to demonstrate the clinical utility of this probe set. This study evaluated urine from 265 patients being evaluated for bladder cancer and found that the overall sensitivity of FISH for detecting bladder cancer (81 %) was significantly higher than urine cytology (59 %) [6]. Two FDA trials followed, the first published by Sarosdy et al. in 2002, which led to the FDA approval of UroVysion for the detection of recurrent bladder cancer [8]. The second trial was published in 2006 and led to the FDA approval of UroVysion for the detection of bladder cancer in patients with gross or microscopic hematuria and no history of bladder cancer [9]. Numerous follow-up studies have compared the sensitivity and specificity of FISH to urine cytology and have consistently shown that FISH is more sensitive than cytology for all grades and stages of urothelial carcinoma. A meta-analysis evaluating 14 different studies found that the sensitivity of FISH and cytology for detecting bladder cancer was 72 and 42 %, while the specificity of FISH and cytology was 83 and 96 %, respectively [10].

There are several additional clinical indications for UroVysion testing [11]. Multiple reports have suggested that FISH can help identify which patients with equivocal cytology diagnoses (atypical or suspicious) are most likely to have bladder cancer [12–16]. The clinical management of patients with equivocal cytology diagnoses is challenging because fewer than half of these patients will have bladder cancer on clinical follow-up. This can lead to unnecessary and expensive clinical investigations [17]. Multiple studies now suggest that patients with an equivocal cytology and positive FISH result are at very high risk for having bladder cancer and should be followed more aggressively [12–16]. FISH is also useful for assessing patients undergoing bacillus Calmette–Guerin (BCG) treatment for noninvasive bladder cancer. A 2005 study by Kipp et al. found that patients with a positive FISH result following intravesical therapy were 4.6 times more likely to have recurrent bladder cancer and 9.4 times more likely to have follow-up muscle-invasive bladder cancer than patients with a negative FISH result [18]. Similar results were obtained by Mengual et al. [19] and Savic et al. [20], who found that patients with a positive post-BCG FISH result had 3.0 and 3.8 times higher risk of tumor recurrence, respectively. Although other tumor markers are currently available for diagnosing bladder cancer (e.g., BTA-STAT, NMP22), due to its high sensitivity and specificity, FISH with the UroVysion probe set continues to be one of the most commonly used molecular markers for detecting this type of cancer in urine cytology specimens.

FISH for the Detection of Pancreatobiliary Tract Malignancy

Hepatobiliary and pancreatic cancers represent over 82,000 newly diagnosed cancers a year in the USA, with pancreatic cancers and liver cancers representing the majority of these cases [4]. Although carcinomas of the pancreatobiliary tract ducts (pancreatic adenocarcinoma or cholangiocarcinoma) comprise only a small fraction of these malignancies, they are often lethal and can occur anywhere along the hepatic and common bile duct system [21]. An earlier diagnosis of pancreatobiliary tract malignancy is critical because it may allow for surgical resection of a tumor. It may also allow patients to become candidates for neoadjuvant chemoradiotherapy followed by a liver transplant, which has shown to decrease mortality in patients with cholangiocarcinoma [22]. However, differentiating pancreatobiliary tract malignancies from nonmalignant etiologies such as primary sclerosing cholangitis, choledocholithiasis, chronic pancreatitis, and surgical trauma can be difficult because pancreatobiliary tumors often grow longitudinally along the bile duct and do not generally present as large masses [23, 24]. Due to the difficulty of obtaining adequate biopsies within the pancreatobiliary ducts, routine cytology brushings or washings are often collected for diagnosing malignancy. Unfortunately, routine cytology has relatively poor sensitivity for detecting malignancy in biliary tract specimens with reports ranging from 6 to 80 %, and many reported sensitivities below 50 % [24–27].

In 2004, our group evaluated the value of FISH and the UroVysion probe set for detecting malignancy using pancreatobiliary tract brushing and bile specimens collected during endoscopic retrograde cholangiopancreatography [28]. Although the UroVysion probe set was not specifically tailored for the detection of pancreatobiliary tract tumors, we found that FISH improved the detection of these tumors when compared to routine cytology. Based on these data, we implemented FISH and the UroVysion probe set as a clinical assay in late 2004. Subsequent reports from our group and others confirmed that FISH is a valuable ancillary test for the evaluation of cytologic specimens obtained from pancreatobiliary tract strictures [23, 29–31]. Fritcher et al. [23] published the most comprehensive study evaluating the role of FISH in the detection of pancreatobiliary tract malignancy. This study included 500 patients undergoing clinical evaluation for suspicious pancreatobiliary tract strictures with clinical cytology and FISH results, as well as extensive clinicopathologic follow-up. The results of this study showed that the sensitivity of FISH was significantly higher than cytology (43 % vs. 20 %, $P<0.001$) for detecting malignancy. This study also found that a patient with a polysomy FISH result was over 77 times more likely to have malignancy than a patient with a negative FISH result. Based on these data, it has become routine practice at our institution to perform both routine cytology and FISH on all pancreatibiliary tract brushing specimens from indeterminate pancreatobiliary strictures when there is a suspicion for carcinoma.

FISH for the Detection of Lung Cancer

Cytology (brushings and washings) and biopsy specimens collected during flexible bronchoscopy are used for the diagnosis of suspected lung cancer in patients with indeterminate pulmonary nodules and endobronchial lesions. The overall diagnostic sensitivity of routine cytology bronchial brushing and washing specimens ranges from 44 to 94 % (mean, 72 %) and 27 to 90 % (mean, 68 %), respectively [32]. Peripheral lung tumors are more difficult to diagnose than centrally located tumors by cytology, with sensitivities ranging from 6 to 83 % (mean, 45 %) in brushings and 4 to 43 % (mean, 28 %) in washings [32]. In addition, the size of the tumor is also important with smaller tumors being more difficult to detect [33]. Data suggest that there remains a clinical need for a molecular marker such as FISH to increase detection rates in small (<2 cm in diameter) peripherally located tumors, where the combined sensitivity of bronchoscopic techniques has been reported to be 34 %, compared to 63 % for larger (>2 cm) tumors [33].

Sokolova et al. have been credited for publishing the first DNA-based FISH probe set to be used clinically to improve the detection of lung cancer on cytology specimens [34]. This FISH probe set (originally called LAVysion, Abbott Molecular, Inc.) consisted of locus specific probes to 5p15, 7p12 (*EGFR*), 8q24 (*C-MYC*), and a CEP to chromosome 1. However, it was suggested in this manuscript that it would be advantageous to substitute CEP6 for CEP1 due to staining quality. Several subsequent studies have evaluated the clinical utility of this FISH probe set (with CEP 6) and have shown that FISH increases the sensitivity of lung cancer detection when combined with routine cytology, as compared to routine cytology alone, while maintaining high specificity [35–40]. Two of the larger studies [35, 36] evaluating this FISH probe revealed similar sensitivity (61–65 %) and specificity (92–95 %) using RC and FISH on brushing specimens. In addition, these studies suggest that FISH may be helpful in detecting early stage and peripheral lung cancers that are difficult to detect using conventional cytology. Subsequent studies by Savic et al. and Schramm et al. have also shown that FISH may be particularly useful in patients with equivocal (atypical or suspicious) cytology results [37, 38].

A recent study by our group [40] found that FISH significantly increased the detection of lung cancer using a reflex algorithm in routine clinical practice. In this algorithm, routine cytology, which is relatively inexpensive and has high specificity, is initially performed. Specimens not found to be positive for cancer (i.e., negative, atypical and suspicious) by routine cytology are then sent on for FISH analysis. Based on data from nearly 300 specimens using this algorithm, FISH detected 32 % more peripheral lung cancers than routine cytology alone. The FISH test was most beneficial for detecting small (<2 cm), peripheral cancers where FISH detected 15 cancers (44 %) that were not detected by cytology.

Other FISH probe sets have also been evaluated with similar success. A group from MD Anderson designed and evaluated a probe set comprising chromosomal loci 3p22.1 (containing the *GC20*, *RPL 14*, *CD39A*, and *PMGB*) and 10q22.3 (surfactant protein A gene, *SP-A*) and showed that loss of either of these chromosomal loci by FISH, when combined with cytologic atypia, is more sensitive than cytology alone for diagnosing lung cancer in sputum specimens [41, 42]. Liu et al. [43] recently developed a FISH assay with probes targeting chromosomes 3, 7, and 8. In their study, the overall sensitivity of FISH on brushing specimens when combined with routine cytology was significantly higher (95 % vs. 76 %; $P<0.001$) than routine cytology alone and detected more squamous cell carcinomas and late stage tumors. However, as with any diagnostic molecular assay, all these new FISH probe sets will need to be validated using specimens from the intended patient population to determine their true clinical utility. In addition, these FISH lung assays should be evaluated as part of a testing algorithm that includes bronchoscopic biopsy, bronchial brushing routine cytology, and other bronchoscopic methods currently used in clinical practice.

FISH Barrett's Esophagus Associated Neoplasia

Barrett's esophagus (BE) is a pre-neoplastic condition in which the squamous epithelium of the distal esophagus undergoes transformation to intestinal metaplasia. Patients with BE have up to a 60-fold increased risk of developing esophageal carcinoma when compared to the general population [44, 45]. Current American College of Gastroenterologists guidelines suggest that patients with BE undergo routine surveillance for the detection of dysplasia or malignancy which includes the collection of four-quadrant biopsy specimens every 1–2 cm of affected esophagus [44]. Limitations to this procedure are that it is time consuming and results in a large number of biopsies. Brush cytology has been suggested as an alternative to endoscopic biopsy since cytology can collect cells from a larger surface area in less time than it takes to collect the numerous biopsies suggested by practice guidelines [46]. Unfortunately, cytology has limited sensitivity for detecting dysplasia or malignancy because it can be difficult to differentiate reactive epithelium from dysplasia by routine cytology and because the cytologic features of early dysplastic cells are not significantly different from non-neoplastic Barrett's cells [47].

As with the other body sites discussed in this chapter, FISH has been shown to increase the sensitivity of detecting esophageal dysplasia and cancer over routine cytology alone [44, 46, 47–51]. Recent studies at our institution suggest that a probe set consisting of probes to 8q24, 9p21, 17q11.2, and 20q13.2 has high sensitivity and specificity for the detection of BE-associated dysplasia and esophageal adenocarcinoma [44]. Fritcher et al. evaluated this four-probe set and found that FISH was significantly more sensitive than routine cytology for detecting low-grade dysplasia, high-grade dysplasia, and adenocarcinoma in patients with BE [49]. The specificity of cytology, digital image analysis, and FISH among patients ($n = 14$) with tissue showing only benign squamous mucosa was 93, 86, and 100 % ($P = 0.22$), respectively. In addition, all 33 patients with a polysomic FISH result had HGD and/or EA within 6 months of the FISH test. Similar results were published by Rygiel et al. who concluded that this probe set (with the exception that the *P16* probe was removed) was useful for predicting BE patients at risk for developing high-grade dysplasia and adenocarcinoma [50].

Methodology

FISH can be performed on many different types of specimens including peripheral blood, paraffin-embedded tissue, and cytology specimens that are fresh or processed with standard (i.e., formalin, ethanol, etc.) or commercially available fixatives [52]. A number of different FISH protocols have been used for clinical testing with varied success. The steps involved in FISH analysis of tissue specimens can be divided into specimen collection, cell harvest, slide preparation, prehybridization, hybridization, washing, and microscopic analysis. Detailed protocols for preparing specimens for clinical testing can be found in previous publications [28, 34, 39] or package inserts from FISH probe kits. In general, the process begins by placing the collected cells or tissue on a glass slide for prehybridization. Prehybridization is a series of chemical treatments of the specimen that enables the FISH probes to efficiently hybridize to their cellular targets without disrupting cell morphology. This includes treatment with a protease such as pepsin to increase the accessibility of the probe to DNA. This is an important step in the process because overdigestion can lead to a decrease in FISH signal intensity and underdigestion can result in inefficient hybridization which makes it difficult to determine the true number of FISH signals in a cell. Following prehybridization, cellular DNA and FISH probe DNA are denatured and the FISH probes are allowed to hybridized to their cellular DNA targets. FISH hybridization is generally performed by placing approximately 1–10 μL of FISH probe on the cells being interrogated, placing a coverslip on top of this area, sealing the edges of the coverslip with rubber cement to prevent dehydration of the probe, and placing the slide in either a humidified chamber or a programmable temperature controlled slide processing system such as the ThermoBrite® Denaturation/Hybridization System (Abbott Molecular, Inc., Des Plaines, IL) [52].

Depending on the specimen being hybridized, co-denaturation of probe and target DNA is performed at approximately 70–75 °C for 3–5 min. The slides are then allowed to incubate at 37 °C overnight. After a minimum of 4 h hybridization time (preferably 8–16 h), slides are washed in a detergent such as 0.4× SSC/0.3 % NP-40 to remove nonspecifically bound probe. A fluorescent nuclear counterstain, such as 4′6′-diamidino-2-phenylindole (DAPI; Abbott Molecular, Inc., Des Plaines, IL) is then placed on the slide and the slide is coverslipped for analysis. Slides are microscopically assessed ("scanned") using a fluorescence microscope equipped with the appropriate filters that allow for visualization of the different colored fluorescent probes. FISH scanning and interpretation will be further discussed later in this chapter.

Regulatory Issues

Two Food and Drug Administration (FDA) trials have been conducted for UroVysion that evaluated different clinical claims for detecting bladder cancer [8, 9]. Minor deviations from the test packet have also been published with good results [11]. FDA trials have not been conducted for FISH probe use in diagnosing malignancies of the pancreatobiliary tract, lung, or Barrett's-associated neoplasia. Laboratories that offer laboratory developed FISH assays, i.e., assays that use non-FDA-approved specimens or methodologies that deviate from the FDA-approved methodology, need to comply with CLIA requirements, and should perform appropriate validation studies before using these tests clinically. This would include establishing test accuracy, precision, analytical sensitivity, analytical specificity, reference range, and reportable range. General recommendations on what is required for the validation of laboratory developed tests have recently been published [53]. In addition, a paper that specifically discusses how to go about validating a lab-developed FISH assay has been published [54]. However, this publication described the validation of a FISH assay that is used to detect MLL rearrangements for leukemia in paraffin-embedded specimens and consequently their may be some differences in the specifics of how to go about validating a FISH assay that is used for the detection of malignant cells in cytologic specimens. The CAP Molecular Pathology checklist also has a useful section that describes many of the regulatory requirments for FISH assays. For instance, the CAP checklist indicates that at least one photograph of a representative normal cell (with FISH signals captured) be kept as part of the

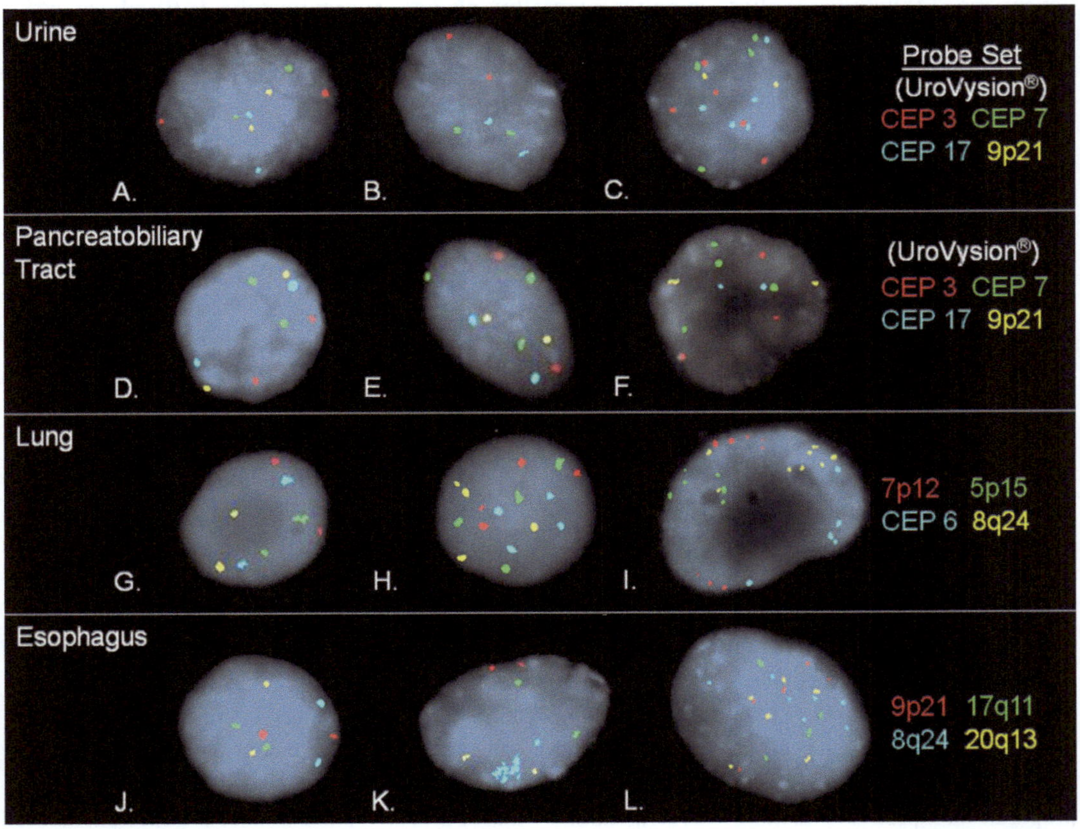

Fig. 1.1 Representative examples of FISH signal patterns observed in cytologic specimens from urine and brushing specimens from bile duct, lung, and esophagus. Normal (disomic) signal patterns (**a**, **d**, **g**, **j**), homozygous 9p21 loss (**b**), tetrasomy (**h**), polysomy (**c**, **f**, **i**, **l**), hypertetrasomy (**i**), trisomy 7 (**e**), and isolated gain (amplification) of 8q24 (**k**)

laboratory record for cases interpreted as normal, whereas at least two pictures be captured and documented for specimens with abnormal results.

Test Interpretation

Subsequent to specimen processing and hybridization, FISH signals are assessed using a fluorescence microscope equipped with the appropriate filters necessary to enumerate specific probe fluororphores. Non-neoplastic cells generally show two copies for each of the FISH probes since each probe targets the two alleles in an individual cell (Fig. 1.1). Occasionally, normal cells will show only one copy of a probe due to signal overlap or incomplete hybridization. Specimens are interpreted as abnormal when the number of cells demonstrating losses or gains of probes exceeds thresholds established in normal value studies. The scanning procedure used to identify aneuploid cells by FISH in cytologic specimens primarily focuses on assessing signal patterns in cells that appear morphologically abnormal (irregular nuclear shape, large nuclei, mottled nuclear staining) with the DAPI nuclear counterstain [55, 56]. Cells with abnormal appearing morphology by the DAPI counterstain are further assessed using the fluorescence microscope filters. Cells with abnormal FISH signal patterns are recorded and if the number of cells with these patterns exceeds predetermined cutoffs, the case is interpreted as abnormal. As illustrated in Fig. 1.1, numerous types of aneuploidy or chromosomal abnormalities are identified by FISH including polysomy (gains of two or more of the four probes in a cell), tetrasomy (four signals for all four probes), trisomy or single gain (gain of a single probe with two or fewer copies of the other probes), and homozygous loss (complete loss of both probes from an individual target). Each of these types of abnormalities can be identified with different FISH probe sets.

Thresholds for different types of chromosomal abnormality depend on the body site and probe set used [55]. In urine specimens that are being evaluated for bladder cancer with UroVysion, two primary types of chromosomal abnormalities are observed, polysomy and homozygous 9p21 (Fig. 1.1). The finding of polysomy generally correlates with the presence of a high-grade tumor, whereas homozygous 9p21 loss often suggests the presence of a low-grade papillary tumor [57]. There are potential pitfalls that one must avoid when interpreting urine specimens by FISH. Urine specimens can contain a wide variety of nonmalignant entities that can impede interpretation such as inflammatory cells, bacteria, proteinaceous debris, sperm, crystals, and lubricant [56]. It is generally still possible to interpret the FISH signals when one or more of these entities are present. However, there are instances where these entities obscure a majority of the epithelial cells causing the specimen to be uninterpretable. These specimens should be interpreted as nondiagnostic. Caution should also be used when evaluating urine specimens from patients receiving immunosuppressive therapy to prevent kidney rejection following transplantation, since these patients can harbor BK virus infected epithelial cells. Data from our group show that BK virus infection can be a rare cause of false-positive FISH results in patients with extremely high titers of the BK virus in their urine [58].

Although biliary and urinary tract specimens are both evaluated with the UroVysion probe set, there are differences in the types of FISH abnormalities that are observed for these two body sites. A large fraction of pancreatobiliary specimens with abnormality demonstrate trisomy 7 (three CEP 7 probes without gains in the other three probes; Fig. 1.1), while this is a rare finding in specimens from the urinary tract. A trisomy 7 result on pancreatobiliary tract specimens is considered an equivocal diagnosis, since only about 50 % of these patients will be diagnosed with malignancy on clinicopathologic follow-up [23]. Additionally, polysomic cells from urine often demonstrate high level gains of individual chromosomes (i.e., up to eight copies for each probe), while polysomic cells from the biliary tract cells infrequently demonstrate more than four or five signals for each of the four probes. However, independent of the degree of chromosomal gains observed, a polysomic result in either specimen is highly specific for malignancy [11, 23].

There are two main types of chromosomal abnormality observed in specimens being analyzed for lung cancer, hypertetrasomy and tetrasomy (Fig. 1.1). Hypertetrasomy refers to cells that show three or more copies in at least two of the four probes, with one or more of the probes exhibiting at least five copies. Tetrasomy is defined as four (or possibly three due to signal overlap) copies of the probe set for each of the probes. This distinction is important because a previous study suggests that 88, 53, and 37 % of patients with a hypertetrasomy, tetrasomy, and negative FISH result, respectively, were found to have lung cancer when FISH was performed on specimens diagnosed as negative or equivocal by routine cytology [40]. These data suggest that a hypertetrasomy FISH result is more specific and therefore more suggestive of lung cancer than a tetrasomy FISH result.

The methodology used to assess esophageal brushing cytology specimens by FISH, and the respective chromosomal abnormalities, is different than what has been described for other body sites. Multiple different chromosomal abnormalities may be observed in esophageal specimens including 9p21 chromosomal loss, single chromosome gain, amplification, and polysomy (Fig. 1.1). A previous report shows that microscopic FISH analysis of esophageal brushing specimens can be carried out by enumerating 100 non-squamous epithelial cells and if the percentage of cells demonstrating chromosomal loss or gain exceeds normal value cutoffs, the case is interpreted as abnormal. However, if no abnormalities are observed in the 100 cell enumeration or if the only abnormality that is observed is 9p21 loss or single gain, then the remainder of the slide should be scanned for polysomic cells. If ≥4 polysomic cells are observed in that additional scan, the specimen should be diagnosed as abnormal [49]. Patient's whose samples exhibit polysomy are likely to have high-grade dysplasia or cancer, while patients with hemizygous or homozygous 9p21 loss alone are likely to have Barrett's esophagus without dysplasia or Barrett's esophagus with low-grade dysplasia [49]. In summary, analysis of specimens by FISH is different based on the probe set used, the diagnostic cutoff values, and the body site analyzed.

How the Test(s) Have Changed Medical Practice

Aneuploidy detection by FISH has revolutionized how we detect tumor cells in cytologic specimens. Nearly all studies to date have suggested that FISH has a significantly higher sensitivity than conventional cytology for the detection of tumor cells in most specimen types. The improved ability to detect tumor offers the possibility of providing therapy at earlier more treatable stages and can reduce healthcare costs by reducing the amount of clinical evaluation required to arrive at a diagnosis. FISH is more time consuming and expensive to perform than conventional cytology and therefore has not replaced cytology. But FISH has become an extremely important ancillary tool for diagnosing selected specimens in cytopathology and cytogenetic laboratories.

Future Directions

We have summarized the success of FISH for detecting aneuploidy in solid tumors and have discussed the role FISH has played in changing clinical practice. As scientists and clinicians forge ahead in the genome era, the technologies used to detect aneuploidy will likely change, and aneuploidy assessment of tumors will likely be just part of large-scale genome analyses of individual tumors including DNA and RNA mutations analyses and epigenetic interrogation. The role that aneuploidy plays in carcinogenesis will also continue to be an active area of research. A recent review article by Gordon et al. [59] discuss this topic in depth and highlight the importance of aneuploidy in cancer development. More importantly, aneuploidy has become a promising target for future cancer therapies. These therapies may target mechanisms involved in tumor cell chromosomal instability (e.g., mutations that trigger instability), target cellular responses to aneuploidy (e.g., targeting specific pathways such as ubiquitin–proteasome pathway), or target specific cancer cells with genetic dependencies owing to recurrent chromosomal gains or losses [59]. No matter what the strategy, future studies uncovering the genetic and epigenetic mysteries of solid tumor will transform what we know about these tumors and will hopefully shed light on how to cure and reduce the mortality associated with cancer.

Disclosure Drs. Kipp and Halling and the Mayo Clinic have patents and receive royalties from the sale of some of the FISH probes discussed in this study. They also receive grant funding from Abbott Molecular, Inc. to develop FISH assays for the detection of neoplastic cells in cytologic specimens.

References

1. Beroukhim R, Mermel CH, Porter D, Wei G, Raychaudhuri S, Donovan J, Barretina J, Boehm JS, Dobson J, Urashima M, Mc Henry KT, Pinchback RM, Ligon AH, Cho YJ, Haery L, Greulich H, Reich M, Winckler W, Lawrence MS, Weir BA, Tanaka KE, Chiang DY, Bass AJ, Loo A, Hoffman C, Prensner J, Liefeld T, Gao Q, Yecies D, Signoretti S, Maher E, Kaye FJ, Sasaki H, Tepper JE, Fletcher JA, Tabernero J, Baselga J, Tsao MS, Demichelis F, Rubin MA, Janne PA, Daly MJ, Nucera C, Levine RL, Ebert BL, Gabriel S, Rustgi AK, Antonescu CR, Ladanyi M, Letai A, Garraway LA, Loda M, Beer DG, True LD, Okamoto A, Pomeroy SL, Singer S, Golub TR, Lander ES, Getz G, Sellers WR, Meyerson M. The landscape of somatic copy-number alteration across human cancers. Nature. 2010;463:899–905.
2. DeVita VT, Lawrence TS, Rosenberg SA. Cancer: principles & practice of oncology: primer of the molecular biology of cancer. Philadelphia, PA: Lippincott Williams & Wilkins; 2011.
3. Weinberg RA. In retrospect: the chromosome trail. Nature. 2008;453:725.
4. Siegel R, Naishadham D, Jemal A. Cancer statistics, 2012. CA Cancer J Clin. 2012;62:10–29.
5. Tanaka MF, Sonpavde G. Diagnosis and management of urothelial carcinoma of the bladder. Postgrad Med. 2011;123:43–55.
6. Halling KC, King W, Sokolova IA, Meyer RG, Burkhardt HM, Halling AC, Cheville JC, Sebo TJ, Ramakumar S, Stewart CS, Pankratz S, O'Kane DJ, Seelig SA, Lieber MM, Jenkins RB. A comparison of cytology and fluorescence in situ hybridization for the detection of urothelial carcinoma. J Urol. 2000;164:1768–75.
7. Sokolova IA, Halling KC, Jenkins RB, Burkhardt HM, Meyer RG, Seelig SA, King W. The development of a multitarget, multicolor fluorescence in situ hybridization assay for the detection of urothelial carcinoma in urine. J Mol Diagn. 2000;2:116–23.
8. Sarosdy MF, Schellhammer P, Bokinsky G, Kahn P, Chao R, Yore L, Zadra J, Burzon D, Osher G, Bridge JA, Anderson S, Johansson SL, Lieber M, Soloway M, Flom K. Clinical evaluation of a multi-target fluorescent in situ hybridization assay for detection of bladder cancer. J Urol. 2002;168:1950–4.
9. Sarosdy MF, Kahn PR, Ziffer MD, Love WR, Barkin J, Abara EO, Jansz K, Bridge JA, Johansson SL, Persons DL, Gibson JS. Use of a multitarget fluorescence in situ hybridization assay to diagnose bladder cancer in patients with hematuria. J Urol. 2006;176: 44–7.
10. Hajdinjak T. Urovysion fish test for detecting urothelial cancers: meta-analysis of diagnostic accuracy and comparison with urinary cytology testing. Urol Oncol. 2008;26:646–51.
11. Halling KC, Kipp BR. Bladder cancer detection using fish (urovysion assay). Adv Anat Pathol. 2008;15:279–86.
12. Bubendorf L. Multiprobe fluorescence in situ hybridization (urovysion) for the detection of urothelial carcinoma - fishing for the right catch. Acta Cytol. 2011;55:113–9.
13. Huysentruyt CJ, Baldewijns MM, Ruland AM, Tonk RJ, Vervoort PS, Smits KM, van de Beek C, Speel EJ. Modified urovysion scoring criteria increase the urothelial carcinoma detection rate in cases of equivocal urinary cytology. Histopathology. 2011;58: 1048–53.
14. Kipp BR, Halling KC, Campion MB, Wendel AJ, Karnes RJ, Zhang J, Sebo TJ. Assessing the value of reflex fluorescence in situ hybridization testing in the diagnosis of bladder cancer when routine urine cytological examination is equivocal. J Urol. 2008;179: 1296–301. discussion 1301.
15. Lotan Y, Bensalah K, Ruddell T, Shariat SF, Sagalowsky AI, Ashfaq R. Prospective evaluation of the clinical usefulness of reflex fluorescence in situ hybridization assay in patients with atypical cytology for the detection of urothelial carcinoma of the bladder. J Urol. 2008;179:2164–9.
16. Schlomer BJ, Ho R, Sagalowsky A, Ashfaq R, Lotan Y. Prospective validation of the clinical usefulness of reflex fluorescence in situ hybridization assay in patients with atypical cytology for the detection of urothelial carcinoma of the bladder. J Urol. 2010; 183:62–7.
17. Voss JS, Kipp BR, Krueger AK, Clayton AC, Halling KC, Karnes RJ, Henry MR, Sebo TJ. Changes in specimen preparation method may impact urine cytologic evaluation. Am J Clin Pathol. 2008;130: 428–33.
18. Kipp BR, Karnes RJ, Brankley SM, Harwood AR, Pankratz VS, Sebo TJ, Blute MM, Lieber MM, Zincke H, Halling KC. Monitoring intravesical therapy for superficial bladder cancer using fluorescence in situ hybridization. J Urol. 2005;173:401–4.
19. Mengual L, Marin-Aguilera M, Ribal MJ, Burset M, Villavicencio H, Oliver A, Alcaraz A. Clinical utility of fluorescent in situ hybridization for the surveillance of bladder cancer patients treated with bacillus calmette-guerin therapy. Eur Urol. 2007;52:752–9.

20. Savic S, Zlobec I, Thalmann GN, Engeler D, Schmauss M, Lehmann K, Mattarelli G, Eichenberger T, Dalquen P, Spieler P, Schoenegg R, Gasser TC, Sulser T, Forster T, Zellweger T, Casella R, Bubendorf L. The prognostic value of cytology and fluorescence in situ hybridization in the follow-up of nonmuscle-invasive bladder cancer after intravesical bacillus calmette-guerin therapy. Int J Cancer. 2009;124:2899–904.
21. Alberts SR, Gores GJ, Kim GP, Roberts LR, Kendrick ML, Rosen CB, Chari ST, Martenson JA. Treatment options for hepatobiliary and pancreatic cancer. Mayo Clin Proc. 2007;82:628–37.
22. Darwish Murad S, Kim WR, Harnois DM, Douglas DD, Burton J, Kulik LM, Botha JF, Mezrich JD, Chapman WC, Schwartz JJ, Hong JC, Emond JC, Jeon H, Rosen CB, Gores GJ, Heimbach JK. Efficacy of neoadjuvant chemoradiation, followed by liver transplantation, for perihilar cholangiocarcinoma at 12 us centers. Gastroenterology. 2012;143(1):88–98.
23. Fritcher EG, Kipp BR, Halling KC, Oberg TN, Bryant SC, Tarrell RF, Gores GJ, Levy MJ, Clayton AC, Sebo TJ, Roberts LR. A multivariable model using advanced cytologic methods for the evaluation of indeterminate pancreatobiliary strictures. Gastroenterology. 2009; 136:2180–6.
24. Yamagata M. Endoscopic diagnosis of extrahepatic bile duct carcinoma: advances and current limitations. World J Clin Oncol. 2011;2:203–16.
25. Howell DA, Beveridge RP, Bosco J, Jones M. Endoscopic needle aspiration biopsy at ercp in the diagnosis of biliary strictures. Gastrointest Endosc. 1992;38:531–5.
26. Volmar KE, Vollmer RT, Routbort MJ, Creager AJ. Pancreatic and bile duct brushing cytology in 1000 cases: review of findings and comparison of preparation methods. Cancer. 2006;108:231–8.
27. Furmanczyk PS, Grieco VS, Agoff SN. Biliary brush cytology and the detection of cholangiocarcinoma in primary sclerosing cholangitis: Evaluation of specific cytomorphologic features and ca19-9 levels. Am J Clin Pathol. 2005;124:355–60.
28. Kipp BR, Stadheim LM, Halling SA, Pochron NL, Harmsen S, Nagorney DM, Sebo TJ, Therneau TM, Gores GJ, de Groen PC, Baron TH, Levy MJ, Halling KC, Roberts LR. A comparison of routine cytology and fluorescence in situ hybridization for the detection of malignant bile duct strictures. Am J Gastroenterol. 2004;99:1675–81.
29. Levy MJ, Baron TH, Clayton AC, Enders FB, Gostout CJ, Halling KC, Kipp BR, Petersen BT, Roberts LR, Rumalla A, Sebo TJ, Topazian MD, Wiersema MJ, Gores GJ. Prospective evaluation of advanced molecular markers and imaging techniques in patients with indeterminate bile duct strictures. Am J Gastroenterol. 2008;103:1263–73.
30. Moreno Luna LE, Kipp B, Halling KC, Sebo TJ, Kremers WK, Roberts LR, Barr Fritcher EG, Levy MJ, Gores GJ. Advanced cytologic techniques for the detection of malignant pancreatobiliary strictures. Gastroenterology. 2006;131:1064–72.
31. Huddleston BJ, Lamb RD, Gopez EV, Adler DG, Collins BT. Cholangiocarcinoma in a 17-year-old boy with primary sclerosing cholangitis and urovysion fluorescent in situ hybridization. Diagn Cytopathol. 2012;40:337–41.
32. Mazzone P, Jain P, Arroliga AC, Matthay RA. Bronchoscopy and needle biopsy techniques for diagnosis and staging of lung cancer. Clin Chest Med. 2002;23:137–58. ix.
33. Rivera MP, Mehta AC. Initial diagnosis of lung cancer: ACCP evidence-based clinical practice guidelines (2nd edition). Chest. 2007;132:131S–48S.
34. Sokolova IA, Bubendorf L, O'Hare A, Legator MS, Jacobson KK, Grilli BSB, Dalquen P, Halling KC, Tamm M, Seelig SA, Morrison LE. A fluorescence in situ hybridization-based assay for improved detection of lung cancer cells in bronchial washing specimens. Cancer. 2002;96:306–15.
35. Bubendorf L, Muller P, Joos L, Grilli B, Vogel S, Herzog M, Barascud A, Feichter G, Dalquen P, Tamm M. Multitarget fish analysis in the diagnosis of lung cancer. Am J Clin Pathol. 2005;123:516–23.
36. Halling KC, Rickman OB, Kipp BR, Harwood AR, Doerr CH, Jett JR. A comparison of cytology and fluorescence in situ hybridization for the detection of lung cancer in bronchoscopic specimens. Chest. 2006;130:694–701.
37. Savic S, Glatz K, Schoenegg R, Spieler P, Feichter G, Tamm M, Bubendorf L. Multitarget fluorescence in situ hybridization elucidates equivocal lung cytology. Chest. 2006;129:1629–35.
38. Schramm M, Wrobel C, Born I, Kazimirek M, Pomjanski N, William M, Kappes R, Gerharz CD, Biesterfeld S, Bocking A. Equivocal cytology in lung cancer diagnosis: improvement of diagnostic accuracy using adjuvant multicolor fish, DNA-image cytometry, and quantitative promoter hypermethylation analysis. Cancer Cytopathol. 2011;119:177–92.
39. Varella-Garcia M, Kittelson J, Schulte AP, Vu KO, Wolf HJ, Zeng C, Hirsch FR, Byers T, Kennedy T, Miller YE, Keith RL, Franklin WA. Multi-target interphase fluorescence in situ hybridization assay increases sensitivity of sputum cytology as a predictor of lung cancer. Cancer Detect Prev. 2004;28:244–51.
40. Voss JS, Kipp BR, Halling KC, Henry MR, Jett JR, Clayton AC, Rickman OB. Fluorescence in situ hybridization testing algorithm improves lung cancer detection in bronchial brushing specimens. Am J Respir Crit Care Med. 2010;181:478–85.
41. Barkan GA, Caraway NP, Jiang F, Zaidi TM, Fernandez R, Vaporcyin A, Morice R, Zhou X, Bekele BN, Katz RL. Comparison of molecular abnormalities in bronchial brushings and tumor touch preparations. Cancer. 2005;105:35–43.
42. Katz RL, Zaidi TM, Fernandez RL, Zhang J, He W, Acosta C, Daniely M, Madi L, Vargas MA, Dong Q, Gao X, Jiang F, Caraway NP, Vaporciyan AA, Roth JA, Spitz MR. Automated detection of genetic abnormalities combined with cytology in sputum is a sensitive predictor of lung cancer. Mod Pathol. 2008;21:950–60.

43. Liu YZ, Wang Z, Fang LL, Li L, Cao J, Xu X, Han YL, Cai Y, Wang LX, Wang MR. A potential probe set of fluorescence in situ hybridization for detection of lung cancer in bronchial brushing specimens. J Cancer Res Clin Oncol. 2012;138(9):1541–9.
44. Brankley SM, Wang KK, Harwood AR, Miller DV, Legator MS, Lutzke LS, Kipp BR, Morrison LE, Halling KC. The development of a fluorescence in situ hybridization assay for the detection of dysplasia and adenocarcinoma in barrett's esophagus. J Mol Diagn. 2006;8:260–7.
45. Cameron AJ, Ott BJ, Payne WS. The incidence of adenocarcinoma in columnar-lined (barrett's) esophagus. N Engl J Med. 1985;313:857–9.
46. Fahmy M, Skacel M, Gramlich TL, Brainard JA, Rice TW, Goldblum JR, Connor JT, Casey G, Legator MS, Tubbs RR, Falk GW. Chromosomal gains and genomic loss of p53 and p16 genes in barrett's esophagus detected by fluorescence in situ hybridization of cytology specimens. Mod Pathol. 2004;17:588–96.
47. Berry AV, Baskind AF, Hamilton DG. Cytologic screening for esophageal cancer. Acta Cytol. 1981;25: 135–41.
48. Falk GW, Skacel M, Gramlich TL, Casey G, Goldblum JR, Tubbs RR. Fluorescence in situ hybridization of cytologic specimens from barrett's esophagus: a pilot feasibility study. Gastrointest Endosc. 2004;60:280–4.
49. Fritcher EG, Brankley SM, Kipp BR, Voss JS, Campion MB, Morrison LE, Legator MS, Lutzke LS, Wang KK, Sebo TJ, Halling KC. A comparison of conventional cytology, DNA ploidy analysis, and fluorescence in situ hybridization for the detection of dysplasia and adenocarcinoma in patients with barrett's esophagus. Hum Pathol. 2008;39:1128–35.
50. Rygiel AM, Milano F, Ten Kate FJ, Schaap A, Wang KK, Peppelenbosch MP, Bergman JJ, Krishnadath KK. Gains and amplifications of c-myc, egfr, and 20.Q13 loci in the no dysplasia-dysplasia-adenocarcinoma sequence of barrett's esophagus. Cancer Epidemiol Biomarkers Prev. 2008;17:1380–5.
51. Rygiel AM, van Baal JW, Milano F, Wang KK, ten Kate FJ, Fockens P, Rosmolen WD, Bergman JJ, Peppelenbosch MP, Krishnadath KK. Efficient automated assessment of genetic abnormalities detected by fluorescence in situ hybridization on brush cytology in a barrett esophagus surveillance population. Cancer. 2007;109:1980–8.
52. Halling KC, Wendel AJ, editors. Molecular pathology of lung diseases. New York, NY: Springer Science and Business Media, LLC; 2008.
53. Halling KC, Schrijver I, Persons DL. Test verification and validation for molecular diagnostic assays. Arch Pathol Lab Med. 2012;136:11–3.
54. Wiktor AE, Van Dyke DL, Stupca PJ, Ketterling RP, Thorland EC, Shearer BM, Fink SR, Stockero KJ, Majorowicz JR, Dewald GW. Preclinical validation of fluorescence in situ hybridization assays for clinical practice. Genet Med. 2006;8:16–23.
55. Halling KC, Kipp BR. Fluorescence in situ hybridization in diagnostic cytology. Hum Pathol. 2007;38:1137–44.
56. Kipp BR, Fritcher EG, del Rosario KM, Stevens CL, Sebo TJ, Halling KC. A systematic approach to identifying urothelial cells likely to be polysomic by fluorescence in situ hybridization. Anal Quant Cytol Histol. 2005;27:317–22.
57. Halling KC. Vysis urovysion for the detection of urothelial carcinoma. Expert Rev Mol Diagn. 2003; 3:507–19.
58. Kipp BR, Sebo TJ, Griffin MD, Ihrke JM, Halling KC. Analysis of polyomavirus-infected renal transplant recipients' urine specimens: correlation of routine urine cytology, fluorescence in situ hybridization, and digital image analysis. Am J Clin Pathol. 2005;124:854–61.
59. Gordon DJ, Resio B, Pellman D. Causes and consequences of aneuploidy in cancer. Nat Rev. 2012; 13:189–203.

Epidermal Growth Factor Receptor Testing in Lung Adenocarcinoma

2

Neal I. Lindeman

Background

Lung cancer is the most lethal cancer in the USA, with an estimated 220,000 new diagnoses in 2011 and a case mortality rate of ~85 % [1]. This combination of high incidence and mortality makes lung cancer the leading cause of cancer-related deaths in American men and women, responsible for more deaths than the next four cancers (breast, prostate, colon, and pancreas) combined [1]. Lung cancer is not restricted to the USA, and lung cancer is a leading cause of cancer morbidity and mortality around the world.

Disease stage is the primary determinant of mortality in lung cancer. Early stage disease (confined to lung or with spread to local lymph nodes) is typically treated surgically and is associated with ~50 % 5-year survival [1]. However, prognosis is more grim in advanced stage disease, which is typically treated with chemotherapy and associated with ~15 % 5-year survival [1]. Moreover, because the lung has great reserve capacity and the symptoms of lung cancer can be somewhat nonspecific—cough, dyspnea, hemoptysis, pleuritic pain—~85 % of patients present with advanced disease [1]. Accordingly, early diagnosis and prevention (~90 % of lung cancer cases are associated with tobacco smoke [1]) are of keen interest to public health programs directed against lung cancer.

The vast majority of lung cancers are carcinomas, classically divided into two types: small cell and non-small cell carcinoma. Small cell carcinomas account for ~15 % of lung carcinomas, are typically centrally located, show neuroendocrine differentiation, and are typically treated with chemotherapy and/or radiation, with poor survival (~5 % at 5 years) [1].

"Non-small cell" carcinomas (NSCLC) account for ~85 % of lung cancers and have better overall survival than small cell carcinomas (~17 % 5-year survival) [1]. Among NSCLC, adenocarcinoma and squamous cell carcinoma subtypes predominate, accounting for approximately 40–45 % each, with additional rare subtypes (large cell carcinoma, salivary duct-like carcinoma) accounting for the remainder. Not uncommonly, NSCLCs contain mixed histology, with patterns of both adenocarcinoma and squamous carcinoma, and regions of small cell/neuroendocrine histology can also be present. Until the recent discovery of the importance of EGFR biology in adenocarcinoma, NSCLCs were all treated with the same chemotherapy regimens, and the distinction between NSCLC subtypes was a largely academic exercise.

In point of fact, clinical trials of therapeutic agents in lung cancer typically did not distinguish between NSCLC subtypes, which proved

N.I. Lindeman, M.D. (✉)
Molecular Diagnostics Laboratory, Harvard Medical School, Brigham and Women's Hospital, Boston, MA 02115, USA
e-mail: nlindeman@partners.org

W.E. Highsmith Jr. (ed.), *Molecular Diagnostics: 12 Tests That Changed Everything*, Molecular and Translational Medicine, DOI 10.1007/978-1-4614-8127-0_2,

problematic. Gefitinib, an oral ATP-mimetic inhibitor of the EGFR cytoplasmic tyrosine kinase, showed promising results in early phase trials, with rare, dramatic responses to treatment, including significant prolongation of disease-free survival of a year or more and radiologic regression of tumors [2, 3]. However, when used in large phase III trials for patients with all types of NSCLC, no clear benefit was demonstrated, and gefitinib was effectively removed from the US market [4]. A similar EGFR tyrosine kinase inhibitor (TKI), erlotinib, did reach the US market after showing a very modest survival benefit in unselected advanced stage NSCLC patients [5].

However, retrospective review of the few patients who showed dramatic clinical responses to gefitinib and erlotinib revealed discriminating characteristics. All of these patients had adenocarcinoma histology. In addition, patients who responded to EGFR TKIs were more likely to have never smoked tobacco products, to be female, to have Asian ancestry, and tended to be younger than patients who did not respond to therapy [2, 3, 6]. Although these clinical associations had value for population studies, they were insufficiently sensitive or specific to use to determine which patients might respond to EGFR TKI therapy. Only adenocarcinoma histology proved to have some value as a sensitive predictor for selecting patients for TKI therapy: functionally all the patients who responded to treatment had some element of adenocarcinoma in their tumor. However, specificity of histology as sole predictor was poor, as most patients with adenocarcinoma still did not respond to treatment.

A search was conducted to find a suitable biomarker within the tumor to predict which patients with adenocarcinoma of the lung were likely to respond to treatment with gefitinib and erlotinib, and several candidates emerged: EGFR protein overexpression by immunohistochemistry (IHC) [7, 8], *EGFR* polysomy by fluorescence in situ hybridization (FISH) [9, 10], and *EGFR* mutation analysis by molecular diagnostic methods [11–13]. Quite often all three of these predictors were present simultaneously, which caused confusion in the published literature. Ultimately, *EGFR* mutation analysis by molecular diagnostic methods was shown to be the superior predictor of response to therapy, and FISH and IHC were shown to be of limited value in this regard [7, 14–16].

The mutations are nonrandomly distributed in exons 18–21, which encode part of the EGFR cytoplasmic tyrosine kinase domain. EGFR (aka HER1) is a transmembrane growth factor receptor of the HER family, whose other members include ERBB2 (aka HER2/neu), which is a critical oncogene and therapeutic target in breast cancer. Upon binding of ligand to the extracellular domain of EGFR, the receptor forms a dimer either by binding with another EGFR molecule (homodimer) or with another HER family protein (heterodimer). Autophosphorylation of the dimerized receptor causes activation of several downstream signaling pathways, including RAS-RAF-MEK, JAK-STAT, and PIK3CA-AKT-mTOR, leading to growth, survival, and proliferation. The activating mutations in EGFR exert their oncogenic effects through ligand-independent constitutive activation of the cytoplasmic tyrosine kinase, leading to dysregulated cell growth, proliferation, and survival [11, 12, 17].

Two mutations are seen in ~90 % of tumors: 65 % of mutant tumors have an in-frame deletion in exon 19 that involves ELREA residues at codons 746–750, and 25 % of mutant tumors have a missense point mutation at codon 858 (L858R) in exon 21. The remaining ~10 % of cases contain primarily missense point mutations at codon 719 in exon 18 (G719C, G719S, G719A), and mutations in exon 20 that include insertion/duplications around codons 770, and two point mutations, S768I and T790M. Importantly, the exon 20 mutations, while oncogenic, confer *resistance* to the TKIs rather than sensitivity. The T790M, in particular, is commonly acquired in patients after successful response to therapy, and heralds acquired secondary resistance [18]. The T790M mutation is also encountered in the germline of rare patients with hereditary cancer syndrome [19].

Clinical Applications

Once a suitable biomarker was available, a better assessment of the patients who respond to treatment could be established. *EGFR* mutations are seen in ~20 % of adenocarcinomas and mixed carcinomas with areas of adenocarcinoma histology, but are not seen in well-characterized squamous carcinomas or small cell carcinomas. Patients with *EGFR*-mutant adenocarcinoma have a ~80 % likelihood of responding to treatment with an EGFR TKI and have a median survival of ~2 years (as opposed to ~8 months without TKI treatment).

Initially, because these drugs are less toxic and better tolerated than standard platinum doublet chemotherapy, patients with adenocarcinoma were empirically treated with erlotinib or gefitinib. However, a series of large prospective studies published between 2009 and 2011 demonstrated that patients with *EGFR*-nonmutant lung adenocarcinomas have better outcome with chemotherapy than with TKIs, establishing *EGFR* mutation testing as a prerequisite for determining treatment and ending the practice of empirical TKI therapy [20–24].

Furthermore, while TKIs were initially studied as second-line agents for lung cancer patients with advanced stage who had progressed after receiving chemotherapy, subsequent studies have shown clinical benefit for their use as first-line treatment in advanced stage *EGFR*-mutant lung adenocarcinoma. This has led to an increased demand for *EGFR* testing for all new diagnoses of advanced stage lung cancer. Moreover, since a high percentage of patients with early stage lung cancer eventually relapse, and the samples obtained at relapse may be small and heterogeneous, some oncologists are advocating testing all new diagnoses of lung adenocarcinoma for *EGFR* mutations, even in early stage patients.

Methodology

Multiple techniques are used in the molecular diagnostics laboratory to detect EGFR mutations, but all begin with PCR. The PCR products can then be analyzed by Sanger dideoxyterminator sequencing, pyrosequencing, oligonucleotide probe hybridization, single nucleotide extension with fluorescent or mass spectrometric detection, real-time PCR, melt curve analysis, restriction digestion, denaturing HPLC, and other techniques. A comprehensive review of these is beyond the scope of this chapter. However, a few points are worth mentioning.

The "gold standard" reference technique used in the studies that first demonstrated the clinical value of testing was Sanger sequencing [11, 12] (Figs. 2.1 and 2.2). While versatile and able to detect mutations in all four of the critical exons

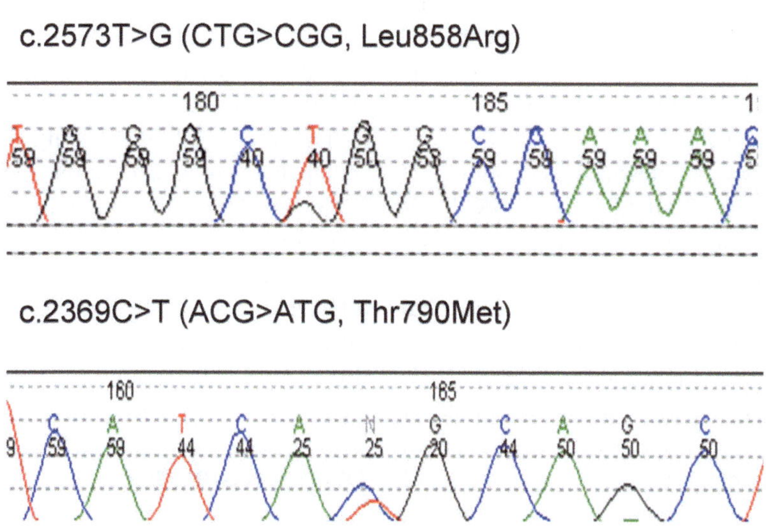

Fig. 2.1 Sanger sequence showing two mutations in a patient with lung adenocarcinoma who relapsed after initial response to treatment with erlotinib. The *top panel* shows the patient's initial sensitizing mutation, L858R (c.2573 T>G) substitution in exon 21. The *bottom panel* shows the secondary resistance mutation, T790M substitution (c.2369C>T) in exon 20. Only the L858R mutation was detected in the pretreatment sample

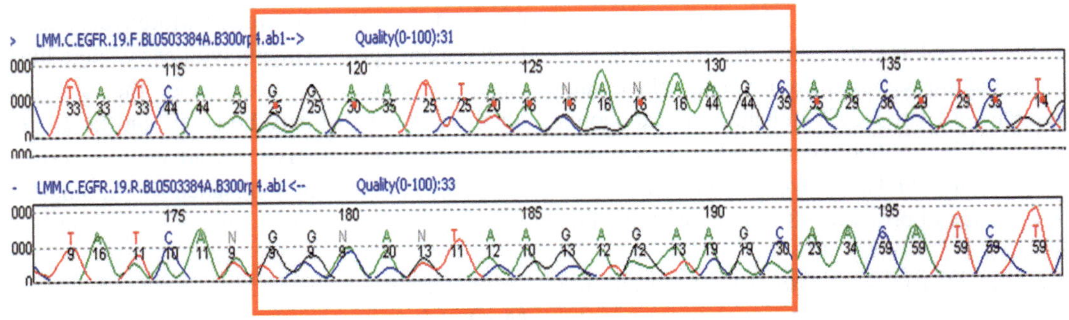

Fig. 2.2 Sanger Sequence result showing an in-frame 15 bp deletion in exon 19 of EGFR. The *top bar* shows the forward sequence, while the *lower bar* shows the reverse sequence. The *orange box* highlights the deleted nucleotides, which encode ELREA residues 746–750. This common EGFR mutation is associated with a favorable response to treatment with gefitinib or erlotinib

(18–21), this method has relatively poor analytical sensitivity and can give false-negative results in the many small and heterogeneous biopsy or cytology specimens that are the mainstay of diagnosis for patients with advanced stage disease. In general, Sanger sequencing can reliably detect mutant DNA at a relative concentration of 20–25 %, which corresponds to ~50 % malignant cell content for diploid tumors. This typically necessitates microdissection of samples by a pathologist or a specially trained technologist prior to analysis, which extends the turnaround time and may still be insufficient. Fortuitously, many of the tumors with mutations also have increased EGFR copy number [15, 25], so the ability to detect a positive case is somewhat better, but establishing the copy number of each case in order to help interpret a negative mutation result is not practical.

Sensitivity may be enhanced by a variety of methods, including allele-specific PCR or sequencing after amplification with suppression of wild-type amplification (e.g., with peptide nucleic acid [PNA] [26] or locked nucleic acid [LNA] probes [27], restriction digestion of wild-type sequence between rounds of PCR, COLD-PCR) or laser capture microdissection of individual cancer cells. These methods can detect mutations in samples with cancer cell contents of 10 % or lower, sometimes even less than 1 %. However, while these methods enable testing of many of the small samples that would be insufficient for unmodified Sanger sequencing, they also confer a risk of false-positive results. Novel mutations of uncertain significance have been reported with these methods, often unable to be confirmed on repeat analysis [28]. Artifactual mutations are a risk as well. Furthermore, these methods can detect minor subpopulations with a mutation in the absence of overall mutant background, and the clinical significance of these is unclear. This is particularly confusing when an untreated patient is discovered to have a sensitizing EGFR mutation alongside a T790M resistance mutation—should such a patient be treated with a TKI, or not?

Regulatory Issues

The US Food and Drug Administration (FDA) has approved commercial assay kits for EGFR testing, although EGFR testing is not listed as a "companion diagnostic" on the labeling for Tarceva (erlotinib) or other EGFR TKIs at the time of this writing.

The College of American Pathologists (CAP) offers a Proficiency Testing challenge for laboratories that perform EGFR testing, consisting of two shipments of samples per year.

Test Interpretation

The exon 19 deletion mutations and exon 21 L858R point mutation confer sensitivity to treatment with targeted EGFR TKIs, and patients with these tumors should be treated with erlotinib in the USA (and/or gefitinib in other countries) if they are in advanced stage and otherwise amenable to treatment (i.e., not being referred for hospice or palliation).

The exon 18 codon 719 mutations and exon 21 L861Q are considered likely to confer sensitivity to EGFR TKIs and should also be treated with erlotinib or gefitinib, although they are less likely to derive as substantial a benefit as patients with the more common sensitizing mutations. These mutations are less well studied.

The exon 20 insertion mutations and T790M point mutation are associated with resistance to erlotinib/gefitinib and should not be treated with these agents. Several clinical trials with so-called irreversible inhibitors of EGFR have been attempted, but results have so far been disappointing. The T790M is typically acquired as a secondary mutation in a patient who has relapsed after initial treatment; when it is encountered in an untreated patient, a possible explanation is a germline mutation, which is associated with hereditary cancer syndrome. Patients with germline T790M should be referred for genetic counseling.

False-negative results may be seen in patients with low tumor content, and it is imperative that the molecular diagnostics laboratory differentiate between a true negative result and an apparently negative result in a suboptimal sample. Rebiopsy may be needed if a patient does not have a sample with adequate tumor content to enable a definitive diagnosis.

How the Test Has Changed Medical Practice

The discovery of EGFR mutations and their role in predicting outcome in lung adenocarcinoma has revolutionized thoracic oncology and, to some extent, oncology in general.

First, this test has provided a viable treatment option and hope to patients with one of the most dismal diagnoses in medicine, a disease that, as mentioned above, kills more patients than the next four cancers combined. While not curative, EGFR TKIs promise an extra year or more of relatively high quality, chemotherapy-free life for the ~20,000 new patients each year diagnosed in the USA with EGFR-mutant lung cancer.

Second, this test has led to a change in clinical trial design. Gefitinib is not available on the US market because the phase III studies looked at all NSCLC and the benefit of this drug in 10 % of NSCLC was too small to be statistically significant. Trials are now designed with biomarkers in mind to select patients most likely to derive a benefit, which should lead to more therapies, effectively targeted to a wider variety of cancer subtypes. 2011 saw the FDA approve an ALK inhibitor for ALK-mutant lung cancer; and, extending beyond lung cancer, a BRAF inhibitor for BRAF mutant melanoma.

Third, this test prompted aggressive search for other defining molecular alterations in cancer, both lung and beyond. Lung cancer has evolved from a histologic-based small-cell/non-small cell classification to a molecular-based classification that contains multiple different molecular subtypes. This same process is being repeated in tumors of all types. Some trials are looking at molecular classification as more important than even tumor of origin as determinant of therapy (i.e., treat any tumor with a PIK3CA mutation, whether it is a breast cancer, an endometrial cancer, or a lung cancer).

Fourth, this test helped usher in an era of commercial development of molecular diagnostics for cancer. Before EGFR, the commercial market for molecular oncology was relatively small, and few companies invested the resources into this area. With the emergence of companion diagnostics and application to common medical problems like lung cancer and melanoma, commercial manufacturers have begun to focus on this field, leading to greater standardization (and cost!).

Fifth, the FDA has shown accelerated approval processes for new targeted therapies. The EGFR story unfolded over several years. By contrast, the next lung cancer subtype to have a targeted treatment, ALK-mutant lung cancer, proceeded rapidly through FDA, with release of a diagnostic and a drug within 4 years of the initial discovery and before phase III trials had been concluded.

Future Directions

While EGFR-mutant lung cancers do respond to treatment, they also do relapse. About half of relapses are associated with acquisition of the T790M mutation in exon 20, which leads to steric hindrance of the binding of the drug in the ATP-binding pocket. New therapeutic options are needed for these patients. Another 20 % of patients who relapse have amplification of another oncogene, MET [29]. Inhibition of MET has similarly proven frustrating. There is still no explanation for the remaining patients who relapse.

KRAS mutations (point mutations in codons 12, 13, 61) are seen in 30 % of lung adenocarcinomas, essentially none of which also have EGFR mutations. No good treatment option exists for KRAS mutant lung cancers, and KRAS testing is of limited use in lung cancer, except as a possible "rule out" for EGFR testing in a multitest algorithm: because KRAS is technically easier to test than EGFR, some laboratories may screen EGFR requests with a KRAS test first.

A variety of mutually exclusive, rare, molecular alterations have been shown in about half of the remaining 50 % of adenocarcinomas of the lung, each accounting for 1–5 % of the total. These include mutations in BRAF, ERBB2, AKT1, NRAS, and MEK, in total accounting for ~20 % of lung adenocarcinomas. Targeted therapies that inhibit these mutant proteins are in development or in clinical trials, but currently not standard of care, nor is testing for these mutations.

Another lung adenocarcinoma subtype with targeted therapy contains a chromosomal abnormality—inversion of chromosome 2 resulting in dysregulation of the ALK (anaplastic lymphoma kinase) gene, typically by fusion with EML4 [30]. Early trials have shown ~60 % of patients with ALK rearrangements, as detected by fluorescence in situ hybridization (FISH) (Fig. 2.3) will respond to a targeted inhibitor of the ALK kinase, crizotinib [31]. Although the frequency of ALK rearrangement in lung adenocarcinoma is only ~5 %, crizotinib has been approved by FDA for tumors

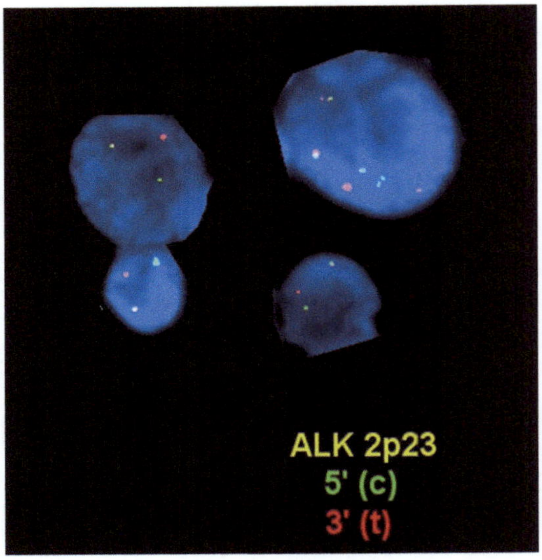

Fig. 2.3 FISH showing EML4-ALK translocation in a lung cancer. The wild-type configuration shows *red* and *green* signals juxtaposed against one another to give a *yellow* fusion signal. The translocation causes a split of the centromeric 5′ *green* signal and the telomeric 3′ *red* signal. This result predicts a favorable clinical response to treatment with crizotinib

that have demonstrated ALK rearrangements, and FISH for ALK is now standard of care, along with EGFR mutation testing, in adenocarcinomas of the lung.

Other subtypes of lung adenocarcinoma with chromosomal abnormalities include those with ROS1 rearrangements, which anecdotally respond to crizotinib, and those with RET rearrangements, which await trials to assess sensitivity in vivo to vandetanib. Each of these subtypes is present in 1–2 % of lung adenocarcinomas [32].

In contrast to adenocarcinomas of the lung, squamous carcinomas have relatively few molecular subtypes with targeted clinical treatment. FGFR1 amplification is a common finding [33] and trials are underway to assess the efficacy of ponatinib in FGFR1 amplified squamous lung cancer, with FISH and IHC as candidate biomarkers. DDR2 [34] and PIK3CA mutations are also common in squamous carcinoma; however, these have yet to develop as diagnostic or therapeutic targets outside the research lab. This is likely to change in the coming years.

References

1. Cancer facts and figures 2011. Atlanta, GA: American Cancer Society. http://www.cancer.org/acs/groups/content/@epidemiologysurveilance/documents/document/acspc-029771.pdf (2011). Accessed 29 May 2012.
2. Fukuoka M, Yano S, Giaccone G, et al. Multi-institutional randomized phase II trial of gefitinib for previously treated patients with advanced non-small-cell lung cancer (the IDEAL Trial). J Clin Oncol. 2003;21:2237–46.
3. Kris MG, Natale RB, Herbst RS, et al. Efficacy of gefitinib, an inhibitor of the epidermal growth factor receptor tyrosine kinase, in symptomatic patients with non-small cell lung cancer: a randomized trial. JAMA. 2003;290:2149–58.
4. Thatcher N, Chang A, Parikh P, et al. Gefitinib plus best supportive care in previously treated patients with refractory advanced non-small-cell lung cancer: results from a randomised, placebo-controlled, multi-centre study (Iressa survival evaluation in lung cancer). Lancet. 2005;366:1527–37.
5. Shepherd FA, Rodrigues Pereira J, Ciuleanu T, et al. Erlotinib in previously treated non-small-cell lung cancer. N Engl J Med. 2005;353(2):123–32.
6. Miller VA, Kris MG, Shah N, et al. Bronchioloalveolar pathologic subtype and smoking history predict sensitivity to gefitinib in advanced non-small-cell lung cancer. J Clin Oncol. 2004;22:1103–9.
7. Dacic S, Flanagan M, Cieply K, et al. Significance of EGFR protein expression and gene amplification in non-small cell lung carcinoma. Am J Clin Pathol. 2006;125:860–5.
8. Hirsch FR, Varella-Garcia M, Bunn Jr PA, et al. Epidermal growth factor receptor in non-small-cell lung carcinomas: correlation between gene copy number and protein expression on impact on prognosis. J Clin Oncol. 2003;21:3798–807.
9. Cappuzzo F, Hirsch FR, Rossi E, et al. Epidermal growth factor receptor gene and protein and gefitinib sensitivity in non-small-cell lung cancer. J Natl Cancer Inst. 2005;97:643–55.
10. Hirsch FR, Varella-Garcia M, McCoy J, et al. Increased epidermal growth factor receptor gene copy number detected by fluorescence in situ hybridization associates with increased sensitivity to gefitinib in patients with bronchioloalveolar carcinoma subtypes: a southwest oncology group study. J Clin Oncol. 2005;23:6838–45.
11. Paez JG, Janne PA, Lee JC, et al. EGFR mutations in lung cancer: correlation with clinical response to gefitinib therapy. Science. 2004;304:1497–500.
12. Lynch TJ, Bell DW, Sordella R, et al. Activating mutations in the epidermal growth factor receptor underlying responsiveness of non-small-cell lung cancer to gefitinib. N Engl J Med. 2004;350:2129–39.
13. Pao W, Miller V, Zakowski M, et al. EGF receptor gene mutations are common in lung cancers from "never smokers" and are associated with sensitivity of tumors to gefitinib and erlotinib. Proc Natl Acad Sci USA. 2004;101:13306–11.
14. Li AR, Chitale D, Riely GJ, et al. EGFR mutations in lung adenocarcinomas: clinical testing experience and relationship to EGFR gene copy number and immunohistochemical expression. J Mol Diagn. 2008; 10:242–8.
15. Sholl LM, Xiao Y, Joshi V, et al. EGFR mutation is a better predictor of response to tyrosine kinase inhibitors in non-small cell lung carcinoma than FISH, CISH, and immunohistochemistry. Am J Clin Pathol. 2010;133(6):922–34.
16. Fukuoka M, Wu YL, Thongprasert S, et al. Biomarker analyses and final overall survival results from a phase III, randomized, open-label, first-line study of gefitinib versus carboplatin/paclitaxel in clinically selected patients with advanced non-small-cell lung cancer in Asia (IPASS). J Clin Oncol. 2011;29(21): 2866–74.
17. Yun CH, Boggon TJ, Li Y, et al. Structures of lung cancer-derived EGFR mutants and inhibitor complexes: mechanism of activation and insights into differential inhibitor sensitivity. Cancer Cell. 2007; 11(3):217–27.
18. Kobayashi S, Boggon TJ, Dayaram T, et al. EGFR mutation and resistance of non-small-cell lung cancer to gefitinib. N Engl J Med. 2005;352(8):786–92.
19. Oxnard GR, Miller VA, Robson ME, et al. Screening for germline EGFR T790M mutations through lung cancer genotyping. J Thorac Oncol. 2012;7(6): 1049–52.
20. Maemondo M, Inoue A, Kobayashi K, North-East Japan Study Group, et al. Gefitinib or chemotherapy for non-small-cell lung cancer with mutated EGFR. N Engl J Med. 2010;362(25):2380–8.
21. Rosell R, Carcereny E, Gervais R, Spanish Lung Cancer Group in collaboration with Groupe Français de Pneumo-Cancérologie and Associazione Italiana Oncologia Toracica, et al. Erlotinib versus standard chemotherapy as first-line treatment for European patients with advanced EGFR mutation-positive non-small-cell lung cancer (EURTAC): a multicentre, open-label, randomised phase 3 trial. Lancet Oncol. 2012;13(3):239–46.
22. Zhou C, Wu YL, Chen G, et al. Erlotinib versus chemotherapy as first-line treatment for patients with advanced EGFR mutation-positive non-small-cell lung cancer (OPTIMAL, CTONG-0802): a multicentre, open-label, randomised, phase 3 study. Lancet Oncol. 2011;12:735–42.
23. Mitsudomi T, Morita S, Yatabe Y, West Japan Oncology Group, et al. Gefitinib versus cisplatin plus docetaxel in patients with non-small-cell lung cancer harbouring mutations of the epidermal growth factor receptor (WJTOG3405): an open label, randomised phase 3 trial. Lancet Oncol. 2010;11(2):121–8.
24. Mok TS, Wu YL, Thongprasert S, et al. Gefitinib or carboplatin-paclitaxel in pulmonary adenocarcinoma. N Engl J Med. 2009;361:947–57.

25. Dahabreh IJ, Linardou H, Siannis F, et al. Somatic EGFR mutation and gene copy gain as predictive biomarkers for response to tyrosine kinase inhibitors in non-small cell lung cancer. Clin Cancer Res. 2010;16:291–303.
26. Nagai Y, Miyazawa H, Huqun, et al. Genetic heterogeneity of the epidermal growth factor receptor in non-small cell lung cancer cell lines revealed by a rapid and sensitive detection system, the peptide nucleic acid-locked nucleic acid PCR clamp. Cancer Res. 2005;65(16):7276–82.
27. Arcila ME, Oxnard GR, Nafa K, et al. Rebiopsy of lung cancer patients with acquired resistance to EGFR inhibitors and enhanced detection of the T790M mutation using a locked nucleic acid-based assay. Clin Cancer Res. 2011;17(5):1169–80.
28. Tsao MS, Sakurada A, Cutz JC, et al. Erlotinib in lung cancer—molecular and clinical predictors of outcome. N Engl J Med. 2005;353:133–44.
29. Engelman JA, Zejnullahu K, Mitsudomi T, et al. MET amplification leads to gefitinib resistance in lung cancer by activating ERBB3 signaling. Science. 2007;316:1039–43.
30. Soda M, Choi YL, Enomoto M, et al. Identification of the transforming EML4-ALK fusion gene in non-small-cell lung cancer. Nature. 2007;448(7153):561–6.
31. Shaw AT, Yeap BY, Solomon BJ, et al. Effect of crizotinib on overall survival in patients with advanced non-small-cell lung cancer harbouring ALK gene rearrangement: a retrospective analysis. Lancet Oncol. 2011;12:1004–12.
32. Takeuchi K, Soda M, Togashi Y, et al. RET, ROS1 and ALK fusions in lung cancer. Nat Med. 2012;18(3):378–81.
33. Dutt A, Ramos AH, Hammerman PS, et al. Inhibitor-sensitive FGFR1 amplification in human non-small cell lung cancer. PLoS One. 2011;6:e20351.
34. Hammerman P, Sos M, Ramos A, et al. Mutations in the DDR2 kinase gene identify a novel therapeutic target in squamous cell lung cancer. Cancer Discov. 2011;1:78–89.

3 The Human Epidermal Growth Factor Receptor 2 (HER2)

Laura J. Tafe and Gregory J. Tsongalis

Background

While the field of pharmacogenomics (PGX) continues to mature and its clinical application gains utility, one aspect of PGX, personalized medicine, is proving to have a major impact on the management of the cancer patient. Our increasing knowledge base of tumor cell biology and our ever increasing abilities to design therapeutics against various biological targets involved in different pathways have resulted in significant advances using these novel-targeted therapies. One such biomarker, the human epidermal growth factor receptor 2 (HER2), was the first to be targeted with a novel humanized monoclonal antibody approach and later with a small molecule tyrosine kinase inhibitor.

This manuscript was modified from a published review article in Clin Chem Lab Med, 2012. (http://www.reference-global.com/doi/abs/10.1515/CCLM.2011.707?prevSearch=%2528tsongalis%2529%2BUND%2B%255Bjournal%253A%2Bcclm%255D&searchHistoryKey=)

L.J. Tafe, M.D. (✉)
Department of Pathology and the Geisel School of Medicine at Dartmouth, Dartmouth-Hitchcock Medical Center, Lebanon, NH 03756, USA
e-mail: Laura.J.Tafe@hitchcock.org

G.J. Tsongalis, Ph.D., F.A.C.B, H.C.L.D., C.C.
Department of Pathology, Geisel School of Medicine at Dartmouth, Dartmouth Hitchcock Medical Center and Norris Cotton Cancer Center, Lebanon, NH 03756, USA

The human epidermal growth factor receptor 2 (HER2) is a proto-oncogene located on chromosome 17p11.2–12 that encodes a 185-kd transmembrane tyrosine kinase receptor ($p185^{HER\text{-}2}$). This gene is a member of the HER gene family which includes HER1 (epidermal growth factor receptor—EGFR/erbB1), HER3 (erbB3), and HER4 (erbB4). Each receptor contains an extracellular domain, a single transmembrane lipophilic domain, and an intracellular tyrosine kinase (TK) domain (Fig. 3.1). The TK domain is nonfunctional in the HER-3 receptor. HER2, unlike the other members of this family, has no identified ligand and is constitutively active with the ability to undergo ligand-independent dimerization. Other HER proteins can preferentially heterodimerize with HER2 which leads to phosphorylation of the tyrosine residues and activation of downstream effectors including the mitogen activating protein kinase (MAPK), phosphatidylinositol 3-kinase (PI3K), and signal transducers and activators of transcription (STAT) pathways that regulate cell proliferation, survival, and other processes important in carcinogenesis. The oncogenic activation of HER2, present in approximately 15–20 % of all breast cancers as well as some other cancer types (discussed later), commonly occurs through gene amplification which results in receptor protein overexpression (Fig. 3.2) [1, 2]. This overexpressed protein has become the target of several novel therapies.

W.E. Highsmith Jr. (ed.), *Molecular Diagnostics: 12 Tests That Changed Everything*, Molecular and Translational Medicine, DOI 10.1007/978-1-4614-8127-0_3,

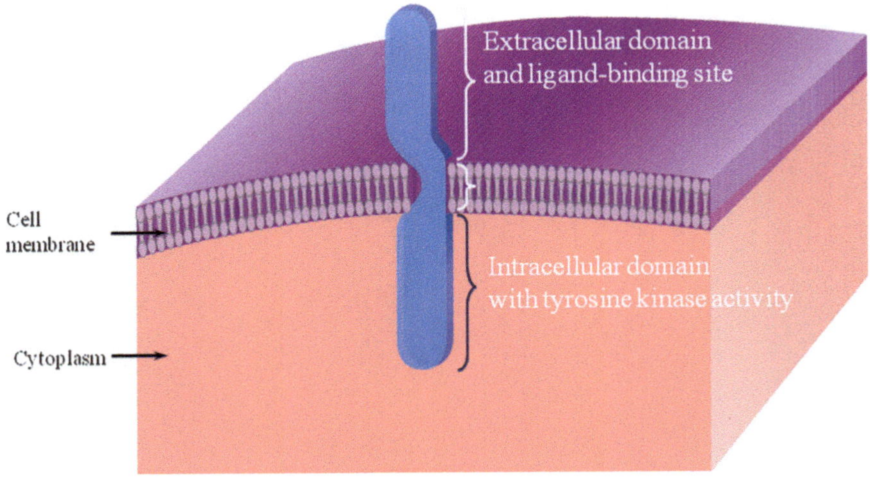

Fig. 3.1 Schematic diagram showing the extra- and intracellular domains of the HER2 receptor

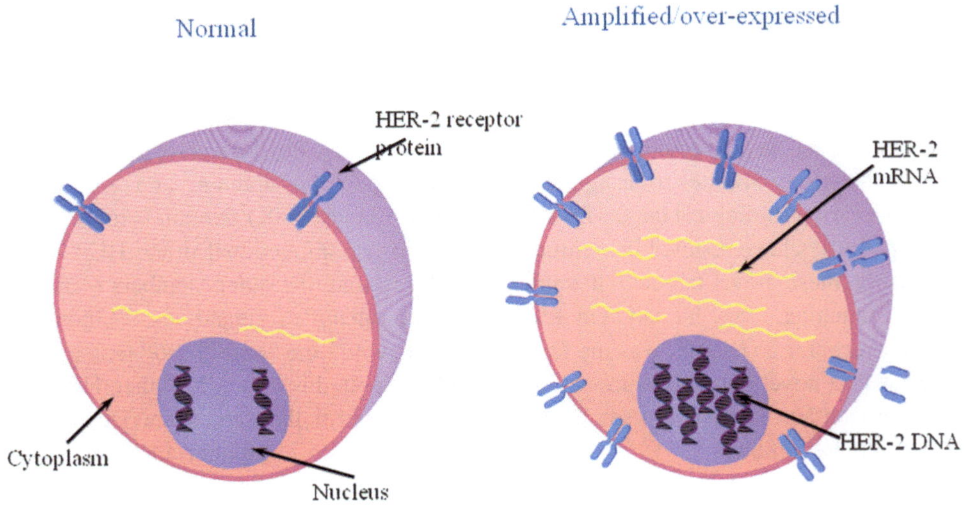

Fig. 3.2 Schematic diagram illustrating gene amplification which results in receptor overexpression

Clinical Applications: Targeting HER2

Currently there are two FDA-approved targeted therapies against HER2 that are available to treat patients with cancers that either overexpress the HER2 protein or have an amplified *HER2* gene. Such targeted therapies can be designed against the extracellular receptor domain or the intracellular tyrosine kinase domain. Trastuzumab (Herceptin; Genetech, South San Francisco, CA) is a recombinant humanized monoclonal antibody which specifically targets the extracellular domain of the HER2 receptor. This was the first monoclonal antibody therapy approved for use in human cancers. Although the exact mechanism of action of the antitumor activity of trastuzumab is unknown, a number of mechanisms have been proposed including (1) activation of antibody-dependent cellular cytotoxicity, (2) blockage of proteolytic cleavage of the HER2 extracellular domain, (3) inhibition of intracellular signal transduction, (4) inhibition of tumor-induced angiogenesis, and (5) inhibition of repair of cancer treatment-induced DNA damage [3, 4].

More recently, lapatinib (Tykerb; Glaxo SmithKline, London, UK), an orally available, small molecule, reversible inhibitor of both HER2 and EGFR tyrosine kinases (TKs) was approved by the FDA. The use of tyrosine kinase inhibitors (TKIs), including the selective EGFR inhibitors, gefitinib (Iressa, AstraZeneca Pharmaceuticals LP, Wilmington, DE), and erlotinib (Tarceva, Genentech/OSI Pharmaceuticals, LLC, Farmingdale, NY), have been used in clinical practice for various human cancers. These compounds are all 4-anilinoquinoline derivatives but have distinct TK targets and mechanisms of action [5]. The binding of lapatinib inhibits phosphorylation thus blocking the downstream effects of the MAPK, PI3K, and STAT pathways. In vitro, lapatinib can effectively inhibit human tumor cell lines that overexpress EGFR or HER2, indicating selectivity for cancers that overexpress these receptors [6].

Methodology: Detecting HER2 Status

An association between *HER2* gene amplification and poor prognosis in breast cancer patients was first demonstrated in 1987 [7]. Subsequently, approval of trastuzamab highlighted the need for companion diagnostics to be available in the clinical laboratory setting. This provided more of a rationale for the need to establish HER2 status in clinical tumor specimens prior to the initiation of therapy. Since an association exists between p185$^{HER\text{-}2}$ protein overexpression and *HER2* gene amplification, quantification can be measured at either the protein level or at the gene level. Numerous technologies and approaches have been evaluated and described for the detection of HER2 gene amplification and/or overexpression with several becoming FDA-cleared assays for use in clinical testing.

Immunohistochemistry (IHC) measures expression of a target gene by utilizing antibodies specific for antigenic epitopes of a given gene product (Fig. 3.3). Because these assays are usually performed on tissue sections with intact cellular architecture, their expression can be localized to a specific cell type or specific region within the cell (i.e., nuclear, cytoplasmic, or membranous). A typical IHC protocol would involve application of a primary antibody against the target protein to the tissue section on a slide. A biotinylated secondary antibody directed against the primary antibody species is then applied. Signal detection is performed utilizing avidin which has a very high affinity for biotin and is conjugated to an enzyme. The presence or absence of the target protein is determined by adding a chromogenic substrate which produces

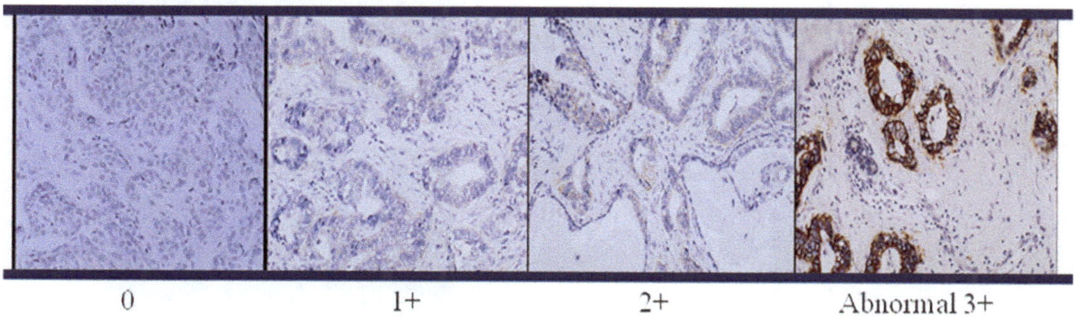

Fig. 3.3 HER2 analysis by IHC. Scoring is based on staining intensity and percent of cells showing expression (0–1+, 2+, 3+). Score 0 (negative) = no membrane staining is observed; score 1+ (negative) = weak, incomplete membrane staining in any proportion of invasive tumor cells, or weak complete membrane staining in <10 % of cells; score 2+ (equivocal) = complete membrane staining that is nonuniform or weak but with obvious circumferential distribution in >10 % of invasive tumor cells, or strong complete membrane staining in no more than 30 % of cells; score 3+ (positive) = complete and uniform strong membrane staining in >30 % of invasive tumor cells

a colorimetric reaction for which the intensity of the color is proportional to the number of target proteins present. A number of HER2 antibodies are commercially available for IHC including the FDA-approved HercepTest (polyclonal, DAKO, Carpinteria, CA) and Pathway/Confirm (clone 4B5, monoclonal, Ventana Medical Systems, Tucson, AZ). The IHC signal is quantified and scored most commonly according to the 2007 ASCO/CAP guidelines on a scale of 0–3+ based on the membranous staining pattern, intensity, and percentage of staining (Fig. 3.3) [8]. The most commonly used testing algorithm of HER2 status includes the use of a semiquantitative immunohistochemistry (IHC) assay to detect HER2 protein overexpression followed by fluorescence in situ hybridization (FISH) if IHC is equivocal (2+). This scoring system has come under intense scrutiny recently due to the lack of precision of this technology. While IHC is a well-recognized technique and is relatively inexpensive, the drawbacks mostly stem from it being an indirect detection method for an unstable target. It is well recognized that protein stability is affected by cold ischemic times, tissue fixation methods, and length of time in fixative [9–11]. Also, background or nonspecific staining can be a result of the indirect detection chemistries used.

Alternatively, laboratories may chose to detect gene copy number as there has been good correlation between p185$^{\text{HER-2}}$ protein overexpression and *HER2* gene amplification. Fluorescence in situ hybridization (FISH) is the technique most commonly used to quantify *HER2* gene copy number or amplification and many labs are now performing FISH as their primary test for *HER2* analysis. Like IHC, this technique detects the target gene in the context of the cellular architecture of a fixed tissue section. FISH uses a single-stranded nucleic acid probe that hybridizes to the denatured *HER2* gene locus (17q21) to form a double-stranded hybrid between probe and target sequence. The probe is labeled with a fluorescent dye so that direct visualization of the probe is possible with a fluorescent microscopy. In FISH assays where the goal is to enumerate gene copy number, a second probe, labeled with a different fluorochrome, is used as a comparative control such as a centromeric enumeration probe (CEP) for

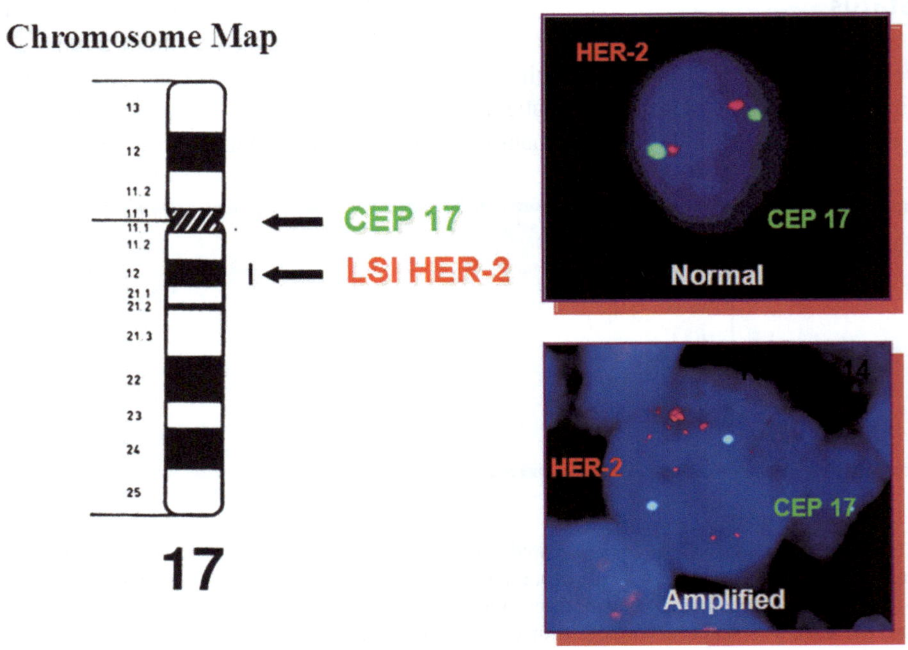

Fig. 3.4 HER2 analysis by fluorescence in situ hybridization (FISH)

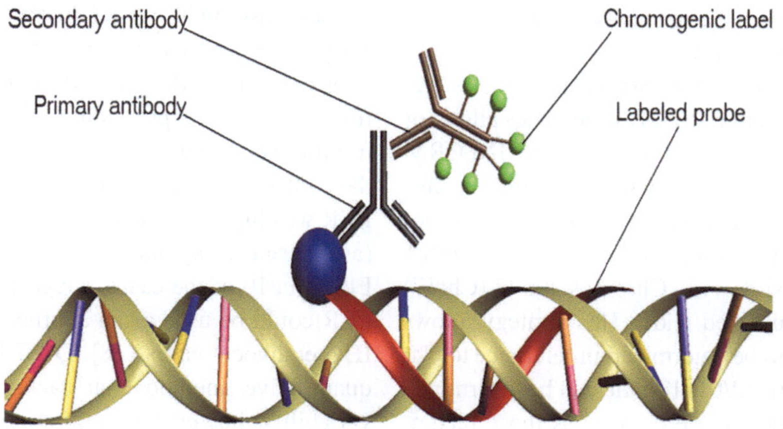

Fig. 3.5 Schematic diagram of chromogenic in situ hybridization (CISH). http://www.histalim.com/.../in-situ-hybridization.php

chromosome 17 (Fig. 3.4). Amplification status is then determined by measuring the HER2/CEP17 signal ratio (positive >2.0 and negative <2.0, according to PathVysion FDA-approved package insert). The PathVysion (Abbott Laboratories, Abbott Park, IL) and pharmDx (DAKO, Glostrup, Denmark) are two examples of dual-colored FISH assays which have received FDA approval. A single color assay (INFORM, Ventana Medical Systems, Tucson, AZ) used HER2 copy number/nucleus enumeration and a separate probe assay to assess chromosome number. While FISH has been reported to be the more accurate of the in situ technologies to determine *HER2* status, it is more costly than IHC and requires fluorescent microscopy capabilities. Guidelines have also been established for HER2 FISH testing [8].

Bright-field IHC has been introduced as an alternative to FISH. Two types are currently available, chromogenic in situ hybridization (CISH) and enzyme metallography with silver deposition (SISH). The main advantages of these techniques are that the signals do not fade and the slides can be archived and retained as part of the pathological record. In addition, CISH and SISH do not require a fluorescent microscope and with the use of bright-field microscopy the viewer is able to evaluate gene status in the context of good morphology and tumor heterogeneity is much easier to view.

CISH, similar to the IHC process, uses a chromogenically labeled complementary DNA or RNA strand (probe) to localize a specific DNA or RNA target sequence in a tissue specimen (Fig. 3.5). The CISH method can be used to evaluate gene amplification, chromosome translocation, gene detection, and chromosome enumeration. CISH utilizes peroxidase or alkaline phosphatase reactions to visualize signals and is applicable to formalin-fixed, paraffin-embedded (FFPE) tissues, blood and bone marrow smears, metaphase chromosome spreads, and fixed cells. The CISH signals can be quantified using a 40× objective. Although CISH does not permit an actual determination of gene copy number, it has been shown to correlate well with FISH [12].

The SPOT-Light HER2 CISH kit (Invitrogen, Carlsbad, CA) is an FDA approved, single HER2 signal assay. The assay results can be visualized as a colored precipitate signal and counted using a 40× objective. The assay interpretation is based on the numbers of signal dots or clusters present in >50 % of tumor cells. The CISH procedure however, is time consuming and takes nearly as long as FISH to prepare the slides.

A dual-colored CISH assay, HER2 CISH pharmDX kit (Dako, Denmark), is also FDA approved. The signals are enumerated with a bright-field microscope similar to the method of counting FISH signals (HER2:CEP17 ratio).

This kit can be used manually or automated on Dako Autostainer instruments.

The other alternative ISH technology is silver in situ hybridization (SISH) which does allow for gene copy number enumeration. The INFORM HER2 SISH (Ventana, Tucson, AZ) assay is also available in the USA. This assay utilizes chromogenic silver deposition to detect a HER2 DNA probe on one slide and a Chromosome 17 (Chr17) probe on a matched slide. This strategy allows HER2 status to be determined in reference to Chr 17 so that a HER2/Chr17 ratio can be determined using the same reported ranges as those recommended by ASCO/CAP for FISH. The silver signals are counted and a ratio is calculated. All steps in this assay are fully automated and can be performed on the Benchmark series of automated strainers (Ventana, Tucson, AZ) which leads to an approximate 6-h turnaround time. The main disadvantages of assays which require two separate slides is the inability to know whether signal counts are being conducted on the same cells. In addition, there is an inherent risk of sectioning through smaller tumors when biopsy material is used for analysis.

In an attempt to overcome this, Ventana has recently introduced, and gained FDA approval for, the INFORM HER2 Dual ISH DNA Probe Cocktail, which combines ISH and IHC staining of HER2 and Chr 17 using SISH and Alk-Phos Red, respectively. This assay is also performed on the Benchmark instruments and is designed such that the HER2 probe and Chr 17 reference probe are visualized on the same slide during one automated run. High concordance rates with FISH have been reported in multiple studies for CISH (81–100 %) and SISH (94–98.9 %) [12–15].

Testing for *HER2* amplification has also been performed using PCR technology [16]. *HER2* gene amplification is associated with mRNA and protein overexpression. Recently, Baehner et al. report a 97 % concordance between central FISH analysis by PathVysion and HER2 mRNA quantitative reverse-transcriptase polymerase chain reaction (RT-PCR) by the Onco*type* DX assay [17]. Lehmann-Che et al. report a similar 97.3 % overall concordance of HER2 overexpression between IHC and quantitative reverse-transcriptase PCR (Q-RT-PCR) in 466 cases. They used TATA binding protein (an endogenous control), to determined a cutoff ratio of >7 for HER2 overexpression with the use of a training set of tumors that had correlative IHC data. Of 14 cases with equivocal 2+ IHC, Q-RT-PCR was highly predictive of final HER2 status (as determined by additional methods including FISH) in 10 of the cases, suggesting that Q-RT-PCR could be used as an alternative to FISH in IHC equivocal cases [18]. Q-RT-PCR is a fast, quantitative method that lacks intraobserver variability; however, careful microscopic selection of tumor prior to extraction is crucial. Quantitative PCR-based assays, although compelling will likely require a great deal more validation before they are accepted into clinical practice.

Currently, the CellSearch (Veridex LCC, Raritan, NJ) immunoassay technology is the only FDA-approved technology for detecting circulating tumor cells (CTCs) in patients with metastatic breast cancer. Ventana has developed a CellSearch Tumor Phenotyping Reagent HER2 which can be used in conjunction with the CTC identification technology to phenotype CTCs for HER2 expression.

However, this assay is still for research use only and the best method of quantifying HER2 expression in CTCs is still being determined [19–21].

Test Interpretation: Breast Cancer

P185^{HER-2} overexpression is associated with a worse clinical outcome [7] but is predictive of response to targeted therapies like trastuzumab and lapatinib. Trastuzumab was approved by the US Food and Drug administration (FDA) in 1998 and is widely used as a standard therapy for patients with HER2-positive metastatic breast cancer [22, 23]; and, as adjuvant therapy in early breast cancer combined with chemotherapeutic agents [24]. Therapy with trastuzumab, however, is not without drawbacks. It has been associated with a small risk of cardiac toxicity in approximately 4 % of patients when combined with doxorubicin-containing protocols [25]. And, although combined chemotherapy regimens have been modified, trastuzumab is an intravenously administered drug and the cost is significant.

In 2007, the FDA approved lapatinib for use in combination with capecitabine for treatment of advanced HER2-positive breast cancer in patients who had previously received chemotherapy or trastuzumab [26]. The role of adjuvant and neoadjuvant lapatinib in early stage disease is currently being studied by the ALTTO (Adjuvant Lapatinib and/or Transuzumab Treatment Optimization) and the NeoALTTO trials.

Accurate HER2-testing strategies are critical for appropriate management of breast cancer patients. In the review by Sauter et al., they conclude that because FISH assays are less dependent on tissue fixation and correlate better than IHC with tumor response to trastuzumab or laptinib, FISH should be used as the primary HER2-testing modality [27]. With approximately 200,000 women in the USA every year developing breast cancer, small discordance rates between HER2 assays can mean thousands of potentially inaccurate findings which could lead to tumors misclassified as false negative and those patients denied trastuzumab or tumors being classified as false positive and those women needlessly receive the $100,000 drug.

Despite there being multiple testing methodologies available, the debate on which testing strategy establishes the most accurate, reproducible, and clinically relevant HER2 status persists. The ASCO/CAP guidelines for breast cancer put forth in 2007 were drafted in part in response to several studies that showed that there was huge discordance between IHC data and FISH data observed between community laboratories and central laboratories (>27 % discordant for IHC—[28]; 23 % discordant for 3+ IHC and 74 % discordant for 2+ IHC—[29], and initial overall concordance of IHC and FISH of 82 %) [30, 31], suggesting the lack of standardization of the assays and interpretation.

The ASCO/CAP guidelines recommend HER2 testing by either IHC or FISH with confirmatory testing for equivocal cases (FISH for IHC equivocal and additional counting and/or repeat if FISH equivocal). These guidelines recommend criteria for accepting and rejecting IHC and FISH results without maintaining that either technique is preferable, emphasizing that there is no "gold standard" testing strategy. In addition, they altered the definition of a positive result (3+ uniform intense membrane staining in >30 % vs. prior >10 % of invasive tumor cells, >6 HER2 copies/nucleus, or HER2/CEP 17 ratio >2.2) and created an equivocal FISH category (HER2/CEP 17 ratio of 1.8–2.2 or average gene copy number between 4.0 and 6.0). The guidelines recommend optimal validation of the tests in which positive and negative HER2 categories are at least 95 % concordant with an alternative validated method or the same validated method performed at another laboratory. They stress the importance of internal quality control (QA) procedures, participation in proficiency testing with at least 90 % correct response rate, and laboratory accreditation with onsite and self inspection [8]. These guidelines do raise a number of issues that are difficult to control, such as preanalytical factors—e.g., variability across laboratories in tissue fixation methods and times which impact the tissue antigenicity. Despite the adherence to and acceptance of these guidelines, some authors still feel they are flawed. Subsequent to the publication of these guidelines, a second manuscript was published by many of the same authors that examined some of the false pretenses presented in the 2007 guideline document. These differences in the 2009 manuscript included the recommendation of FISH testing as a more accurate methodology, the lack of data to support an equivocal zone for FISH testing, and the lack of data to support a FISH cutoff ratio of >2.2 [27].

Another potential inherent issue with HER2 testing is tumor HER2 heterogeneity (either protein overexpression or amplification) which is seen in approximately 1 % of tumors [32] and is defined by CAP as more than 5 % but less than 50 % of infiltrating tumor cells with a FISH ratio higher than 2.2 [33]. The clinical significance and implications for targeted HER2 therapy are not clearly defined [34], but ASCO/CAP guidelines recommend documenting the presence of heterogeneity in the patient's report [33].

Polysomy 17 (p17) is another biological variable that's significance is unclear and incidence is dependent on how it is defined. According to the ASCO/CAP guidelines, polysomy is when a tumor has increased HER2 and CEP17 signals with a ratio of less than 1.8 [8]. Downs-Kelly et. al. report that in their patient population using a definition of CEP17 of ≥2.1, >2.5, or >3 would correlate with a p17 incidence of 35.4, 17.7, and 8 %, respectively. This same group found in a cohort of HER2 nonamplified/p17 cases (defined as a mean CEP17 of ≥2.1) that most of these cases are not associated with HER2 mRNA or protein overexpression. In addition, they noted no correlation with tumor size, ER/PR status, grade or lymph node status, but they did identify a correlation with p17 and women >50 years of age ($P=0.02$) [35]. The report by Perez et al. on associations between tumor characteristics and disease-free survival in the N9831 adjuvant trastuzumab trial defines p17 as ≥3 CEP17 signals in more than 30 % of nuclei. They found that in patients with *HER2* amplification, p17 did not predict for trastuzumab benefit [i.e., the benefit seen in patients with *HER2*-amplified tumors was not significantly different between *HER2* amplified/p17 and *HER2* amplified/normal 17 ($P=0.36$)]. However, they did observe that in HER2-positive patients treated with chemotherapy alone, those with p17 seemed to benefit more than those with normal 17, suggesting that polysomy may have some prognostic value for those treated with chemotherapy [36].

Recent array CGH studies have shown that complete polysomy 17 is rare and that CEP17 copy numbers >3 in dual-colored FISH assays are actually due to gains/amplification of the centromeric region in addition to *HER2* [37–39]. With co-amplification, the *HER2*/CEP17 ratio may be normal masking the fact that some of these are *HER2*-amplified tumors. Therefore, several authors now recommend reporting the average number of *HER2* genes per nucleus in addition to the *HER2*/CEP17 ratio in these complex cases [39, 40]. Further investigation is required to clarify the importance of these findings and to reach consensus on reporting them.

Regulatory Issues

HER2 testing either by IHC or FISH was one of the first true companion diagnostics approved by the FDA. The concept of having a novel therapeutic available that acted against a specific target also required knowledge of whether that target was present in the patient's tumor. Targeted therapies tend to be more expensive and not without potential side effects. In this case, Herceptin was known to be associated with cardiotoxicity; in order for breast cancer patients to be eligible for treatment, the tumor must have an amplified target gene or overexpress the target. The FDA initially approved an IHC assay followed by a FISH-based assay.

Two companion diagnostics, using different technologies and detecting different types of biological information, has led to much controversy as to which test is best for patient management. IHC detects HER2 protein expression, while FISH detects HER2 gene amplification, a mechanism by which cells overexpress protein. The need for testing guidelines was supported by studies that identified a very high false-positive rate in HER2 IHC testing, preanalytical variables such as tissue processing, and analytical variables such as test validation, calibration, competency, etc. This controversy lingers and two sets of competing guidelines have since been introduced [8, 27].

How the Test Has Changed Medical Practice

The emergence of targeted therapy for HER+ breast cancers has improved patient outcomes significantly. HER2 overexpression is observed in a significant percentage of breast cancers (up to 30 %), with gene amplification being the most significant mechanism of overexpression. This biological phenomenon is associated with tumors that have a higher risk for recurrence and worse overall survival. However, it also plays a significant role in determining which patients will be eligible for newer targeted therapies. Treatment with these novel therapies has been shown to improve response rates, time to progression, and survival. Testing breast cancers for HER2 amplification and/or overexpression status is critical as negative results identify individuals who will gain no benefit from costly and potentially toxic therapy, whereas, positive results identify patients who are eligible for potentially life-saving therapy.

Future Directions

HER2 overexpression or amplification has been reported in many other tumor types including, ovarian, gastric, lung, head and neck, prostate, and bladder carcinoma. Tuefferd et. al. report that in a multicenter series of 320 patients with advanced ovarian cancer, 6.6 % of tumors had HER2 overexpression and amplification [41]. In a study of 1,005 patients with invasive bladder carcinoma, 5.1 % had *HER2* amplification [42]. Clearly, there is the possibility that patients with other cancers besides breast cancer may benefit from HER2-targeted therapies. This potential has been perhaps been best brought to fruition to date in gastric carcinomas.

In October 2010, trastuzumab was approved by the FDA for use in combination with cysplatin and either capecitabine or 5-fluorouracil in patients with metastatic gastric or gastroesophageal junction cancer (GC/GEJ) who had not previously received treatment for metastatic disease. This approval was granted following the results of the ToGA (Trastuzumab for Gastric Cancer) phase III, international, randomized controlled trial which were recently published. This trial enrolled 594 patients with GC/GEJ with tumors overexpressing HER2 protein by IHC or gene amplification by FISH and they were randomized 1:1 into chemotherapy alone versus chemotherapy plus trastuzumab arms. The overall survival was clinically significant ($P=0.0046$) in those receiving trastuzumab (13.8 months at trial termination; 1- year follow-up—13.1 months) versus those treated with chemotherapy only (11.1 months at trial termination; 1-year follow-up—11.7 months) [43]. The tumors were evaluated at a central laboratory by IHC (HercepTest, Dako, Denmark) and FISH (pharmDx, Dako). They found HER2 positivity rate of 22.1 % with IHC/FISH concordance of 87.3 %. They used new IHC scoring criteria which are essentially modified HercepTest criteria that were based on a study by Hofmann et al. that suggested differences in the staining pattern in gastric tumors vs. breast cancers thus necessitating the modified criteria [44]. Patients were eligible for the trial if their tumor samples were either IHC 3+ or FISH positive with a HER2:CEP17 ratio ≥2. The results of this trial are expected to make significant impact on clinical practice. However, this trial did not include patients from North America and there is still no consensus on the optimal HER2-testing strategies in patients with gastric cancer. It is not clear if the ASCO/CAP guidelines created for breast cancer are applicable to GC, or if what Hofmann et al. suggest, modified criteria are necessary. At least one study evaluating HER2 testing within a US cohort suggests that the ASCO/CAP guidelines are applicable to GC/GEJ carcinoma [45]. However, additional validation studies from North America are needed to help address these questions.

In this era of personalized medicine, the development of targeted therapeutics has had a major impact on the treatment of cancer patients. Paired with this is the need for accurate and clinically relevant companion diagnostics available in clinical laboratories.

References

1. Yarden Y, Sliwkowski MX. Untangling the ErbB signalling network. Nat Rev Mol Cell Biol. 2001;2(2): 127–37.
2. De P, Smith BR, Leyland-Jones B. Human epidermal growth factor receptor 2 testing: where are we? J Clin Oncol. 2010;28(28):4289–92.
3. Spector NL, Blackwell KL. Understanding the mechanisms behind trastuzumab therapy for human epidermal growth factor receptor 2-positive breast cancer. J Clin Oncol. 2009;27(34):5838–47.

4. Hudis CA. Trastuzumab–mechanism of action and use in clinical practice. N Engl J Med. 2007; 357(1):39–51.
5. Wood ER, Truesdale AT, McDonald OB, Yuan D, Hassell A, Dickerson SH, et al. A unique structure for epidermal growth factor receptor bound to GW572016 (Lapatinib): relationships among protein conformation, inhibitor off-rate, and receptor activity in tumor cells. Cancer Res. 2004;64(18):6652–9.
6. Rusnak DW, Affleck K, Cockerill SG, Stubberfield C, Harris R, Page M, et al. The characterization of novel, dual ErbB-2/EGFR, tyrosine kinase inhibitors: potential therapy for cancer. Cancer Res. 2001;61(19): 7196–203.
7. Slamon DJ, Clark GM, Wong SG, Levin WJ, Ullrich A, McGuire WL. Human breast cancer: correlation of relapse and survival with amplification of the HER-2/neu oncogene. Science. 1987;235(4785):177–82.
8. Wolff AC, Hammond ME, Schwartz JN, Hagerty KL, Allred DC, Cote RJ, et al. American Society of Clinical Oncology/College of American Pathologists guideline recommendations for human epidermal growth factor receptor 2 testing in breast cancer. Arch Pathol Lab Med. 2007;131(1):18–43.
9. Khoury T, Sait S, Hwang H, Chandrasekhar R, Wilding G, Tan D, et al. Delay to formalin fixation effect on breast biomarkers. Mod Pathol. 2009;22(11): 1457–67.
10. Oyama T, Ishikawa Y, Hayashi M, Arihiro K, Horiguchi J. The effects of fixation, processing and evaluation criteria on immunohistochemical detection of hormone receptors in breast cancer. Breast Cancer. 2007;14(2):182–8.
11. Hammond ME, Hayes DF, Dowsett M, Allred DC, Hagerty KL, Badve S, et al. American Society of Clinical Oncology/College of American Pathologists guideline recommendations for immunohistochemical testing of estrogen and progesterone receptors in breast cancer (unabridged version). Arch Pathol Lab Med. 2010;134(7):e48–72.
12. Penault-Llorca F, Bilous M, Dowsett M, Hanna W, Osamura RY, Ruschoff J, et al. Emerging technologies for assessing HER2 amplification. Am J Clin Pathol. 2009;132(4):539–48.
13. Bartlett JM, Campbell FM, Ibrahim M, Wencyk P, Ellis I, Kay E, et al. Chromogenic in situ hybridization: a multicenter study comparing silver in situ hybridization with FISH. Am J Clin Pathol. 2009;132(4):514–20.
14. Papouchado BG, Myles J, Lloyd RV, Stoler M, Oliveira AM, Downs-Kelly E, et al. Silver in situ hybridization (SISH) for determination of HER2 gene status in breast carcinoma: comparison with FISH and assessment of interobserver reproducibility. Am J Surg Pathol. 2010;34(6):767–76.
15. Carbone A, Botti G, Gloghini A, Simone G, Truini M, Curcio MP, et al. Delineation of HER2 gene status in breast carcinoma by silver in situ hybridization is reproducible among laboratories and pathologists. J Mol Diagn. 2008;10(6):527–36.
16. Capizzi E, Gruppioni E, Grigioni AD, Gabusi E, Grassigli A, Grigioni WF, et al. Real time RT-PCR approach for the evaluation of ERBB2 overexpression in breast cancer archival samples: a comparative study with FISH, SISH, and immunohistochemistry. Diagn Mol Pathol. 2008;17(4):220–6.
17. Baehner FL, Achacoso N, Maddala T, Shak S, Quesenberry Jr CP, Goldstein LC, et al. Human epidermal growth factor receptor 2 assessment in a case-control study: comparison of fluorescence in situ hybridization and quantitative reverse transcription polymerase chain reaction performed by central laboratories. J Clin Oncol. 2010;28(28):4300–6.
18. Lehmann-Che J, Amira-Bouhidel F, Turpin E, Antoine M, Soliman H, Legres L, et al. Immunohistochemical and molecular analyses of HER2 status in breast cancers are highly concordant and complementary approaches. Br J Cancer. 2011; 104(11):1739–46.
19. Ignatiadis M, Rothe F, Chaboteaux C, Durbecq V, Rouas G, Criscitiello C, et al. HER2-positive circulating tumor cells in breast cancer. PLoS One. 2011;6(1):e15624.
20. Riethdorf S, Muller V, Zhang L, Rau T, Loibl S, Komor M, et al. Detection and HER2 expression of circulating tumor cells: prospective monitoring in breast cancer patients treated in the neoadjuvant GeparQuattro trial. Clin Cancer Res. 2010;16(9): 2634–45.
21. Fehm T, Muller V, Aktas B, Janni W, Schneeweiss A, Stickeler E, et al. HER2 status of circulating tumor cells in patients with metastatic breast cancer: a prospective, multicenter trial. Breast Cancer Res Treat. 2010;124(2):403–12.
22. Slamon DJ, Leyland-Jones B, Shak S, Fuchs H, Paton V, Bajamonde A, et al. Use of chemotherapy plus a monoclonal antibody against HER2 for metastatic breast cancer that overexpresses HER2. N Engl J Med. 2001;344(11):783–92.
23. Vogel CL, Cobleigh MA, Tripathy D, Gutheil JC, Harris LN, Fehrenbacher L, et al. Efficacy and safety of trastuzumab as a single agent in first-line treatment of HER2-overexpressing metastatic breast cancer. J Clin Oncol. 2002;20(3):719–26.
24. Romond EH, Perez EA, Bryant J, Suman VJ, Geyer Jr CE, Davidson NE, et al. Trastuzumab plus adjuvant chemotherapy for operable HER2-positive breast cancer. N Engl J Med. 2005;353(16):1673–84.
25. Tan-Chiu E, Yothers G, Romond E, Geyer Jr CE, Ewer M, Keefe D, et al. Assessment of cardiac dysfunction in a randomized trial comparing doxorubicin and cyclophosphamide followed by paclitaxel, with or without trastuzumab as adjuvant therapy in node-positive, human epidermal growth factor receptor 2-overexpressing breast cancer: NSABP B-31. J Clin Oncol. 2005;23(31):7811–9.
26. Geyer CE, Forster J, Lindquist D, Chan S, Romieu CG, Pienkowski T, et al. Lapatinib plus capecitabine for HER2-positive advanced breast cancer. N Engl J Med. 2006;355(26):2733–43.

27. Sauter G, Lee J, Bartlett JM, Slamon DJ, Press MF. Guidelines for human epidermal growth factor receptor 2 testing: biologic and methodologic considerations. J Clin Oncol. 2009;27(8):1323–33.
28. Roche PC, Suman VJ, Jenkins RB, Davidson NE, Martino S, Kaufman PA, et al. Concordance between local and central laboratory HER2 testing in the breast intergroup trial N9831. J Natl Cancer Inst. 2002; 94(11):855–7.
29. Reddy JC, Reimann JD, Anderson SM, Klein PM. Concordance between central and local laboratory HER2 testing from a community-based clinical study. Clin Breast Cancer. 2006;7(2):153–7.
30. Dybdal N, Leiberman G, Anderson S, McCune B, Bajamonde A, Cohen RL, et al. Determination of HER2 gene amplification by fluorescence in situ hybridization and concordance with the clinical trials immunohistochemical assay in women with metastatic breast cancer evaluated for treatment with trastuzumab. Breast Cancer Res Treat. 2005;93(1): 3–11.
31. Mass RD, Press MF, Anderson S, Cobleigh MA, Vogel CL, Dybdal N, et al. Evaluation of clinical outcomes according to HER2 detection by fluorescence in situ hybridization in women with metastatic breast cancer treated with trastuzumab. Clin Breast Cancer. 2005;6(3):240–6.
32. Hanna W, Nofech-Mozes S, Kahn HJ. Intratumoral heterogeneity of HER2/neu in breast cancer–a rare event. Breast J. 2007;13(2):122–9.
33. Vance GH, Barry TS, Bloom KJ, Fitzgibbons PL, Hicks DG, Jenkins RB, et al. Genetic heterogeneity in HER2 testing in breast cancer: panel summary and guidelines. Arch Pathol Lab Med. 2009;133(4): 611–2.
34. Cottu PH, Asselah J, Lae M, Pierga JY, Dieras V, Mignot L, et al. Intratumoral heterogeneity of HER2/neu expression and its consequences for the management of advanced breast cancer. Ann Oncol. 2008;19(3):595–7.
35. Downs-Kelly E, Yoder BJ, Stoler M, Tubbs RR, Skacel M, Grogan T, et al. The influence of polysomy 17 on HER2 gene and protein expression in adenocarcinoma of the breast: a fluorescent in situ hybridization, immunohistochemical, and isotopic mRNA in situ hybridization study. Am J Surg Pathol. 2005; 29(9):1221–7.
36. Perez EA, Reinholz MM, Hillman DW, Tenner KS, Schroeder MJ, Davidson NE, et al. HER2 and chromosome 17 effect on patient outcome in the N9831 adjuvant trastuzumab trial. J Clin Oncol. 2010; 28(28):4307–15.
37. Yeh IT, Martin MA, Robetorye RS, Bolla AR, McCaskill C, Shah RK, et al. Clinical validation of an array CGH test for HER2 status in breast cancer reveals that polysomy 17 is a rare event. Mod Pathol. 2009;22(9):1169–75.
38. Marchio C, Lambros MB, Gugliotta P, Di Cantogno LV, Botta C, Pasini B, et al. Does chromosome 17 centromere copy number predict polysomy in breast cancer? A fluorescence in situ hybridization and microarray-based CGH analysis. J Pathol. 2009; 219(1):16–24.
39. Vranic S, Teruya B, Repertinger S, Ulmer P, Hagenkord J, Gatalica Z. Assessment of HER2 gene status in breast carcinomas with polysomy of chromosome 17. Cancer. 2011;117(1):48–53.
40. Varga Z, Tubbs RR, Wang Z, Sun Y, Noske A, Kradolfer D, et al. Co-amplification of the HER2 gene and chromosome 17 centromere: a potential diagnostic pitfall in HER2 testing in breast cancer. Breast Cancer Res Treat. 2012;132(3):925–35.
41. Tuefferd M, Couturier J, Penault-Llorca F, Vincent-Salomon A, Broet P, Guastalla JP, et al. HER2 status in ovarian carcinomas: a multicenter GINECO study of 320 patients. PLoS One. 2007;2(11):e1138.
42. Lae M, Couturier J, Oudard S, Radvanyi F, Beuzeboc P, Vieillefond A. Assessing HER2 gene amplification as a potential target for therapy in invasive urothelial bladder cancer with a standardized methodology: results in 1005 patients. Ann Oncol. 2010;21(4): 815–9.
43. Bang YJ, Van Cutsem E, Feyereislova A, Chung HC, Shen L, Sawaki A, et al. Trastuzumab in combination with chemotherapy versus chemotherapy alone for treatment of HER2-positive advanced gastric or gastro-oesophageal junction cancer (ToGA): a phase 3, open-label, randomised controlled trial. Lancet. 2010;376(9742):687–97.
44. Hofmann M, Stoss O, Shi D, Buttner R, van de Vijver M, Kim W, et al. Assessment of a HER2 scoring system for gastric cancer: results from a validation study. Histopathology. 2008;52(7):797–805.
45. Tafe LJ, Janjigian YY, Zaidinski M, Hedvat CV, Hameed MR, Tang LH, et al. Human epidermal growth factor receptor 2 (HER2) testing in gastroesophageal cancer: correlation between immunohistochemistry (IHC) and fluorescence in-situ hybridization (FISH). Arch Pathol Lab Med. 2011;135(11): 1460–5.

4 Tamoxifen and Irinotecan Pharmacogenomics

John Logan Black III

Background

Pharmacogenomics is defined as the use of a person's genetic information to individualize treatment. This is a burgeoning field which is starting to have a major impact on many areas in medicine. Notable examples are the following: The use of cytochrome P450 2C9 (*CYP2C9*) and vitamin K epoxide reductase complex subunit 1 (*VKORC1*) genotyping to predict response to warfarin, the use of serotonin transporter (*SLC6A4*) promoter length polymorphism for prediction of response to serotonin reuptake inhibitors, the use of *CYP2C19* genotyping to predict response to clopidogrel, the use of HLA-B*5701 genotyping to predict hypersensitivity reactions to abacavir, and the use of HLA-B*1502 genotyping to identifying individuals of Asian ancestry who are at risk of developing Stevens–Johnson syndrome and toxic epidermal necrolysis when administered carbamazepine, phenytoin, or fosphenytoin therapy.

In some ways, the implementation of these and other pharmacogenomic tests into clinical practice has been disappointingly slow. This appears to be due to (1) lack of clear clinical outcomes data derived from prospective studies showing medical economic benefit, (2) a physician workforce which is inadequately trained to handle the complexities of the genotyping results that are obtained, and (3) slow FDA acceptance of pharmacogenomic data plus reluctance to generate clear drug label changes which mandate pharmacogenomic testing prior to use of specific drugs.

This chapter will focus on pharmacogenomic applications involving two drugs used in Oncology: *CYP2D6* testing for postmenopausal estrogen receptor-positive breast cancer patients receiving tamoxifen and *UGT1A1* testing for oncology patients receiving irinotecan. In the case of *CYP2D6*, acceptance has been deterred by inconsistent results between studies so the clinical impact has not been so great. In the case of *UGT1A1*, however, there is greater acceptance and an FDA black box warning which is driving acceptance of the testing in clinical settings.

CYP2D6 Genotyping for Tamoxifen and Breast Cancer

Clinical Applications

Breast cancer remains one of the most commonly diagnosed cancers. An estimated 230,480 new cases of breast cancer and 39,520 breast cancer deaths are expected in 2011 despite the fact that incidence rates are stable and death rates have been

J.L. Black III, M.D. (✉)
Nucleotide Polymorphism Laboratory, Division of Clinical Biochemistry and Immunology, Department of Laboratory Medicine and Pathology, Mayo Clinic, 200 1st Street SW, Rochester, MN 55905, USA
e-mail: black.john@mayo.edu

W.E. Highsmith Jr. (ed.), *Molecular Diagnostics: 12 Tests That Changed Everything*, Molecular and Translational Medicine, DOI 10.1007/978-1-4614-8127-0_4,

declining for all women except American Indians/ Alaska Natives [1]. Overall trends in 5-year survival rates have been improving from 75 % in 1974–1976 to 88 % in 1995–2001 in the USA [2].

Tamoxifen, a selective estrogen receptor modulator, has been a mainstay in therapy for this condition since 1977 when it was first approved for postmenopausal metastatic breast cancer. Subsequently, the list of indications has grown to include postmenopausal, node-positive, adjuvant therapy for breast cancer; premenopausal metastatic breast cancer; postmenopausal node-negative breast cancer; metastatic breast cancer in males; reduction in breast cancer incidence in high-risk women; and ductal carcinoma in situ. There is insufficient data available regarding the effect of tamoxifen on breast cancer incidence in women with inherited mutations (*BRCA1*, *BRCA2*) to be able to make specific recommendations on the effectiveness of tamoxifen citrate in these patients [3].

Tamoxifen-Mechanism of Action

Tamoxifen is the *trans*-isomer of a triphenylethylene derivative and is a nonsteroidal agent with potent estrogenic antagonist and partial estrogenic agonist activity. Tamoxifen demonstrates anticancer action, anticarcinogenic potential, and an ability to reverse multidrug resistance. The drug has been shown to upregulate both estrogen and progesterone receptors in breast cancer. It is also known as a selective estrogen receptor modulator (SERM). Tamoxifen's anticancer activity was thought to be due to its ability to compete with estrogen at the estrogen receptor (ER) in target tissues such as the breast. However, the drug is also an inhibitor of protein kinase C and Ca^{2+}-calmodulin-dependent cAMP phosphodiesterase, induces cells surrounding the cancer cells to secrete the negative growth factor transforming growth factor-beta (TGF-beta), and suppresses insulin-like growth factor I (IGF-1), which is a potent mitogen for breast cancer cell in vitro [3].

Tamoxifen Metabolism

Tamoxifen is extensively metabolized by the cytochrome P450 system to several primary and secondary metabolites, some which exhibit more antiestrogenic effect in breast cancer cells than tamoxifen itself. For example, 4-hydroxytamoxifen has approximately 30- to 100-fold more potent antiestrogen effect than tamoxifen. The major metabolic pathway of tamoxifen is *N*-demethylation to *N*-desmethyltamoxifen. This pathway is primarily catalyzed by CYP3A4 and CYP3A5. N-Desmethyltamoxifen is further oxidized to a number of metabolites that appear important to tamoxifen activity including hydroxylated by the *CYP2D6* enzyme to endoxifen [4]. See Fig. 4.1 for a more complete discussion of tamoxifen metabolism.

Why Individualized Treatment Is Important in Breast Cancer Management

There are strong incentives for seeking an individualized treatment approach for patients with breast cancer. Not all patients respond to tamoxifen equally and the hope is to find a genetic etiology for this. Secondly, tamoxifen is commonly used and is fairly inexpensive compared to other medications partly because it is available in a generic form. This makes the drug attractive to insurance companies, if it is effective in place of aromatase inhibitors, which are much more expensive. Third, there is a high cost of nonresponse to tamoxifen in terms of morbidity and mortality so focusing treatment on patients who can respond to the drug is highly relevant.

Review of the Literature

The role of *CYP2D6* genotype in tamoxifen response in breast cancer patients has been under examination since the metabolic pathways of tamoxifen were described as detailed by Destra et al. [4] (Fig. 4.1). Goetz et al. [5] did the initial retrospective study to examine outcomes related to *CYP2D6* genotype in postmenopausal women with early-stage ER-positive breast cancers who were treated with tamoxifen alone for 5 years. Follow-up for these patients was a median of 11.4 years and only the *CYP2D6*4* allele was studied. Even though the sample size was 223 patients, homozygosity for the **4* genotype was associated with worse recurrence-free time and

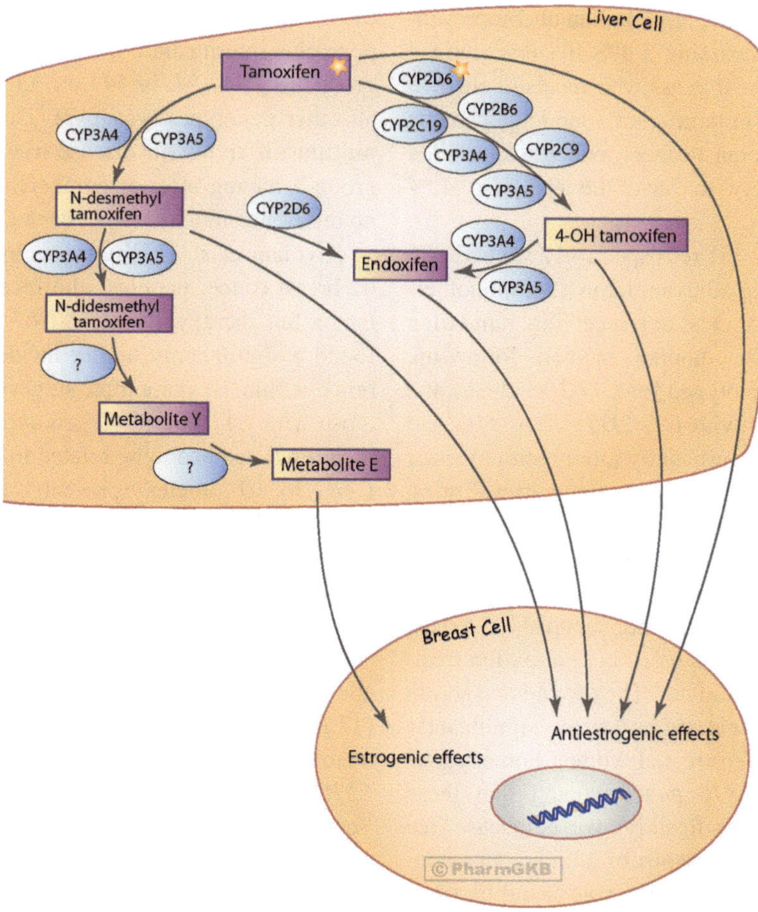

Fig. 4.1 Tamoxifen, a selective estrogen receptor modulator (SERMs), is important for the treatment and prevention of breast cancer. Tamoxifen is extensively metabolized predominantly by the cytochrome P450 system to several primary and secondary metabolites. Some of these metabolites exhibit more antiestrogenic effect in breast cancer cells than tamoxifen itself. This pathway depicts major pathways of tamoxifen metabolism that might have relevance to tamoxifen activity. Tamoxifen 4-hydroxylation is the most studied because it has been shown that 4-hydroxy-tamoxifen is approximately 30- to 100-fold more potent antiestrogen than tamoxifen. Tamoxifen 4-hydroxylation is catalyzed by *CYP2D6* and other isoforms. The major metabolic pathway of tamoxifen is *N*-demethylation to *N*-desmethyltamoxifen. This pathway is primarily catalyzed by CYP3A4 and CYP3A5. *N*-Desmethyltamoxifen is further oxidized to a number of metabolites that appear important to tamoxifen activity. First, *N*-desmethyltamoxifen is hydroxylated by the *CYP2D6* enzyme to endoxifen. This metabolite is as potent as 4-hydroxytamoxifen in terms of antiestrogenic activity, while its plasma concentrations in breast cancer patients are much higher than that of 4-hydroxytamoxifen. Second, *N*-desmethyltamoxifen undergoes sequential metabolism to metabolite E, which exhibits in vitro estrogenic activity. Details of tamoxifen primary and sequential metabolism have been published by Desta et al. [4]. Image and legend are from the Pharmacogenomic Knowledge Base (http://www.pharmgkb.org/index.jsp), are copyrighted to PharmGKB and Stanford University, and are used with permission from PharmGKB and Stanford University [69]

disease-free survival compared to women with either the **1/*4* or **1/*1* genotypes. Further analyses revealed that patients who were placed on *CYP2D6* inhibitors such as selective serotonin reuptake inhibitors also did more poorly and experienced shorter time to recurrence and worse recurrence-free survival leading to the conclusion that decreased *CYP2D6* function, whether due to drug inhibition or genotype, was a predictor of response to tamoxifen in this patient population [6].

Research from the large Italian chemoprevention trial, encompassing 5,408 hysterectomized women aged 35–70 years who received either 5 years of placebo or tamoxifen, found that patients who developed breast cancer while on tamoxifen were more likely to have the *CYP2D6*4/*4* genotype [7].

Schroth et al. [8] retrospectively studied 206 patients receiving adjuvant tamoxifen monotherapy and 280 patients not receiving tamoxifen therapy with 71 months median follow-up. Patients were genotyped for *CYP2D6* alleles and found that those with *CYP2D6*4*, *5*, *10*, and *41* alleles had significantly more recurrences of breast cancer, shorter relapse-free survival rates, and worse event-free survival rates compared with carriers of functional alleles.

Xu et al. [9] examined the association between *CYP2D6*10* genotype and survival of breast cancer in 152 patients receiving tamoxifen treatment vs. 141 who did not. They found that serum 4-OH-Tam concentrations were significantly lower in tamoxifen-treated women homozygous for the *CYP2D6*10* genotype and that these women had a significantly worse disease-free survival than heterozygous or homozygous non-*10* patients. No association was found between genotype and those patients not treated with tamoxifen.

Schroth et al. [10] conducted another retrospective study of 1,325 German and US patients treated with adjuvant tamoxifen for early-stage breast cancer (Stage I through III) who were mainly postmenopausal with a median follow-up of 6.3 years. Inclusion criteria required that the patients be hormone receptor positive without metastatic disease and on adjuvant tamoxifen therapy and no chemotherapy. The patients were genotyped for *CYP2D6*3*, *4*, *5*, *10*, and *41* to predict *CYP2D6* phenotype. Compared with extensive metabolizers, those with decreased *CYP2D6* activity had worse event-free survival and disease-free survival but no significant differences in overall survival.

Ramon y Cajal et al. [11] evaluated the impact of *CYP2D6* genotyping in predicting disease-free survival and toxicity in patients treated with adjuvant tamoxifen. Ninety-one samples were tested for 27 alleles and patients were grouped into a poor plus intermediate metabolizer group called group1 (e.g., *4/*4*, *4/*41*, *1/*5*, and *2/*5*) vs. all other genotypes (group 2). There was a significant difference in disease-free survival with group 1 having inferior numbers, but there was no difference in toxicity between groups.

Kiyotani et al. [12] retrospectively evaluated 67 breast cancer patients who received adjuvant tamoxifen therapy for *CYP2D6*10* alleles and found a significantly higher incidence of recurrence within 10 years after surgery compared to those with *CYP2D6*1/*1* genotype. The risk of recurrence seemed to be related to the number of *CYP2D6*10* alleles present. Patients with *CYP2D6*10/*10* had a significantly shorter recurrence-free survival period after adjustment for other prognostic factors.

Newman et al. [13] conducted a chart review and genotyping for *CYP2D6*3*, *4*, *5*, and *41* alleles in 115 patients with familial breast cancer (47 *BRCA1* and 68 *BRCA2*) treated with 20 mg tamoxifen per day following surgery. Use of *CYP2D6*-inhibiting medications was evaluated. Poor metabolizer status for *CYP2D6* predicted worse overall survival in patients with familial breast cancer, especially those with BRCA2 mutations.

Nowell et al. [14] found no association between *CYP2D6*4* genotype and overall survival in a retrospective study of 162 tamoxifen-treated ER-positive patients and Wegman [15, 16] similarly found no association between *CYP2D6*4* and disease-free interval and overall survival in a retrospective study. Okishiro et al. [17] also did not find a positive association.

Lammers et al. [18] conducted a cohort study of 102 patients using *CYP2D6* genotype and concomitant use of *CYP2D6*-inhibiting medication on time to breast cancer progression and overall survival in women using 40 mg tamoxifen per day for metastatic breast cancer. *CYP2D6*3*, *4*, *5*, *6*, *10*, and *41* were evaluated. Overall survival was shorter in patients with a poor metabolizer phenotype compared to extensive metabolizer phenotype. Use of *CYP2D6* inhibitors was also associated with worse overall survival.

493 patients of the Austrian TIGER study receiving adjuvant tamoxifen therapy were evaluated for *CYP2D6*4* genotype [19]. The study included patients with previous chemotherapy. No significant differences in time to tumor progression or progression-free survival between the *CYP2D6*4* genotype groups were found overall. However, in a subgroup of patients treated with chemotherapy, the *CYP2D6*4* poor metabolizers had a tendency toward shorter mean time to progression. The study suggested that *CYP2D6*4* genotyping might be particularly valuable for patients who previously received chemotherapy.

Lim et al. [20] studied 165 Asian breast cancer patients receiving 20 mg of tamoxifen daily and 228 healthy Asian subjects to determine the impact of *CYP2D6*, *CYP3A5*, *CYP2C9*, and *CYP2C19* genotype on tamoxifen pharmacokinetics. Focusing on the *CYP2D6* results, *CYP2D6*5* and **10* were associated with significantly lower endoxifen and higher *N*-desmethyltamoxifen concentrations. The role of the other genes studied here appeared to be minor.

Similarly, Madlensky et al. [21] determined tamoxifen metabolite concentration in reference to *CYP2D6* genotype and breast cancer outcomes from 1,370 patients with ER-positive breast cancer participating in the Women's Healthy Eating and Living Study. Breast cancer outcomes were not associated with concentrations of tamoxifen, 4-OH-Tam, and ND-tamoxifen. However, women in the upper four quintiles of endoxifen concentration had a lower recurrence rate than women in the bottom quintile and being a poor/intermediate metabolizer genotype was one predictor of being in the lower quintile. The study suggests that the minimal concentration threshold above which endoxifen is effective against breast cancer recurrence can be achieved by 80 % of those given the drug.

Seruga and Amir [22] conducted a meta-analysis which included ten studies in the analysis. When compared to reduced function, normal function was associated with a trend toward improved disease-free survival but not overall survival. Pooled data from studies involving the use of *CYP2D6* inhibitors revealed that use with tamoxifen was associated with nonsignificant association with decreased disease-free survival. Overall, the effect of *CYP2D6* genotype on breast cancer outcomes appeared small and the authors concluded that *CYP2D6* testing may not be warranted, although avoidance of the use of potent inhibitors of *CYP2D6* seemed reasonable.

Lash et al. [23] conducted a review of the ten epidemiological studies which examined the association between *CYP2D6* genotype and breast cancer recurrence with relative-risk estimates outside of the range of reasonable bounds including several already cited above. The authors reviewed the epidemiological evidence and found issues with study heterogeneity caused by study design, selection bias, uncontrolled confounders, and potential information bias or misclassification. Taken together, their conclusion was that more evidence should be collected before any decision is reached on the need for *CYP2D6* genotyping for patients receiving tamoxifen for breast cancer treatment.

Limitations of Studies

There are many limitations to the studies to date. Most of the studies are retrospective. Medication compliance was not assessed except in those where metabolite levels were obtained. No studies examined for all of the known variants of *CYP2D6*; indeed, this is exceedingly difficult as will be discussed below. Ethnicity also plays a role in the frequency of *CYP2D6* alleles and might impact the actual expressed phenotype of some alleles, none of which has been adequately studied to date. There is inadequate research as to what should be done when a patient is known to have deficiency alleles: e.g., should the patient be switched to another agent or should the dose of tamoxifen be altered? Studies do not address what potency of *CYP2D6* inhibitor should be avoided when a patient is receiving tamoxifen therapy. Finally, there is considerable heterogeneity between the various studies to date including: tumor, stage, chemotherapy programs, use of radiation therapy, ethnicity, tamoxifen dose, and medical economic outcomes. These limitations likely account for the inconsistent findings that have been reported and these issues will only be addressable using a carefully designed prospective study involving very large numbers of patients.

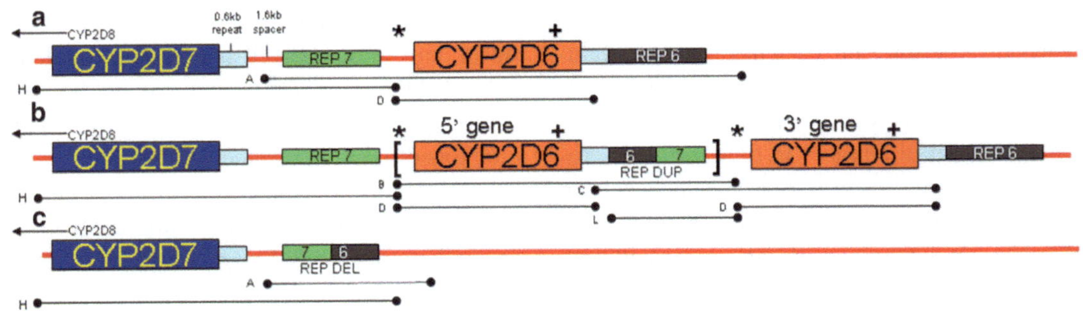

Fig. 4.2 *CYP2D* locus structures for single, typical duplicated and deleted arrangements. (a) Single *CYP2D6* arrangement. *CYP2D8* (not shown) and *CYP2D7* pseudogenes are located 5′ to the *CYP2D6* gene. Similar 0.6 kb repeats follow the *CYP2D7* and *CYP2D6* sequences as do rep 7 and rep 6, respectively, which differ by just a few nucleotides in the rep's 5′ and 3′ regions. Note a 1.6 kb spacer is located 3′ to the *CYP2D7* pseudogene but is normally absent downstream of the *CYP2D6* gene. (b) Typical *CYP2D6* duplication arrangement or multiplication. The first *CYP2D6* gene is followed by rep dup, a hybrid containing a 5′ rep 6 sequence and a 3′ rep 7 sequence. Multiplications of the sequence shown between the *brackets* are known to exist. (c) *CYP2D6* deletion arrangement (*CYP2D6*5*) where *CYP2D7* is followed by a rep del which is a hybrid containing a 5′ rep 7 sequence and a 3′ rep 6 sequence. PCR fragments that can be used in genotyping are depicted as *lettered lines* under the structures (see the following references for methods [25, 27]). Probe locations for Taqman® copy number assays are designated as *asterisk* and *plus sign* for the 5′ flanking *CYP2D6* assay and the *CYP2D6* intron 6 assay, respectively

CYP2D6 Structure and Variation

The *CYP2D6* gene is located on chromosome 22q13.1. *CYP2D6* is one of the most polymorphic CYP isoforms with nomenclature ranging from *CYP2D6*1A* to *CYP2D6*105* (http://www.cypalleles.ki.se/*CYP2D6*.htm) (Fig. 4.2). *CYP2D6* may be duplicated and duplications of up to 13 copies on a single chromosome have been described [24]. CYP2D7 pseudogene is located adjacent to *CYP2D6* and it is highly homologous to *CYP2D6* which has led to many recombinant events between these two alleles in ancestry which has given rise to many hybrid alleles with little or no function (e.g., *CYP2D6*4*N, **13*, **16*, **36*, and others) (Figs. 4.3 and 4.4). The gene can also be deleted as in the case of **5*. Allelic frequencies and consequently the incidence of phenotypes (poor, intermediate, extensive, and ultrarapid) vary widely among ethnic groups.

CYP2D6 is involved in phase I drug metabolism of many medications; plus it is involved in the bioactivation of tamoxifen and codeine among others. *CYP2D6* is one of the prototypic examples of pharmacogenomic targets and was listed as one of only two "valid pharmacogenomic biomarkers" in the 2003 Food and Drug Administration (FDA) Draft Guidance for Pharmacogenomic data.

An issue in *CYP2D6* genotyping is the presence of recombinant or hybrid genes in addition to the deletions, duplications, and multiplications already mentioned. These hybrid genes are the result of recombinant events that have occurred between *CYP2D6* and *CYP2D7* pseudogene and they can occur as single hybrid genes on a chromosome or as tandem hybrid alleles. Figure 4.3 shows the known hybrid gene arrangements of the *CYP2D6-2D7* variety and Fig. 4.4 shows the known hybrid gene arrangements of the *CYP2D7-2D6* variety.

CYP2D6 Substrates, Inducers, Inhibitors, and Probes

The following is a list of substrates, inducers, and inhibitors. Due to the rapid advance in knowledge in this arena, this list may not be complete at the time of publication. An accurate listing of inducers, inhibitors, and substrates for the Human Cytochrome P450 enzymes is maintained by Indiana University at http://medicine.iupui.edu/clinpharm/ddis/.

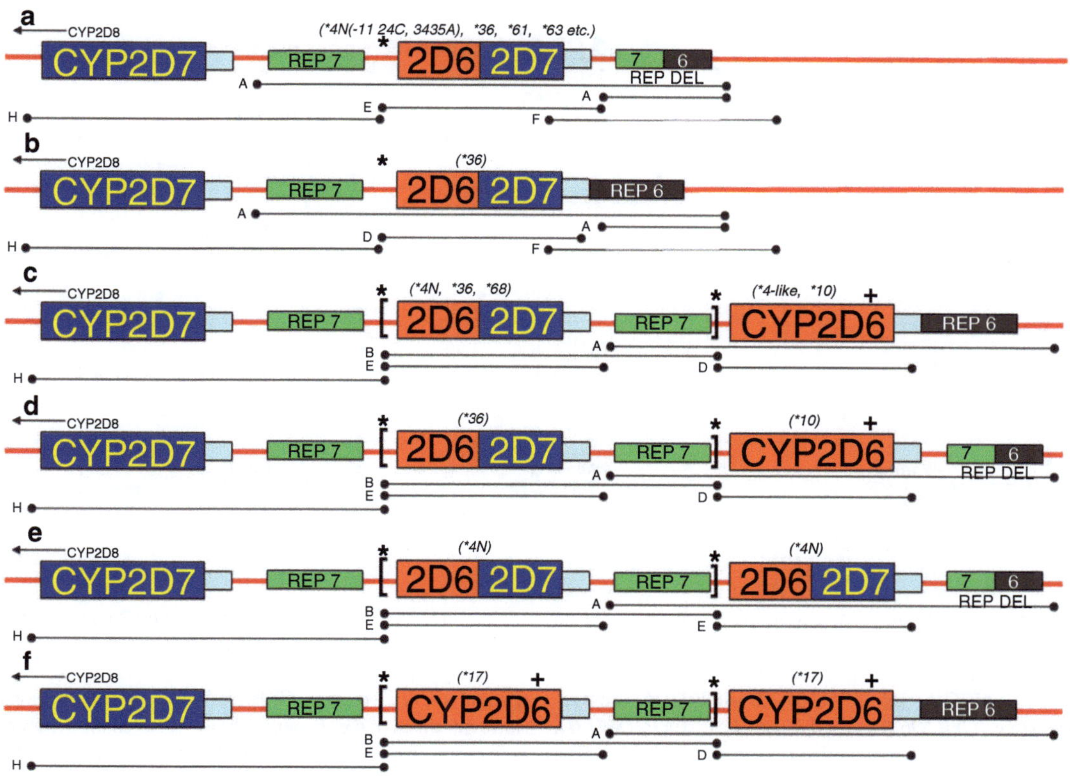

Fig. 4.3 *CYP2D* locus structures for single and hybrid tandems of *CYP2D6-2D7*. (a) When a chromosome has a single *CYP2D6-2D7* gene, the allele is usually followed by the 1.6 kb spacer sequence before transitioning into rep del. (b) Rarely, as in the case of this *CYP2D6*36*, conversion back to CYP2D6-like sequence occurs in the 0.6 kb repeat and this is followed by the typical rep 6 region. (c) The most frequently encountered *CYP2D6-2D7* hybrid tandem is depicted here. A 5′ recombinant allele is trailed by a spacer sequence and rep 7 before the 3′ *CYP2D6* allele. (d) This hybrid tandem is identical to C except for a transition back to CYP2D7-like sequence in the 0.6 kb repeat 3′ to the 3′ **10* allele which is followed by the expected 1.6 bp spacer and rep del. (e) (*CYP2D6-2D7*) *X N* arrangement involving **4N*. (f) *CYP2C6*17* duplication arrangement which lacks the rep dup sequence. This duplication will not yield a duplication signal in many genotyping platforms which detect the presence of a duplication on the basis of the rep dup sequence. PCR fragments that can be used in genotyping are depicted as *lettered lines* under the structures (see the following references for methods [25, 27]). Probe locations for Taqman® copy number assays are designated as *asterisk* and *plus sign* for the 5′ flanking *CYP2D6* assay and the *CYP2D6* intron 6 assay, respectively. Note that *CYP2D8* is thought to be present in all of the structures but is not shown for simplicity

The medications that are metabolized by *CYP2D6* can be broadly classified into analgesics and antitussives: codeine, dextromethorphan, lidocaine, oxycodone, phenacetin, promethazine, and tramadol; the antihistamine chlorpheniramine; cardiac and antihypertensive drugs alprenolol, bufuralol, carvedilol, debrisoquine, encainide, flecainide, S-metoprolol, mexiletine, nebivolol, perhexiline, propafenone, propranolol, sparteine, and timolol; the estrogen antagonist tamoxifen; gastrointestinal and metabolic drugs dexfenfluramine, metoclopramide, ondansetron, and phenformin; the psychotropics amitriptyline, amphetamine, aripiprazole, atomoxetine, chlorpromazine, clomipramine, desipramine, duloxetine, fluoxetine, fluvoxamine, haloperidol, imipramine, minaprine, nortriptyline, paroxetine, perphenazine, risperidone, thioridazine, venlafaxine, and zuclopenthixol; and the memory sparing agent donepezil.

Inhibitors can be classified according to potency. The most potent are bupropion, cinacalcet, fluoxetine, paroxetine, and quinidine.

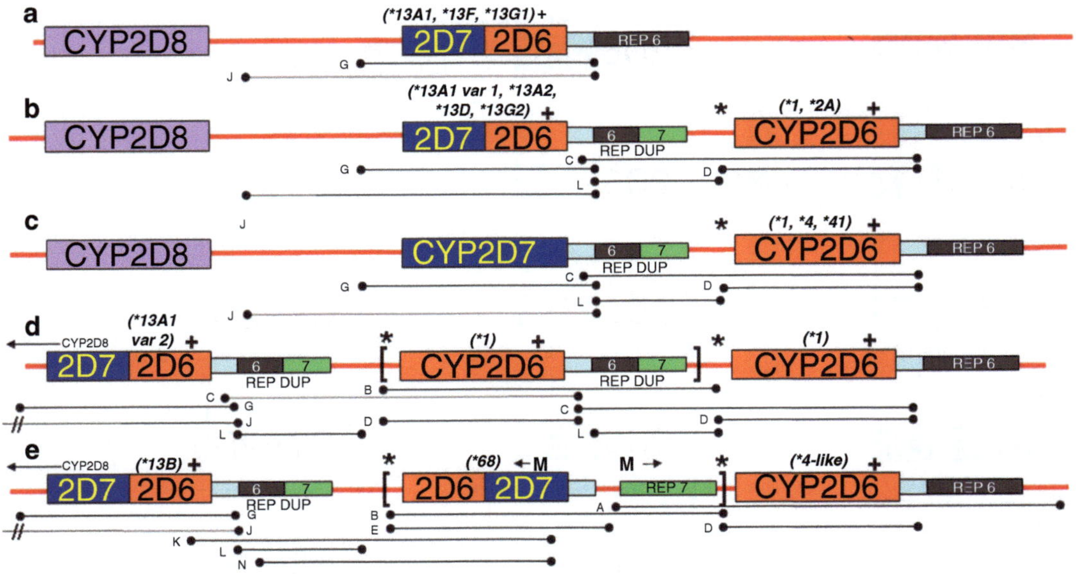

Fig. 4.4 *CYP2D* locus structures for single and hybrid tandems of *CYP2D7-2D6*. (a) Single *CYP2D7-2D6* arrangement (e.g., *CYP2D6*13A1*, *CYP2D6*13F*, *CYP2D6*13G1*). (b) *CYP2D7-2D6+CYP2D6* arrangement (e.g., *CYP2D6*13A1*, *CYP2D6*13A2*, *CYP2D6*13D*, *CYP2D6*13G2* with a tandem *CYP2D6*1*, *CYP2D6*2A*). Notice that the hybrid gene is followed by rep dup which will yield a false positive for the typical duplication arrangement (see Fig. 4.2b) using most genotyping platforms. (c) *CYP2D7* gene in a duplication arrangement that is followed by rep dup upstream of the tandem *CYP2D6* gene (e.g., *CYP2D6*1*, *CYP2D6*4*, *CYP2D6*41*). (d) *CYP2D7–2D6+CYP2D6 X N* hybrid tandem multiplication arrangement. In this case the *CYP2D7-2D6* hybrid is a *CYP2D6*13A1 variant 2* and the *CYP2D6* alleles are *CYP2D6*1*. (e) *CYP2D7-2D6* hybrid (*CYP2D6*13B*) followed by rep dup, *CYP2D6-2D7* hybrids (*CYP2D6* 68 X 2*), and a *CYP2D6* gene (*CYP2D6*4*-like). Multiplications have multiples of the sequence shown between the *brackets* and were observed in (d, e). PCR fragments that can be used in genotyping are depicted as *lettered lines* under the structures (see the following references for methods [25, 27]). Probe locations for Taqman® copy number assays are designated as *asterisk* and *plus sign* for the 5′ flanking *CYP2D6* assay and the *CYP2D6* intron 6 assay, respectively. Note that *CYP2D8* is thought to be present in all of the structures but is only shown in structures (Fig. 4.2a–c) for simplicity

Moderate potency inhibitors are duloxetine, sertraline, and terbinafine. Weak inhibitors are amiodarone and cimetidine. There is also a large list of other agents which have not been clearly classified as inhibitors including celecoxib, chlorpheniramine, chlorpromazine, citalopram, clemastine, clomipramine, cocaine, diphenhydramine, doxepin, doxorubicin, escitalopram, halofantrine, histamine H1 receptor antagonists, hydroxyzine, levomepromazine, methadone, metoclopramide, mibefradil, midodrine, moclobemide, perphenazine, ranitidine, haloperidol, ritonavir, ticlopidine, and tripelennamine.

CYP2D6 can be induced by dexamethasone and rifampin.

Pharmacologic probe drugs which can be used to phenotype a given individual for *CYP2D6* include debrisoquine, dextromethorphan, sparteine, and bufuralol.

Methodology

Several *CYP2D6* genotyping platforms exist today, but only two of them are FDA-approved in vitro diagnostics (IVD). The gold standard by which all platforms are compared is DNA sequencing which is a bit ironic since very few laboratories can accurately sequence this gene due to the complexities presented by the *CYP2D* loci. Ours is one of the few labs which currently has the capacity to provide complete genotyping services for this complicated gene.

IVD Tests

The two FDA-approved IVDs are the Roche AmpliChip CYP450 test and the Luminex xTAG® *CYP2D6* v3 test.

The Roche AmpliChip CYP450 test was the first FDA-approved IVD which genotypes *CYP2D6* and *CYP2C19*. 33 *CYP2D6* alleles and 3 *CYP2C19* alleles can be identified with this microarray-based test. In addition, duplications and deletions are detected, but the array cannot determine which alleles are duplicated in all cases. The integrated software enables generation of customized reports containing the genotype and phenotype. The microarray was not designed to detect multiplications of genes or hybrid genes and it is not capable of detecting tandem hybrids, which, when present often, generates incorrect phenotype calls [25]. The fact that phenotype prediction is incorporated into the software is not ideal given that the phenotype prediction based upon genotype is somewhat controversial as will be discussed below and changes as the function of the various alleles is further defined.

The Luminex xTAG® *CYP2D6* v3 IVD was recently released for clinical use but was withdrawn due to technical issues. The kit will likely be reissued in the near future and it evaluates samples for 15 *CYP2D6* alleles plus duplications and deletions. Proprietary software generates a genotype but the phenotype prediction is left to the clinician which is desirable due to controversies associated with phenotype prediction with *CYP2D6* and research redefining some of the functionality of some alleles. The kit was not designed to detect hybrid alleles nor hybrid tandems and it is not cleared to predict which allele is duplicated when a duplication signal is present, although this can be done on a limited basis by comparing the mean signal intensive for heterozygous calls ±2 standard deviations to the signal intensity derived from a heterozygous sample with a duplication signal. One advantage to the use of this kit is that the kit will yield "no calls" or signal variation in such a way as to lead the experienced user to suspect that a hybrid allele is present. These samples can be further studied using methods defined below to derive an accurate genotype.

Non-IVD Tests

The remaining *CYP2D6* assays fall within the laboratory developed test (LDT) category and are not FDA-approved IVDs. These include real-time PCR assays, PCR fragment analysis, allele-specific amplification, and DNA sequencing of all of the above except TaqMan® assays.

Real-time PCR (rtPCR) (TaqMan® assay, ABI) can be used to detect *CYP2D6* polymorphisms in a sample thus deriving genotype and it can be used to determine copy number.

In the case of SNP detection, *CYP2D6* polymorphisms are targeted using PCR primer pairs which amplify a region of DNA containing the polymorphism of interest. Labeled Taqman® probes targeting both the wild-type and mutant alleles are also used to detect the present of wild-type or mutant allele in the amplicon. During PCR, each probe anneals specifically to its complementary sequence between the forward and reverse PCR primer sites. When the oligonucleotide probe is intact, the proximity of the reporter dye to the quencher results in quenching of the reporter fluorescence. Taq polymerase extends the primers bound to the template DNA. The polymerase cleaves only probes that are hybridized to the target, separating the reporter dye from the quencher dye resulting in increased fluorescence by the reporter. Thus, the fluorescence signal generated by PCR amplification indicates which alleles are present in the sample.

Similarly, *CYP2D6* copy number and hybrid genes including tandem hybrids can be detected using rtPCR. This method relies upon determining copy number of two positions located in widely different positions in *CYP2D6*. For example, probe Hs04502391_cn which detects copy number of intron 6 (Applied Biosystems, Inc) can be used with a separate assay which targets the 5′-flanking region as described by Hosono et al. [26]. Both assays are performed in triplicate with an internal control-RNaseP TaqMan® copy number reference and TaqMan® Genotyping PCR Master Mix as directed by the manufacturer (ABI). Relative quantification is then performed using CopyCaller® Software (ABI) following the comparative $\Delta\Delta C_T$ method. If copy number calls for both probes are equal, the number of alleles present in the sample is easily interpreted into no duplications, duplications, or multiplications of *CYP2D6*. If copy number calls for both probes are unequal, it is likely that there is a hybrid present which can be elucidated using methods mentioned below.

Fragment analysis is most useful for detecting the presence or absence of a duplication, a deletion, or a hybrid allele. Primers are designed, as we have described [25, 27], which allow the unique PCR amplification of any part of the CYP2D locus that is of interest. Specifically, a sample can be interrogated for the presence or absence of a rep dup, rep del, *CYP2D6-2D7* hybrid, or *CYP2D7-2D6* hybrid (see Figs. 4.2, 4.3, and 4.4). The PCR product can be detected and sized using agarose gel, Agilent chip (Agilent Technologies), or QIAxcel (Qiagen). The PCR product can then be sequenced, if needed, to determine the exact hybrid allele present in the case of *CYP2D6-2D7* hybrid or *CYP2D7-2D6* hybrid.

Similarly, the problem of determining which allele is duplicated in ambiguous samples can be managed by PCR amplifying the alleles present [25, 27] and then sequencing them, thus removing any uncertainty about genotype. This can be combined with an rtPCR assay to determine the number of copies of *CYP2D6* present to further determine the actual genotype and, thus, the predicted phenotype.

Regulatory Issues: FDA Guidance on Tamoxifen Dosing

The FDA has not changed the label for tamoxifen but does state that tamoxifen is metabolized by *CYP2D6* to its active state and recommends against the use of *CYP2D6* inhibitors while on tamoxifen.

Test Interpretation

Phenotype prediction is generally based on the genotype and the activity listed for a given allele on the *CYP2D6* Allele Nomenclature Webpage (http://www.cypalleles.ki.se/*CYP2D6*.htm) as well as the extensive literature that exists on this gene. Phenotype prediction is often binned into four categories in a manner similar to that reviewed by Ingelman-Sundberg [28] and Kirchheiner et al. [29]. It should be noted that other methodologies for phenotype prediction have been described and this is a controversial area of pharmacogenomics [30, 31]. In particular, there is controversy about where to classify the *CYP2D6**2A* vs. other *CYP2D6**2* alleles. There is evidence that the *CYP2D6**2* alleles (except *CYP2D6**2A*) have reduced function, although this is somewhat substrate dependent [32–36]. However, the c.-1584C>G polymorphism found in *CYP2D6**2A* increases protein production, possibly through increased induction, which compensates for the reduced function caused by the other polymorphisms found in the *CYP2D6**2* alleles, resulting in a function similar to and possibly greater than *CYP2D6**1* [37, 38].

The classification used in our laboratory is as follows: an ultrarapid metabolizer (UM) has more than two normally functioning alleles (*CYP2D6**1* or *CYP2D6**2A*). An extensive metabolizer (EM) has two normally functioning alleles or one normally functioning allele and two reduced function alleles (e.g., *CYP2D6**2*, *CYP2D6**10*, *CYP2D6**17*, *CYP2D6**41*) or two normally functioning alleles and a reduced function allele. An intermediate metabolizer (IM) has one normally functioning allele and either a reduced function allele or a null allele (e.g., *CYP2D6**4*, *CYP2D6**5*, *CYP2D6**6*, or single *CYP2D7-2D6* gene). Samples with two or three reduced function alleles are also considered intermediate metabolizers. A poor metabolizer (PM) has only null alleles or a null allele plus a reduced function allele.

In summary, from the genotype, phenotype is predicted and from phenotype the clinician determines whether tamoxifen therapy is appropriate for a given patient. The literature supports the use of tamoxifen in individuals with UM, EM, or IM phenotypes; the uncertainty at present lies in the use of tamoxifen in PM individuals.

How the Test(s) Have Changed Medical Practice

CYP2D6 genotyping is not yet widely accepted due to conflicting literature and conflicting guidance from professional organizations. Nonetheless, the testing is available for those clinicians who wish to use this information in their decision-making.

Future Directions

For the use of tamoxifen, there are several trends for the future. There is a clear need for tightly controlled, prospective studies showing medical economic benefit of changing the practice. These should include data across a broad range of *CYP2D6* metabolizers and *CYP2D6* alleles, be multiracial in nature, be inclusive of tamoxifen and tamoxifen metabolite serum levels, and should control for *CYP2D6* inhibitors which might confound results. At the same time there should be ongoing research to determine the role of aromatase inhibitors vs. tamoxifen in the various *CYP2D6* metabolizer categories. Pharmaceutical manufacturers will be likely to move away from drugs that are metabolized and possibly to the use of endoxifen so as to avoid the complications of drug metabolism, although it seems impossible to completely remove the impact of an individual's pharmacogenomics in drug treatment since essentially every aspect of the pharmacokinetics and pharmacodynamics of a drug is under some genetic control.

In terms of technological advances, the use of next generation sequencing is likely to be the most fruitful next step. However, sequencing of *CYP2D6* is a special challenge given the high degree of homology between *CYP2D6* and CYP2D7 pseudogene and the rich array of hybrid alleles that exist. The most likely approach to succeed is the use of single molecule sequencing with long reads. Alternatively, use of allele and recombinant specific PCR followed by DNA sequencing of products has been shown to be an effective method for obtaining accurate results which will reveal otherwise undetected recombinants especially in samples containing *CYP2D6*4* and **10* and duplication signals [25].

UGT1A1 Genotyping for Irinotecan

Background

The American Cancer Society estimates that in 2011 about 141,210 will receive a diagnosis of colorectal cancer and 49,380 people will die of the disease. In the USA, it is the third most commonly diagnosed cancer and cause of cancer death [39]. Colorectal cancer death rates have decreased since 1998 for men and women and every racial/ethnic group, although not in a statistically significant way among American Indian/Alaska Native men and women.

Irinotecan (Camptosar, Pfizer) is a chemotherapeutic agent used in the treatment of colorectal cancer. It is a topoisomerase I inhibitor which has FDA approval for use in adults with (1) metastatic colorectal cancer as a first-line therapy in combination with 5-fluorouracil and leucovorin and (2) metastatic colorectal cancer in patients whose disease has recurred/progressed after initial 5-fluorouracil-based therapy. It has non-FDA indications for use in (3) extensive stage small cell lung cancer as a first-line treatment in combination with cisplatin (4) non-small cell lung cancer and (5) ovarian cancer with is either platinum refractory or platinum resistant [3].

Following primary metabolism by the phase I enzymes (by oxidation, reduction, dealkylation, and cleavage in the intestines and liver), many drugs and their metabolites are further modified for excretion by a group of conjugative, phase II enzymes. One of these phase II enzymes, uridine diphosphate (UDP)-glucuronosyltransferase 1A1 (*UGT1A1*), is responsible for bilirubin conjugation with glucuronic acid. This renders the bilirubin water soluble and permits excretion of the bilirubin–glucuronide conjugates in urine.

UGT1A1 is involved in the metabolism of irinotecan (Fig. 4.5). It is a prodrug that forms an active metabolite, SN-38. SN-38 is normally inactivated by conjugation with glucuronic acid

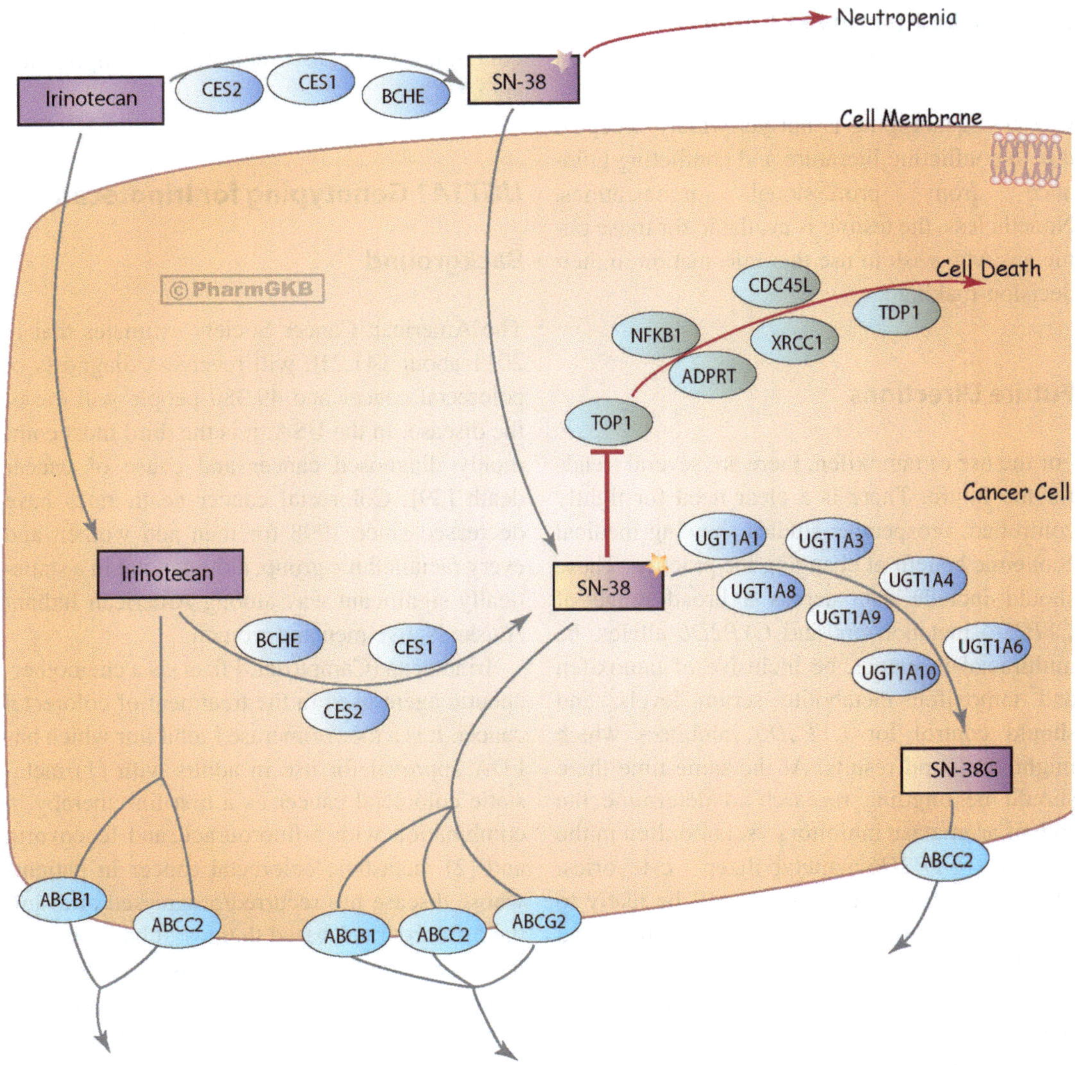

Fig. 4.5 This pathway shows the biotransformation of the chemotherapy prodrug irinotecan to form the active metabolite SN-38, an inhibitor of DNA topoisomerase I. SN-38 is primarily metabolized to the inactive SN-38 glucuronide by *UGT1A1*. Irinotecan is used in the treatment of metastatic colorectal cancer, small cell lung cancer, and some other solid tumors. There is large variability between patients in response to irinotecan, as well as severe side effects such as diarrhea and neutropenia, which might be explained in part by genetic variation in the metabolic enzymes and transporters depicted here. The best known variant to effect this pathway is the promoter polymorphic repeat in *UGT1A1* (*UGT1A1**28*) which has been associated with toxicity (neutropenia). Image and legend are from the Pharmacogenomic Knowledge Base (http://www.pharmgkb.org/index.jsp), are copyrighted to PharmGKB and Stanford University, and are used with permission from PharmGKB and Stanford University [69]

followed by biliary excretion into the gastrointestinal tract. If *UGT1A1* activity is impaired or deficient due to mutations in the coding region or promoter TA (thymine, adenine) repeat polymorphisms located in the promoter region of the gene, SN-38 fails to become conjugated with glucuronic acid, increasing the concentration of SN-38. This can result in severe neutropenia. The combination of neutropenia with diarrhea can be life-threatening.

Mechanism of Action

Irinotecan (CPT-11) is a camptothecin analogue which displays antitumor activity by inhibiting the intranuclear enzyme topoisomerase I. Irinotecan is water soluble and less toxic than camptothecin. The antitumor mechanism of irinotecan is related to inhibition of the topoisomerase I, an intranuclear enzyme that mediates the relaxation of supercoiled DNA, thus enabling replication and transcription to proceed. Some malignant tissues may have higher levels of topoisomerase I than normal cells, suggesting greater susceptibility of neoplasms to these agents, and as a result, reduced expression of topoisomerase I is a mechanism of resistance to irinotecan.

Some of irinotecan's metabolites are active; thus, irinotecan is essentially a prodrug, being converted in vivo to an active metabolite, SN-38 (7-ethyl-10-hydroxycamptothecin), which has 100- to 1,000-fold greater antitumor activity in vitro than irinotecan itself. Carboxylesterase is responsible for conversion of irinotecan to SN-38. SN-38 is responsible for the majority of in vivo antitumor activity of irinotecan [3].

Metabolism

Irinotecan is a prodrug which is metabolized to form the active metabolite SN-38, an inhibitor of DNA topoisomerase I. SN-38 is primarily metabolized to the inactive SN-38 glucuronide by *UGT1A1*. See Fig. 4.5 for additional discussion on the metabolism of irinotecan.

Clinical Application

Why Individualized Treatment Is Important in Colorectal Cancer Management

As in the case of breast cancer, there are many reasons to seek methods to individualized treatment of patients with metastatic colorectal cancer who will be treated with irinotecan. For this discussion, individualized treatment will hinge upon genotyping of *UGT1A1*, although other genes are being studied. Key reasons for striving to individualize irinotecan treatment are as follows: there is interindividual variation in response to irinotecan and the cost of nonresponse is often fatal. Furthermore, the side effect profile for this drug is costly in terms of morbidity and mortality because one of the key side effects is neutropenia and diarrhea which makes the patient susceptible to infection and other complications. Irinotecan is commonly used given that it is a first-line treatment for metastatic colorectal cancer or after disease progression following 5-fluorouracil treatment. Proper management of patients with genetic profiles that will predict either side effects or lack of response would advance the treatment of this cancer substantially especially if effective alternative treatments are identified. Finally, there is the financial cost of treatment of colorectal cancer. If patients can be screened for risk of side effects or nonresponse effectively and these risks can be managed, the overall cost of treatment should be lessened.

Review of the Literature

The first indication that impaired *UGT1A1* function relates to severe toxicity in irinotecan-based chemotherapy may have been Wasserman et al.'s [40] report that patients with Gilbert syndrome had severe side effects to irinotecan. Subsequent research showed that irinotecan (CPT-11) is essentially a prodrug which is converted to SN-38, a compound with increased efficacy and toxicity when compared to irinotecan by carboxylesterases. SN-38 undergoes glucuronidation by *UGT1A1* and is excreted into the bile. Bacterial β-glucuronidase in the gut converts some of the excreted SN-39 glucuronide to SN-39 again [41]. The area under the curve (AUC) of SN-38 and intestinal concentrations are associated with severity of delayed diarrhea, neutropenia, and fever [42].

An early report by McLeod et al. [43] described an association between the *UGT1A1* promoter polymorphism $(TA)_7$, also known as *UGT1A1*28*, and irinotecan toxicity. The researchers showed that homozygous **28* was associated with risk of neutropenia but did not predict response, time to progression, or overall survival. Subsequently, many studies have been published on the relationship between *UGT1A1*28* and hematotoxicity, delayed diarrhea, and overall survival as reviewed by Schulz et al. [41] and the results are mixed. The preponderance of studies that evaluated grade 3 and 4 hematotoxicity found a significant relationship with the **28* [43–51], although some did not [52–54]. Delayed diarrhea was not as strongly associated with approximately half of the cited studies reporting no association [43, 48, 51, 52, 54, 55] and half finding an association [44, 45, 47, 49, 50, 53]. None of the studies that evaluated overall survival found an association with *UGT1A1*28* [43, 47, 50, 52, 53, 55]. Subsequent work by Schulz [56] found no significant influence of the TA repeat *UGT1A1* gene polymorphism across these three dimensions.

UGT1A1 gene polymorphism frequencies vary widely per ethnic and racial group. Furthermore, this gene has several other polymorphisms that may impact gene function and SN-38 metabolism which could alter side effects and response. Innocenti et al. [57] evaluated several pharmacogenetically relevant genes for relationship to irinotecan neutropenia and pharmacokinetics including the *UGT1A1*28*, **6 (c.211G>A, G71R)*, **27 (c.686C>A, P229Q)*, **60 (c.-3279T>G)*, and **93 c.-3156G>A*. These researchers reported that, in their univariate analysis, *UGT1A1*28* and *93 were associated with decreased absolute neutrophil count nadir (ANC) as well as SN-38 glucuronide/SN-38 area under the curve (AUC) and SN-38 AUC. *UGT1A1*60* was also associated with decreased SN-38 glucuronide/SN-38 area under the curve and ANC nadirs. Similarly, Cecchin et al. [58] studied the role of UGT1A variants and found that *UGT1A1*28*, **60*, and **93* as well as *UGT1A7*3* and *UGT1A9*22* may impact outcomes of metastatic colorectal cancer patients treated with irinotecan, fluorouracil, and leucovorin. A key finding of this research was that *UGT1A1**60 and **93* were associated with hematologic effects and response **93*. But the best predictor of severe hematologic toxicity after the first cycle of treatment was *UGT1A7*3/*3*, not *UGT1A1*28/*28*. This observation could be partly accounted for by strong linkage disequilibrium between the *UGT1A1* variants but less so between *UGT1A1* and the *UGT1A7*3* allele. These findings suggest that some of conflicting results from previous studies might be due to incomplete genotyping.

Studies of Japanese subjects have examined the role of ethnicity on *UGT1A1*-related toxicity and outcomes. Specifically, the **28* allele is found in Caucasians and Japanese, but **6* is found in Japanese subjects frequently [59]. Given that **6* is a deficiency allele which has been associated with irinotecan-related side effects [60–62], the Ministry of Health and Labor and Welfare in Japan approved genetic testing for *UGT1A1*28* and *UGT1A1*6*.

Limitations of Studies

The study limitations that exist for *UGT1A1* genotyping associated with irinotecan use are very similar to what exists for *CYP2D6* genotyping for tamoxifen. However, the literature appears to be more mature and some important positive reviews examining this association have been published. The challenges of clinical application of *UGT1A1* genotyping for irinotecan were addressed by Ikediobi et al. [63] and Palomaki et al. [64]: the latter as part of a major review prepared for the Evaluation of Genomic Applications in Practice and Prevention (EGAPP) group. Cited limitations are familiar and include the following: Most of the studies were of a retrospective nature, studies were inclusive of only a few of the possible *UGT1A1* variants that are known to exist, differences in response and side effects in multiple ethnic groups have not been studied adequately, the impact of dose changes on neutropenia, delayed diarrhea, tumor response, and survival has not been adequately studied, and the medical economic benefit of doing testing is unknown. The conclusions by EGAPP were that analytic validity exists for the common *UGT1A1* variant **28* but not for uncommon *UGT1A1* variants. Indeed, most testing platforms are specifically designed for **28* alone and only those labs which offer DNA sequencing will detect the presence of other alleles and those will be limited by the extent of the gene which is sequenced. EGAPP also found that there was adequate clinical validity for the association between *UGT1A1*28* genotype and SN-38 levels, severe diarrhea, and neutropenia, but not for *UGT1A1*

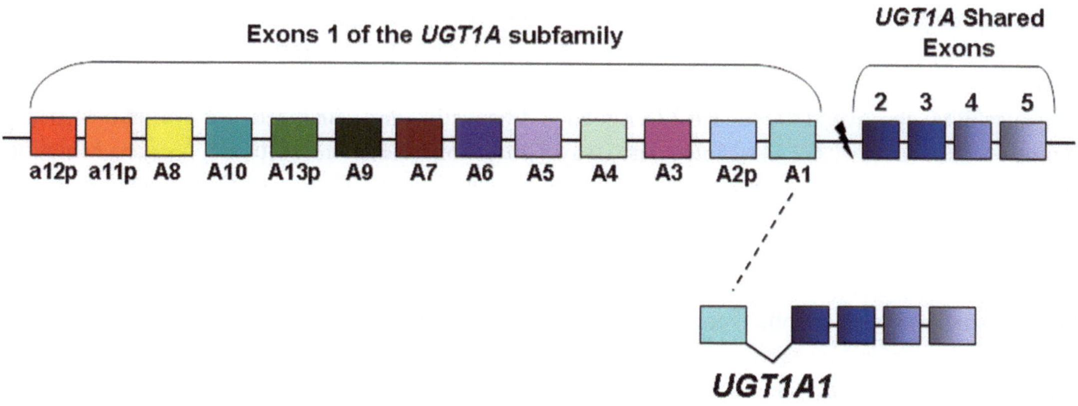

Fig. 4.6 The UGT1A gene complex has 13 tandemly arrayed first exons, 4 of which are pseudogenes as depicted with a "p" suffix. Independent splicing of the first exon to the 4 shared UGT1A exons 2–5 results in enzymes of different specificity. The UGT1A1 enzyme results from splicing of the A1 exon to the shared exons

uncommon variants and clinical outcomes. Clinical utility of the impact of testing was inadequate both in reduction of severe neutropenia and in responsiveness of tumors. The concern is that if the dose of irinotecan is reduced due to the genotype, no prospective study has shown that the risk of severe neutropenia is reduced and no prospective study has shown that tumors respond as well and patient survival is similar to using a full dose. Thus, the fear that dose reduction harms the patient continues to be an issue. Finally, the dosing guidelines for patients heterozygous and homozygous for **28* alleles remain vague.

UGT1A1 Structure and Variation

UDP-glycosyltransferase 1 family, polypeptide A1 (*UGT1A1*) is a gene located at cytogenetic location 2q37.1. The gene has clinical utility in two realms: (1) variations of the gene have diagnostic value for Crigler–Najjar syndrome, types I and II (CN1, CN2), familial transient neonatal hyperbilirubinemia, and Gilbert Syndrome, all of which are conditions of unconjugated hyperbilirubinemia. (2) The gene is useful in predicting severity of side effects in patients treated with irinotecan for metastatic colon cancer.

The UGT1A gene complex is interesting in that the 5′ region of the complex contains 13 tandemly arrayed first exons, of which 4 are pseudo exons, that are linked to 4 common exons in the UGT1A 3′ region (Fig. 4.6). Each first exon has its own promoter and the functional first exons are independently spliced to the common exons to generate 9 UGT1A transcripts each with unique 5′ ends but identical 3′ ends. The 5′ end encodes the N terminus of each UGT1A which determines substrate specificity and the encoded C terminus determines the interaction with the common donor substrate, UDP-glucuronate [65].

UGT1A1 has considerable molecular variability with over 113 alleles described to date. The UGT Alleles Nomenclature Committee maintains a website which displays the haplotypes and known SNPs for *UGT1A1* and the other UGTs (http://www.pharmacogenomics.pha.ulaval.ca/cms/ugt_alleles). The haplotype page includes phenotype information when available including CN1 and CN2 and Gilbert syndrome. One would expect that if a patient has an allele associated with any of these conditions, the patient would be sensitive to irinotecan, but this cannot be assumed since there might be some level of substrate specificity for the alleles. In other words, a variation that cannot conjugate bilirubin might still be able to conjugate SN-38 adequately to prevent associated side effects, although this is not the case with the **28* homozygote associated with Gilbert syndrome.

As with many genes, race and ethnicity impact the frequency of the alleles present in a given population [45, 66].

Methodology

IVD Tests

The only FDA-approved IVD for *UGT1A1* genotyping is the Invader® *UGT1A1* Molecular Assay (Hologic™) which determines only the *UGT1A1*28* allele. This chemistry platform is a homogeneous, isothermal DNA probe-based system which can detect insertions and deletions on PCR products as well as other polymorphisms. The method uses an "invader" sequence, a proprietary cleavase enzyme, and a fret cassette in conjunction with a two-color detection system to detect both alleles of a target sequence in a single reaction, thus yielding genotype calls.

Non-IVD Tests

Other testing methods are non-IVD and are LDTs. The major methods in use today are *UGT1A1* promoter genotyping by fragment analysis and, for whole gene analysis, DNA sequencing.

In *UGT1A1* promoter genotyping by fragment analysis, a portion of the promoter region of the *UGT1A1* gene is amplified by polymerase chain reaction (PCR) using one labeled primer. The labeled PCR products are separated on a genetic analyzer (e.g., ABI3130xl; Applied Biosystems™) and the resulting trace files can be analyzed for TA repeats using GeneMarker software (SoftGenetics) fragment sizing software and verified through visual inspection. Having the ability to distinguish between product sizes differing by 2 bp is essential to the success of the assay and this is often best done using relatively small PCR product sizes in the range of 200–300 bp in length. An advantage is that this method allows for the detection of rarer TA repeat sizes such as TA_5 (*36*) and TA_8 (*37*). The major disadvantage is that only the TA repeat region is interrogated using this method so any other variations will be undetected.

DNA sequencing is the comprehensive method for determining the presence of all known (and frequently novel) variations of *UGT1A1*. In this procedure, *UGT1A1* amplification by PCR is followed by purified products from unincorporated primers and nucleotides by enzymatic digestion and then sequenced in both directions using sequencing primers usually by fluorescent-dye terminator chemistry. Sequencing products are separated on an automated sequencer and trace files are analyzed for variations using mutation-detection software (e.g., Mutation Surveyor, SoftGenetics LLC; Sequencher; Gene Codes Corp.) and visual inspection. The advantage of DNA sequencing is that it will allow for the detection of all variations in a given sample. Sometimes this is also a disadvantage because many variations seen in clinical practice have yet to be compiled into the allelic nomenclature and novel mutations generally are of unknown significance given that no information is available about their phenotype. Also, *cis-* and *trans-relationship* information cannot be easily determined when more than one variation is found, thus compounding the difficulty of precise phenotype prediction. Parenthetically, if full gene sequencing is done, this method will allow the user to determine all known mutations associated with Gilbert syndrome and CN1 and CN2. The presence of these mutations may be an indicator of increased risk of irinotecan side effects, although, as mentioned above, these conclusions should be considered speculative and are not stated by FDA in the irinotecan label.

Regulatory Issues: FDA Guidance on *UGT1A1* Clinical Genotyping for Patients Receiving Irinotecan

FDA recommends that clinicians reduce the dose of irinotecan in patients getting first-line treatment for metastatic colorectal cancer and for patients getting irinotecan treatment for metastatic colorectal cancer which progressed despite 5-fluoruracil treatment if the patient has the homozygous *UGT1A1*28* allele. The agency does not make recommendations about reducing the dose for patients who are heterozygous for the **28* allele, although there is a 5.3–12.5 % risk of neutropenia (see Pfizer package insert, LAB-0134-17.0, revised August 2010). The agency does not comment at all upon the **6* allele which was found to be most predictive of neutropenia in Japanese patients [67] nor does it caution about the many other alleles that have been shown to impair the function of *UGT1A1* probably because no clinical validation exists for their importance in predicting irinotecan toxicity or response.

Test Interpretation

Test interpretation is relatively straightforward. Regardless of the platform used, samples are examined for the presence of *UGT1A1*28*. If present in a homozygous state, irinotecan product labeling recommends consideration of dose reduction due to the risk of grade 4 neutropenia. "When administered in combination with other agents, or as a single-agent, a reduction in the starting dose by at least one level of CAMPTOSAR should be considered for patients known to be homozygous for the UGT1A1*28 allele. However, the precise dose reduction in this patient population is not known and subsequent dose modifications should be considered based on individual patient tolerance to treatment" (see Pfizer package insert, LAB-0134-17.0, revised August 2010). If present in the heterozygous state, the product literature notes an increased risk of neutropenia but does not recommend a dose reduction. Similarly, despite the fact that the Japanese patients with *UGT1A1*6* are at risk for severe neutropenia and the Ministry of Health and Labor and Welfare in Japan approved genetic testing for *UGT1A1*28* and *UGT1A1*6* in patients getting irinotecan, the US FDA has not followed suit leaving clinicians to draw their own conclusions on how to manage the patient.

Test interpretation is relatively simple when only the **28* allele can be detected by the genotyping method in use because other alleles are not seen even if they are present. When more comprehensive genotyping is done, additional alleles are seen and the clinician has a more complicated task of determining the relevance of these alleles. For example, in PCR fragment analysis, the $(TA)_5$ (**36*) and $(TA)_8$ (**37*) alleles can be detected. The number of TA repeats is inversely related to gene expression. Individuals with normal levels of *UGT1A1* expression have six copies of the TA repeat in the promoter or more rarely five copies of the TA repeat (referred to as **36*). Individuals with decreased expression of *UGT1A1* have seven TA repeats (**28* allele) or 8 TA repeats (**37*) [68].

In addition, labs that do partial or full *UGT1A1* gene sequencing can detect any of the alleles identified to date plus any novel mutations. It seems prudent to exercise caution for individuals with alleles that are associated with Gilbert syndrome and CN1 and CN2, but without clear guidance from the FDA on this matter, it is left to the clinician to determine how to use irinotecan in this setting.

How the Test Has Changed Medical Practice

FDA labeling has forced oncologists to think about *UGT1A1*28* testing in the USA. This has resulted in adoption of this test by many clinicians. However, some still do not use the test either because they do not have clear guidance on dosing of irinotecan when **28* is present or out of concern that reducing the dose will result in a lack of response of the tumor. Still, with FDA guidance on the medication label, it seems that it is now standard of care to offer this testing when use of irinotecan is contemplated.

Future Directions

Future research should focus on determining additional alleles associated with irinotecan side effects and response. The risks and benefits of dose reduction for carriers of these alleles also must be clearly established. As we move toward next generation sequencing of specific genes like *UGT1A1* and whole genomes, the amount of data available will become overwhelming. Algorithms that inform clinicians on the correct approach to take with patients possessing specific genotypes also will be necessary especially as the field of pharmacogenomics matures and additional genes and their variations are identified as being relevant to drug selection and dosing. It is also anticipated that pharmaceutical houses will look for medications that are not metabolized or conjugated and thus not as susceptible to individual genetic variation, although it is unlikely that any medication will be completely free from the genetic influences of either the patient taking the drug or the tumor being treated. The medical–legal environment will eventually become a factor in the USA given that genotyping for the *UGT1A1*28* allele is becoming the standard of care after FDA label changes to irinotecan.

Conclusions

This chapter reviews the present data available for the pharmacogenomic management of patients taking tamoxifen and irinotecan. As this review indicates, there are more questions than answers. In the case of tamoxifen, there is still no clear directive that pharmacogenomic testing of the *CYP2D6* gene is indicated in the management of patients with breast cancer. There is more support, mainly via FDA-mandated changes in drug labeling, for the pharmacogenomic management of irinotecan. However, limitations include the fact that only the *UGT1A1*28* allele is considered when it is likely that other alleles should be included in the cautionary statements.

Future research will need to deal with the overwhelming amount of genomic information that will be the result of whole gene and/or whole genome sequencing, the impact of variations on drug response, drug-induced morbidity and mortality, as well as the impact of changing doses to modify risk from these issues. At the same time, it is hoped that new medications will become available that will use genomic data to target breast and colorectal cancer more precisely.

References

1. DeSantis C, Siegel R, Bandi P, Jemal A. Breast cancer statistics, 2011. CA Cancer J Clin. 2011;61(6):409–18. doi:10.3322/caac.20134.
2. Jemal A, Siegel R, Ward E, et al. Cancer statistics, 2006. CA Cancer J Clin. 2006;56:106–30.
3. Micromedex® Healthcare Series [intranet database] version 5.1. Greenwood Village, Colo: Thomson Reuters (Healthcare) Inc.
4. Desta Z, Ward B, Soukhova N, Flockhart DA. Comprehensive evaluation of tamoxifen sequential biotransformation by the human cytochrome P450 system in vitro: prominent roles for CYP3A and CYP2D6. J Pharmacol Exp Ther. 2004;310:1062–75.
5. Goetz MP, Rae JM, Suman VJ, et al. Pharmacogenetics of tamoxifen biotransformation is associated with clinical outcomes of efficacy and hot flashes. J Clin Oncol. 2005;23:9312–8.
6. Goetz M, Knox S, Suman V, et al. The impact of cytochrome P450 2D6 metabolism in women receiving adjuvant tamoxifen. Breast Cancer Res Treat. 2007;101:113–21.
7. Bonanni B, Macis D, Maisonneuve P, et al. Polymorphism in the CYP2D6 tamoxifen-metabolizing gene influences clinical effect but not hot flashes: data from the Italian Tamoxifen Trial. J Clin Oncol. 2006;24:3708–9.
8. Schroth W, Antoniadou L, Fritz P, et al. Breast cancer treatment outcome with adjuvant tamoxifen relative to patient CYP2D6 and CYP2C19 genotypes. J Clin Oncol. 2007;25:5187–93.
9. Xu Y, Sun Y, Yao L, et al. Association between CYP2D6*10 genotype and survival of breast cancer patients receiving tamoxifen treatment. Ann Oncol. 2008;19:1423–9.
10. Schroth W, Goetz M, Hamann U, et al. Association between CYP2D6 polymorphisms and outcomes amoung women with early stage breast cancer treated with tamoxifen. JAMA. 2009;302:1429–36.
11. Ramon y Cajal T, Altes A, Pare L, et al. Impact of CYP2D6 polymorphisms in tamoxifen adjuvant breast cancer treatment. Breast Cancer Res Treat. 2010;119:33–8.
12. Kiyotani K, Mushiroda T, Sasa M, et al. Impact of CYP2D6*10 on recurrence-free survival in breast cancer patients receiving adjuvant tamoxifen therapy. Cancer Sci. 2008;99:995–9.
13. Newman W, Hadfield K, Latif A, et al. Impaired tamoxifen metabolism reduces survival in familial breast cancer patients. Clin Cancer Res. 2008;14:5913–8.
14. Nowell S, et al. Association of genetic variation in tamoxifen-metabolizing enzymes with overall survival and recurrence of disease in breast cancer patients. Breast Cancer Res Treat. 2005 Jun;91(3):49–58.
15. Wegman P, Elingarami S, Carstensen J, Stal O, Nordenskjold B, Wingren S. Genetic variants of CYP3A5, CYP2D6, SULT1A1, UGT2B15, and tamoxifen response in postmenopausal patients with breast cancer. Breast Cancer Res. 2007;9:R7.
16. Wegman P, Vainikka L, Stal O, et al. Genotype of metabolic enzymes and the benefit of tamoxifen in postmenopausal breast cancer patients. Breast Cancer Res. 2005;7:R284–90.
17. Okishiro M, Taguchi T, Jin K, Shimazu K, Tamaki Y, Noguchi S. Genetic polymorphisms of CYP2D6*10

and CYP2C19*2, *3 are not associated with prognosis, endometrial thickness, or bone mineral density in Japanese breast cancer patients treated with adjuvant tamoxifen. Cancer. 2009;115:952–61.
18. Lammers L, Mathijssen R, Van Gelder T, et al. The impact of CYP2D6-predicted phenotype on tamoxifen treatment outcome in patietns with metastatic breast cancer. Br J Cancer. 2010;103:765–71.
19. Stingl J, Parmar S, Huber-Weschselberger A, et al. Impact of *CYP2D6*4* genotype on progression free survival in tamoxifen breast cancer treatment. Curr Med Res Opin. 2010;26:2535–42.
20. Lim J, Chen X, Singh O, et al. Impact of CYP2D6, CYP3A5, CYP2C9, and CYP2C19 polymorphisms on tamoxifen pharmacokinetics in Asian breast cancer patients. Br J Clin Pharmacol. 2011;71:737–50.
21. Madlensky L, Natarajan L, Tchu S, et al. Tamoxifen metabolite concentrations, CYP2D6 genotype, and breast cancer outcomes. Clin Pharmacol Ther. 2011;89:718–25.
22. Seruga B, Amir E. Cytochrome P450 2D6 and outcomes of adjuvant tamoxifen therapy: results of a meta-analysis. Breast Cancer Res Treat. 2010;122: 609–17.
23. Lash T, Lien E, Sorensen H, Hamilton-Dutoit S. Genotype-guided tamoxifen therapy: time to pause for reflection? Lancet Oncol. 2009;10:825–33.
24. Lundqvist E, Johansson I, Ingelman-Sundberg M. Genetic mechanisms for duplication and multiduplication of the CYP2D6 gene and methods for detection of duplicated CYP2D6 genes. Gene. 1999;226:327–38.
25. Black J, Walker D, O'Kane D, Harmandayan M. Frequency of undetected CYP2D6 hybrid genes in clinical samples: impact on phenotype prediction. Drug Metab Dispos. 2012;40(1):111–9. doi:10.1124/dmd.111.040832.
26. Hosono N, Kato M, Kiyotani K, et al. CYP2D6 genotype for functional-gene dosage analysis by allele copy number detection. Clin Chem. 2009;55:1546–54.
27. Kramer W, Walker D, O'Kane D, et al. CYP2D6: novel genomic structures and alleles. Pharmacogenet Genomics. 2009;19:813–22.
28. Ingelman-Sundberg M. Genetic polymorphisms of cytochrome p450 2D6 (CYP2D6) clinical consequences, evolutionary aspects and functional diversity. Pharmacogenomics J. 2005;5:6–13.
29. Kirchheiner J, Nickchen K, Bauer M, et al. Pharmacogenetics of antidepressants and antipsychotics: the contribution of allelic variations to the phenotype of drug response. Mol Psychiatry. 2004;9:442–73.
30. Steimer W, Zopf K, Von Amelunxen S, et al. Allele-specific change of concentration and functional gene dose for the prediction of steady-state serum concentrations of amitriptyline and nortriptyline in CYP2C19 and CY2D6 extensive and intermediate metabolizers. Clin Chem. 2004;50:1623–33.
31. Gaedigk A, Simon S, Pearce R, Bradford L, Kennedy M, Leeder J. The CYP2D6 activity score: translating genotype information into a qualitative measure of phenotype. Clin Pharmacol Ther. 2008;83:234–42.
32. Raimundi S, Fischer J, Eichelbaum M, Griese E, Schwab M, Zanger U. Elucidation of the genetic basis of the common 'intermediate metabolizer' phenotype for drug oxidation by CYP2D6. Pharmacogenetics. 2000;10:577–81.
33. Bapiro T, Hasler J, Ridderstrom M, Masimirembwa C. The molecular and enzyme basis for the diminished activity of the cytochrome P450 2D6.17 variant. Biochem Pharmacol. 2002;64:1387–98.
34. Yu A, Kneller B, Rettie A, Haining R. Expression, purification, biochemical characterization, and comparative function of human cytochrome P450 2D6.1, 2D6.2, 2D6.10, and 2D6.17 allelic isoforms. J Pharmacol Exp Ther. 2002;303:1291–300.
35. Raimundo S, Toscano C, Klein K, et al. A novel intronic mutation, 2988G>A, with high predictivity for impaired function of cytochrome P450 2D6 in white subjects. Clin Pharmacol Ther. 2004;76:128–38.
36. Abduljalil K, Frank D, Gaedigk A, et al. Assessment of activity levels for CYP2D6*1, CYP2D6*2, and CYP2D6*41 genes by population pharmacokinetics of dextromethorphan. Clin Pharmacol Ther. 2010;88:643–51.
37. Lovlie R, Daly AK, Matre GE, Molven A, Steen VM. Polymorphisms in CYP2D6 duplication-negative individuals with the ultrarapid metabolizer phenotype: a role for the CYP2D6*35 allele in ultrarapid metabolism? Pharmacogenetics. 2001;11:45–55.
38. Zanger U, Fischer J, Raimundo S, et al. Comprehensive analysis of the genetic factors determining expression and function of hepatic CYP2D6. Pharmacogenetics. 2001;11:573–85.
39. American Cancer Society. Colorectal cancer facts and figures 2011–2013. Atlanta: American Cancer society; 2011.
40. Wasserman E, Myara A, Lokiec F, et al. Severe CPT-11 toxicity in patients with Gilbert's syndrome: two case reports. Ann Oncol. 1997;8:1049–51.
41. Schulz C, Boeck S, Heinemann V, Stemmler H-J. UGT1A1 genotyping: a predictor of irinotecan-associated side effects and drug efficacy? Anticancer Drugs. 2009;20:867–79.
42. Xie R, Mathijssen R, Sparreboom A, Verweij J, Karlsson M. Clinical pharmacokinetics of irinotecan and its metabolites in relation with diarrhea. Clin Pharmacol Ther. 2002;72:265–75.
43. McLeod HL, Parodi L, Sargent D, et al. UGT1A1*28, toxicity and outcome in advanced colorectal cancer: results from trial N9741. ASCO Annual Meeting Proceedings Part I. J Clin Oncol. 2006;24:18S; Abstract 3520.
44. Iyer L, Das S, Janisch L, et al. UGT1A1*28 polymorphism as a determinant of irinotecan disposition and toxicity. Pharmacogenomics J. 2002;2:43–7.
45. Innocenti F, Undevia S, Iyer L, et al. Genetic variants in the UDP-flucuronosyltransferase 1A1 gene predict the risk of severe neutropenia of irinotecan. J Clin Oncol. 2004;22:1382–8.
46. Ando Y, Saka H, Ando M, et al. Polymorphisms of UDP-glucuronosyltransferase gene and irinotecan

toxicity: a pharmacogenetic analysis. Cancer Res. 2000;60:6921–6.
47. Toffoli G, Cecchin E, Corona G, et al. The role of UGT1A1*28 polymorphism in the pharmacodynamics and pharmacokinetics of irinotecan in patients with metastatic colorectal cancer. J Clin Oncol. 2006;24:3061–8.
48. Rouits E, Boisdron-Celle M, Dumont A, Guerin O, Morel A, Gamelin E. Relevance of different UGT1A1 polymorphisms in irinotecan-induced toxicity: a molecular and clinical study of 75 patients. Clin Cancer Res. 2004;10:5151–9.
49. Roth A, Yan P, Dietrich D, et al. Does UGT1A1*28 homozygosity predict for severe toxicity in patients treated with 5-fluorouracil (5-FU)-irinotecan (IRI)? Results of the PETACC 3-EORTC 40993-SAKK 60/00 trial comparing IRI/5-FU/folinic acid (FA) to 5-FU/FA in stage II-III colon cancer. Gastrointestinal Cancers Symposium 2008:Abstract No. 277.
50. Liu C, Chen P, Chiou T, et al. UGT1A1*28 polymorphism predicts irinotecan-induced severe toxicities without affecting treatment outcome and survival in patients with metastatic colorectal carcinoma. Cancer. 2008;112:1932–40.
51. Kweekel D, Gelderblom H, Van der Straaten T, Antonini N, Punt C, Guchelaar H. UGT1A1*28 genotype and irinotecan dosage in patients with metastatic colorectal cancer: a Dutch Colorectal Cancer Group study. Br J Cancer. 2008;99:275–82.
52. Cote J, Kirzin S, Kramar A, et al. UGT1A1 polymorphism can predict hematologic toxicity in patients treated with irinotecan. Clin Cancer Res. 2007; 13:3269–75.
53. Marcuello E, Altes A, Menoyo A, Del Rio E, Gomez-Pardo M, Baiget M. UGT1A1 gene variations and irinotecan treatment in patients with metastatic colorectal cancer. Br J Cancer. 2004;91:678–82.
54. Seymour M, Braun M, Richman S, et al. Association of molecular markers with toxicity in a randomized trial of chemotherpya for advanced colorectal cancer (FOCUS). ASCO Annual Meeting Proceedings Part I. J Clin Oncol. 2006;24:18S; (June 20 Supplement), Abstract No. 2022.
55. Font A, Sanchez J, Taron M, et al. Weekly regimen of inirotecan/docetaxel in previously treated non-small cell lung cancer patients and correlation with uridine diphosphate glucuronosyltransferase 1A1 (UGT1A1) polymorphism. Invest New Drugs. 2003;21:435–43.
56. Schulz C, Heinemann V, Schalhorn A, et al. UGT1A1 gene polymorphisms: impact on toxicity and efficacy of irinotecan-based regimens in metastatic colorectal cancer. World J Gastroenterol. 2009;15:5058–66.
57. Innocenti F, Kroetz D, Schuetz E, et al. Comprehensive pharmacogenetic analysis of irinotecan neutropenia and pharmacokinetics. J Clin Oncol. 2009;27: 2604–14.
58. Cecchin E, Innocenti F, D'Andrea M, et al. Predictive role of the UGT1A1, UGT1A7, and UGT1A9 genetic variants and their haplotypes on the outcome of metastatic colorectal cancer patients treated with fluorouracil, leucovorin and irinotecan. J Clin Oncol. 2009;27:2457–65.
59. Akiyama Y, Fujita K, Nagashima F, et al. Genetic testing for UGT1A1*28 and *6 in Japanese patients who receive irinotecan chemotherapy. Ann Oncol. 2008;19:2089–94.
60. Nakamura Y, Soda H, Oka M, et al. Randomized phase II trial of irinotecan with Paclitaxel or Gemcitabine for non-small cell lung cancer. J Thorac Oncol. 2011;6:121–7.
61. Takane H, Kawamoto K, Sasaki T, et al. Life-threatening toxicities in a patient iwth *UGT1A1*6/*28* and *SLCO1B1*15/*15* genotypes after irinotecan-based chemotherapy. Cancer Chemother Pharmacol. 2009;63:1165–9.
62. Saito Y, Sai K, Maekawa K, et al. Close association of UGT1A9 IVS1+399C>T with UGT1A1*28, *6, or *60 haplotype and its apparent influence on 7-ethyl-10-hydroxycamptothecin (SN-38) glucuronidation in Japanese. Drug Metab Dispos. 2009;37:272–6.
63. Ikediobi O, Shin J, Nussbaum R, et al. Addressing the challenges of the clinical application of pharmacogenetic testing. Clin Pharmacol Ther. 2009;86:28–31.
64. Palomaki G, Bradley L, Douglas M, Kolor K, Dotson W. Can UGT1A1 genotyping reduce morbidity and mortality in patietns with metastatic colorectal cancer treated with irinotecan? An evidence-based review. Genet Med. 2009;11:21–34.
65. Gong Q-H, Cho J, Huang T, et al. Thirteen UDP-glucuronosyltransferase genes are encoded at the human UGT1 gene complex locus. Pharmacogenomics. 2001;11:357–68.
66. Beutler E, Gelbart T, Demina A. Racial variability in the UDP-glucuronosyltransferase 1 (UGT1A1) promoter: a balanced polymorphism for regulation of bilirubin metabolism? Proc Natl Acad Sci USA. 1998;95:8170–4.
67. Onoue M, Terada T, Kobayashi M, et al. UGT1A1*6 polymorphism is most predictive of severe neutropenia induced by irinotecan in Japanese cancer patients. Int J Clin Oncol. 2009;14:136–42.
68. Innocenti F, Grimsley C, Das S, et al. Haplotype structure of the UDP-glucuronosyltransferase 1A1 promoter in different ethnic groups. Pharmacogenetics. 2002;12:725–33.
69. Klein T, Chang J, Cho M, et al. Integrating genotype and phenotype information: an overview of the PharmGKB project. Pharmacogenomics J. 2001;1: 167–70.

Part II

Infectious Disease

Hepatitis C Virus Testing

5

Hassan M.E. Azzazy and Karim M. Abdel-Hady

Background

Viral hepatitis, the most common form of liver inflammation, is caused by five main viruses denoted hepatitis A, B, C, D, and E. Hepatitis C is caused by the hepatitis C virus (HCV) and is considered a serious form of the disease [1]. HCV is a blood-borne RNA virus that is transmitted mainly via the parenteral route from an infected individual to a healthy one [2]. It is estimated to infect around 170 million people worldwide, with 3.2 million patients chronically infected in the USA alone [2, 3]. Hepatitis C is also the main cause of death from liver disease and the leading cause of liver transplants in the USA [4]. Following exposure to the virus, the disease starts with an acute phase in which approximately 80 % of the cases remain asymptomatic. The remaining 20 % may develop nonspecific symptoms such as fever, fatigue, loss of appetite, nausea, abdominal pain, dark urine, gray-colored feces, and/or jaundice [2]. Although in some patients the disease is self-limiting, 70–85 % of the patients become chronically infected. Of those, 60–70 % are at risk of developing chronic liver disease, 5–20 % are at risk of developing cirrhosis and/or hepatocellular carcinoma (HCC), and 1–5 % die from cirrhosis or HCC [2–4].

The HCV genome is approximately 9,600 bases long comprised in a single positive strand of RNA. The RNA harbors one open reading frame (ORF) flanked by 5′ and 3′ untranslated regions (UTRs). The ORF encodes a single polyprotein nearly 3,010–3,030 amino acids in size. The polyprotein is processed and cleaved with the aid of host cellular machinery and viral enzymes into structural and nonstructural proteins [5]. The viral RNA polymerase (one of the nonstructural proteins) lacks an efficient proofreading capability which results in a high rate of mutation in the HCV genome which allows HCV to evade the host's immune system. Owing to its wide genetic diversity, HCV is classified into six major genotypes, each exhibiting ~30 % sequence variation from one another. Viral sequences that differ by 20–25 % are termed subtypes, and those that have genetic variability <10 %—and sometimes more—are termed quasi-species [6].

The optimal treatment for HCV infection is a combination therapy of pegylated interferon alpha and ribavirin [4, 7, 8]. The treatment is costly and has severe side effects such as depression,

H.M.E. Azzazy, Ph.D. (✉)
Department of Chemistry, The American University in Cairo, AUC Avenue, P.O. Box 74, New Cairo 11835, Egypt

Yousef Jameel Science & Technology Research Center, The American University in Cairo, AUC Avenue, P.O. Box 74, New Cairo 11835, Egypt
e-mail: hazzazy@aucegypt.edu

K.M. Abdel-Hady, B.Sc.
Yousef Jameel Science & Technology Research Center, The American University in Cairo, AUC Avenue, P.O. Box 74, New Cairo 11835, Egypt

W.E. Highsmith Jr. (ed.), *Molecular Diagnostics: 12 Tests That Changed Everything*, Molecular and Translational Medicine, DOI 10.1007/978-1-4614-8127-0_5,

anemia, and flu-like symptoms, and its duration and chances of success depend upon the HCV genotype, its quantity (viral load), and a number of host factors. The aim of treatment is to achieve a sustained virological response (SVR), clinically defined as the absence of HCV RNA from the patient's serum 24 weeks after the discontinuation of therapy. For patients infected with genotypes 2 or 3, the optimum duration of therapy is 24 weeks, with an 80 % chance for achieving SVR. For those infected with genotypes 1, 4, 5, and 6, the optimum duration is 48 weeks, with a 40–50 % chance of achieving SVR for genotype 1. SVR data for the other genotypes is currently limited. The optimal treatment regimen for genotype 1 patients, however, has recently been altered with the advent of protease inhibitor direct acting antiviral agents to include one protease inhibitor to be taken in combination with peginterferon alpha and ribavirin, a regimen that has improved the chances of achieving SVR in those patients [9]. Despite multiple attempts, with several vaccine candidates currently in clinical trials, no vaccine has been developed against HCV.

To diagnose a patient with HCV, physicians cannot rely on the symptoms of the disease since they are scarce and nonspecific. Even biochemical markers, such as alanine aminotransferase (ALT) and aspartate aminotransferase (AST), are of little use in diagnosis, for although they may be elevated in the blood of the patient, 40 % of the patients may exhibit normal levels of those enzymes [7, 10]. Instead, two sensitive and specific classes of laboratory assays are used for the diagnosis of HCV which are *Immunoassays* and *molecular assays* [4]. Immunoassays detect mixtures of anti-HCV IgG antibodies directed against various epitopes of the virus in the patients' serum or plasma upon seroconversion, which occurs 8–12 weeks following exposure to the virus [3, 11, 12]. They are used for the primary screening of patient plasma and serum for HCV infection. However, due to the considerable percentage of false-positive results associated with these assays in low-risk populations, anti-HCV screening assay results require verification with an independent confirmatory (supplemental) molecular assay of higher specificity. Molecular assays detect HCV RNA in the patients' serum or plasma, which on average becomes detectable 1–3 weeks post-exposure (Fig. 5.1) [3, 13]. Unlike immunoassays, molecular HCV assays can confirm the presence or absence of *active* HCV infection, since the detection of anti-HCV antibodies can also be an indication of a *resolved* infection. However, it should be noted that at certain stages of the infection, the levels of viremia may transiently drop below the detection limit of the utilized assay, which is why a single negative molecular HCV assay result does not exclude the possibility of active infection [13]. In this chapter, the role of the different kinds of molecular HCV assays in HCV testing and their methodologies will be discussed.

Clinical Applications

Molecular assays play a very important role in the diagnosis of HCV infection, the determination and monitoring of the appropriate treatment regimen, and the screening of donated blood or blood products, applications which will be discussed in this section. They do not however—according to the American Association for the Study of Liver Diseases (AASLD)—have a role in assessing the severity or the prognosis of HCV yet [4]. Clinical studies are needed to investigate these possibilities.

Diagnosis of HCV Infection

According to the recent clinical practice guidelines of the AASLD and the European Association for the Study of the Liver (EASL), the diagnosis of HCV infection requires the detection of both anti-HCV antibodies by a screening immunoassay and HCV RNA by a sensitive molecular assay [4, 14]. A person suspected of having acute or chronic infection must be first tested for anti-HCV antibodies. A positive test necessitates the confirmation of the results with a supplemental molecular assay. Also if a patient tests negative for anti-HCV antibodies, but has an unexplained liver disease and/or is immunocompromised, or

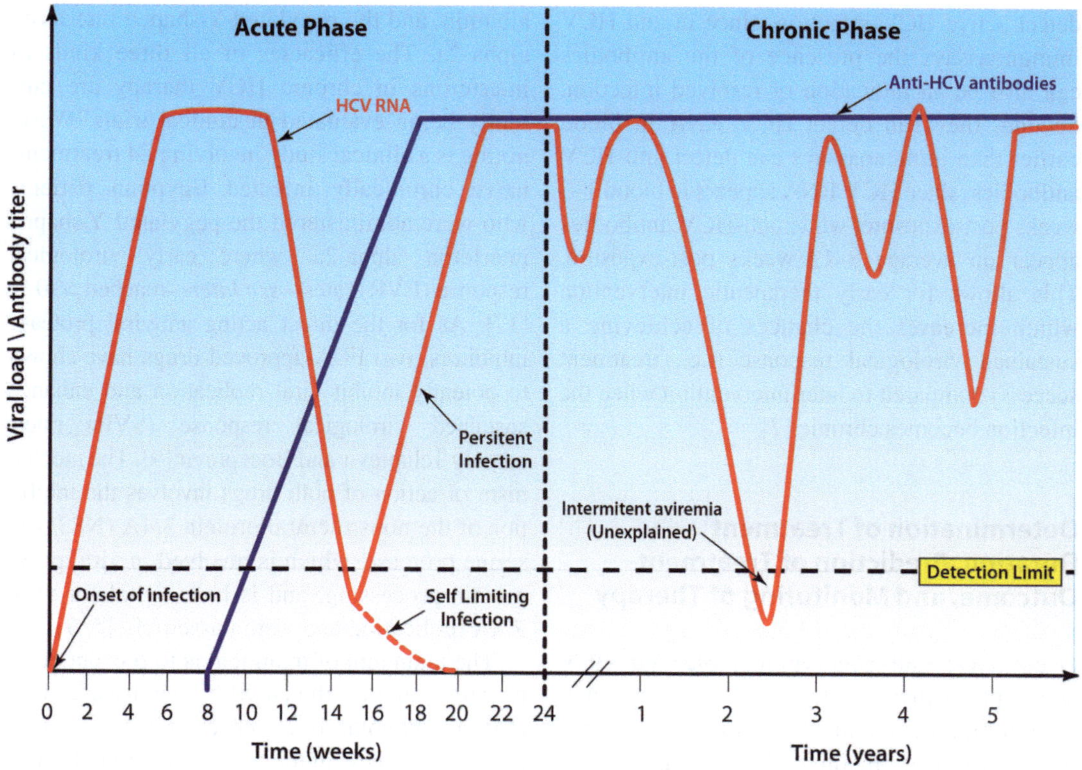

Fig. 5.1 HCV viral load and anti-HCV antibody titer following HCV infection. HCV RNA becomes detectable in blood on average 1–3 weeks after infection onset, and its quantity fluctuates throughout the infection. Sometimes HCV RNA may become undetectable, especially when the anti-HCV antibody titer starts to rise. Antibodies to HCV become detectable on average 8–12 weeks following infection, and remain detectable for life

if the patient is suspected of having acute HCV infection, he or she should also be required to test for HCV RNA. A negative anti-HCV test result for a patient from a low-risk population is enough to rule out the infection [15]. If the patient belongs to a high risk population, he or she may be prompted to repeat the anti-HCV test in 1–3 months [16]. While molecular HCV assays can efficiently diagnose the presence or absence of active infection, a single negative result does not rule out the presence of infection. This is because the level of HCV viremia does not stay constant and may sometimes decrease below detection limit (periods of unexplained aviremia). A single negative HCV RNA test result calls for the repetition of the assay in a 4–6 months time according to the AASLD guidlines [3, 4, 11].

Despite the importance of the supplemental assays, some laboratories do not perform them and report the results of the screening anti-HCV antibody assays directly. The reasons behind this could be either the lack of financial ability to meet the high cost of molecular assays, the absence of established laboratory standards for the assays, the lack of understanding concerning the interpretation of the results of the immunoassays and molecular assays, or a combination thereof. Therefore, in order to facilitate the practice of supplemental assays, the CDC has expanded its recommended anti-HCV antibody testing algorithm to optionally include the signal-to-cut off ratio of the screening anti-HCV assay results in order to minimize the number of test samples that require supplemental testing; where only samples exhibiting low s/co ratios are required to undergo supplemental assays prior to test result reporting [11].

Qualitative and quantitative molecular HCV assays have two advantages over immunoassays testing for anti-HCV antibodies. First, they can detect active HCV infection, since in anti-HCV immunoassays the presence of the antibodies can also be an indication of resolved infection. Second, they can detect HCV RNA in blood earlier than immunoassays can detect anti-HCV antibodies, since HCV RNA appears in blood 1–3 weeks post-exposure, while anti-HCV antibodies appear on average 8–12 weeks post-exposure. This allows for early therapeutic intervention which increases the chances of achieving a sustained virological response (i.e., treatment success) compared to later intervention when the infection becomes chronic [7].

Determination of Treatment Duration, Prediction of Treatment Outcome, and Monitoring of Therapy

Quantitative and genotyping molecular HCV assays play a pivotal role in the determination of the duration of treatment and in the prediction of the treatment outcome. The standard of care (SOC) therapy for the treatment of chronic HCV is a combination therapy of pegylated interferon alpha and ribavirin. Recently, however, with the development of protease inhibitor direct acting antiviral agents, the optimal treatment regimen for genotype 1 chronically infected patients was altered to a triple therapy involving the novel protease inhibitors (PI) in combination with pegylated interferon alpha and ribavirin [4, 9, 14]. Several kinds of interferons were developed for chronic HCV therapy, of which only two can be used in combination with ribavirin in the SOC therapy according to the AASLD and EASL guidelines. These are peginterferon alpha-2a and peginterferon alpha-2b, which are composed of the standard interferon alpha-2a and 2b molecules covalently attached to polyethylene glycol (PEG) molecules of different sizes serving the function of increasing the biological half-life of the interferons in circulation [4, 14]. Other new kinds of interferons include the synthetic interferon alfacon-1 (or consensus interferon, CIFN), albinterferon alpha-2b, which is composed of a standard interferon alpha-2b molecule covalently attached to human albumin, and the pegylated Y-shaped interferon alpha-2a. The efficacies of all three kinds of interferons in chronic HCV therapy are currently being evaluated in clinical trials. Worth noting is a clinical study involving 84 treatment-naïve chronically infected Egyptian patients who were administered the pegylated Y-shaped interferon alpha-2a, where early virological response (EVR) rates—*see later*—reached >90 % [17]. As for the direct acting antiviral protease inhibitors, two FDA-approved drugs have shown to potently inhibit viral replication and enhance sustained virological response (SVR) rates, namely Telaprevir and Boceprevir [9]. The mechanism of action of both drugs involves the inhibition of the nonstructural protein 3/4A (NS3/4A) serine protease, which is involved in viral polyprotein processing, and is hence vital for viral RNA replication and virion assembly [5, 9].

The main aim of treatment is to prevent complications and death caused by the disease. This clinical endpoint however cannot be used to assess the success of the antiviral treatment, since liver problems such as fibrosis, cirrhosis, and HCC take decades before they would occur. Instead, other short-term outcomes can be used; these include the serum levels of liver enzymes (biochemical assessment), the extent of hepatic inflammation (histological assessment), and the changes in HCV viral load in the blood in response to treatment [4]. The main indicator for treatment success is the absence of HCV RNA from the patient's blood 24 weeks after the cessation of therapy measured using a sensitive assay with a limit of detection (LOD) less than or equal to 50 IU/mL; what is called *sustained virological response (SVR)*. Not all patients diagnosed with active HCV infection, however, are required to receive therapy; in some cases where infection is associated with no or slight liver function abnormalities (as reflected by changes in liver enzymes), the physician may not prescribe treatment since the risk of developing future liver problems may be minimal [18]. Once initiated, chronic HCV therapy has several drawbacks. The SOC combination therapy between pegylated interferon alpha and ribavirin is very costly, causes severe side effects including anemia and depression, and has a variable cure rate. The same is true for the novel protease inhibitors, which despite their ability to enhance SVR rates have demonstrated to be associated with higher adverse event occurrences, in addition to their high costs and limited application to patients chronically infected with genotype 1 only [9].

Before initiating therapy, quantitative and genotyping molecular HCV assays must be performed, and their results are used to determine the appropriate duration of treatment and predict its outcome. Studies showed that the optimal duration of treatment with SOC combination therapy with peginterferon alpha and ribavirin for patients infected with HCV genotype 2 or 3 is 24 weeks, with an 80 % chance of achieving SVR. For patients infected with genotypes 1, 4, 5, and 6, the optimum treatment duration is 48 weeks with a smaller chance of success, where only 40–50 % of the patients infected with genotype 1 achieve SVR [4, 7, 19]. On the other hand, regardless of genotype, patients with viral load levels below a baseline of 800,000 IU/mL before the initiation of treatment have a better chance at treatment success than those with a viral load above this baseline [4, 10, 20]. As for the new genotype 1 therapy involving the protease inhibitors, clinical studies have shown that SVR rates increased from 40 to 50 % with peginterferon alpha and ribavirin therapy to 60–80 % with triple therapy [9]. The optimal duration of treatment with triple therapy varies according to the PI drug used and the viral kinetics during treatment [9].

After the initiation of treatment, genotyping molecular HCV assays are no longer performed since the HCV genotype does not change along the course of treatment and the infection with a new HCV genotype is very rare. Quantitative assays, however, continue to be performed during therapy for monitoring the rate of viral clearance from the patient's blood in response to treatment. This can be very helpful in the prediction of the likelihood of achieving SVR at the end of treatment and in deciding whether treatment should be continued for the entire recommended duration (per each genotype) or could be stopped earlier. The early cessation of treatment is beneficial in limiting the exposure to the antiviral drugs, which leads to reduced toxicity and cost savings [4, 7, 10].

Screening Blood and Blood Products for Transfusion

Although anti-HCV antibody screening assays can be used to determine whether a donated blood sample is potentially infected with HCV, the fact that seroconversion occurs on average 8–12 weeks after the onset of infection may cause infected samples to pass by unnoticed; increasing the likelihood of disease transmission through blood transfusion. On the other hand, screening donated blood samples using a qualitative molecular assay effectively lowers the rate of HCV transmission through this route. Compared to immunoassays, molecular assays are able to determine infected blood samples donated from patients in the early acute phase of infection who have not yet achieved seroconversion, unaffected by genotype variations [7, 21]. They are also effective in situations where seroconversion occurs partially or does not occur as in immuno-compromised patients [22].

Methods

HCV molecular assays include qualitative, quantitative, and genotyping assays. Qualitative assays are used to confirm the presence or absence of active infection in the blood of the patient, and quantitative assays are used to determine the amount of HCV particles per milliliter of blood (viral load). In this section, the different molecular methodologies used for detection of HCV will be discussed.

Qualitative and Quantitative Assays

Qualitative and quantitative molecular HCV assays can be carried out using commercially available kits or home-brewed methods. In both cases, the assays are based on one of the following

Table 5.1 Commercial FDA approved qualitative molecular HCV RNA assays

Assay	Amplification technology	Limit of detection (IU/mL)	FDA approved clinical application
Amplicor HCV 2.0	RT-PCR	50	Confirming the presence of active HCV infection
COBAS®Amplicor HCV 2.0	RT-PCR	50	Confirming the presence of active HCV infection
COBAS®Ampliscreen HCV 2.0	RT-PCR	<50	Blood screening
Versant HCV RNA	TMA	≤10	Confirming the presence of active HCV infection
Procleix Ultrio	TMA	≤10	Blood screening
Cobas® TaqScreen MPX Test 2.0	Real time RT-PCR	<50	Blood screening

Table 5.2 Commercially available quantitative molecular HCV RNA assays intended for use in the determination of HCV viral load and as an aid in anti-HCV therapy management

Assay	Amplification technology	Linear quantification range (IU/mL)
COBAS® Amplicor HCV Monitor 2.0[b]	RT-PCR	600–500,000
SuperQuant™	RT-PCR	30–1,470,000
LCx® HCV RNA[b]	RT-PCR	23–2,300,000
COBAS AmpliPrep™/COBAS®Taqman® HCV[a]	Real time RT-PCR	43–69,000,000
Abbott RealTime™ HCV[a]	Real time RT-PCR	12–100,000,000
Artus HCV QS-RGQ	Real time RT-PCR	67.6–17,700,000
Versant HCV RNA 3.0[a]	bDNA	615–7,700,000

[a]FDA approved assays
[b]Phased-out assays

technologies: conventional or real time reverse transcriptase polymerase chain reaction (RT-PCR), transcription-mediated amplification (TMA), and branched DNA technology (bDNA). The first three are based on target-amplification, whereas bDNA is a signal-amplification technology [13].

Reverse Transcriptase-PCR Assays

RT-PCR-based assays can be used for both the qualitative detection of HCV and the quantitative determination of viral load in serum or plasma [13, 23]. The region of HCV RNA that is most commonly amplified in RT-PCR assays is the 5′UTR, because it is highly conserved across all HCV genotypes [24]. Several commercial kits for the detection and quantification of HCV and most of the home-brewed molecular HCV assays are based on RT-PCR [7]. However, with the advent of real time RT-PCR technology to the HCV molecular diagnostic market, many of the assays based on conventional RT-PCR have been phased out. Examples of commercial RT-PCR-based assays include the manual qualitative assays Amplicor®HCV v2.0 and Ampliscreen® HCV v2.0 (Roche Molecular Systems) and their semi-automated versions COBAS®Amplicor®HCV v2.0 and COBAS®Ampliscreen® HCV v2.0. Examples of quantitative assays include the manual Amplicor®HCV Monitor v2.0 and its semi-automated version COBAS Amplicor®HCV Monitor v2.0 (Roche Molecular Systems), LCx® HCV RNA (Abbott Laboratories), and SuperQuant™ (National Genetics Institute) [4, 7, 10, 12]. Characteristics of these assays are listed in Tables 5.1 and 5.2.

Real Time RT-PCR Assays

These assays allow for both detection of HCV RNA and the quantitative measurement of the HCV viral load in a patient's plasma or serum with very high sensitivity and a wider linear range of quantification [4, 10, 23]. Unlike conventional RT-PCR that depends on the end-point detection and quantification of HCV amplicons, real time RT-PCR involves the detection and quantification of HCV amplicons produced from each PCR cycle in real time by detecting and measuring the intensity of fluorescence produced from special fluorochromes utilized in the reaction. In real time RT-PCR assays, amplicons can be detected using DNA-binding dyes, hybridization probes, molecular beacons, or hydrolysis probes (Taqman® probes) [7, 25]. Detection using DNA-binding dyes is the only method that involves the *nonspecific* detection of DNA amplicons, where fluorescent dyes such as SYBR®Green (Molecular Probe Inc., CA, USA) bind to double-stranded DNA produced in the elongation step of the reaction. The remaining three methods involve the *specific* hybridization of fluorescence-labeled probes to their target amplicons.

In the hybridization probes method, two probes, one labeled with an "acceptor" fluorochrome at its 5′ end and the other with a "donor" fluorochrome at its 3′ end bind in close proximity to adjacent target sites on the DNA amplicons in the annealing step of the RT-PCR. The fluorescence emitted from the donor fluorochrome will excite the acceptor fluorochrome by a phenomenon called fluorescence resonance energy transfer (FRET), leading to the emission of light from the acceptor fluorochrome at a longer wavelength than that emitted from the donor. The intensity of light emitted from the acceptor flurochrome is used to quantify the amount of DNA synthesized during the reaction. Molecular beacons are special probes that form stem-and-loop (hairpin) structures in solution, where both ends of each probe are labeled with a "quencher" chromphore and a "reporter" fluorochrome. In the absence of the target amplicons, the hairpin structure of the probes brings the quencher chromophore and reporter fluorochrome in close proximity, resulting in the quenching of the fluorescence of the reporter fluorochrome. In the presence of the target amplicon, the probe binds to its complementary sequence on the amplicon, separating the quencher and reporter and causing the restoration of the reporter's fluorescence, which is then measured to quantify the amount of target amplicons in the sample. A similar concept is applied in the hydrolysis probes method, where the probes contain a reporter fluorochrome at their 5′end whose fluorescence is quenched by a quencher chromophore at their 3′end. The probe hybridizes to its target sequence in the annealing step of RT-PCR, and then during the elongation step a special DNA polymerase hydrolyzes and displaces the probe, separating the quencher from the reporter. This leads to the restoration of the fluorescence of the reporter fluorochrome and the detection of the target amplicons [7, 25]. A schematic representation of detection using hybridization probes and hydrolysis (Taqman®) probes is depicted in Fig. 5.2.

Real time RT-PCR-based assays are fast and have limits of detection (LODs) that can reach down to 10 IU/mL. They also have a very wide linear range of quantification exceeding 6 logs. Furthermore, they are less prone to producing false-positive results caused by contamination arising in gel-based analysis of the conventional RT-PCR amplicons. Such advantages allowed these types of assays to become more popular and to displace the need for qualitative HCV molecular assays [7, 10, 23]. Examples of commercially available real time RT-PCR-based assays include the COBAS®Taqman® HCV test produced by Roche, the Abbott RealTime™ HCV test, and the Artus HCV QS-RGQ (Qiagen, Hilden, Germany). The three assays quantitatively detect HCV RNA in two steps: *extraction* of HCV RNA from the patient's serum or plasma followed by *amplification and real time detection*. In the COBAS Taqman® and the Abbott RealTime™ assays, extraction is performed using the COBAS AmpliPrep™ (Roche Molecular Systems) and m2000sp™ (Abbott Laboratories) systems, respectively. Samples are first mixed with chaotropic lysis buffers to extract HCV RNA from the virions; in this step, an internal control is added to the samples to assess the efficiency of the RT-PCR reaction. Magnetic microparticles are then added to the samples, where the extracted HCV RNA molecules would adsorb onto the microparticles to be washed and then collected by elution with aqueous buffer. The samples are then transferred into optical microplates where they are combined with the RT-PCR master mix. The Real time RT-PCR step

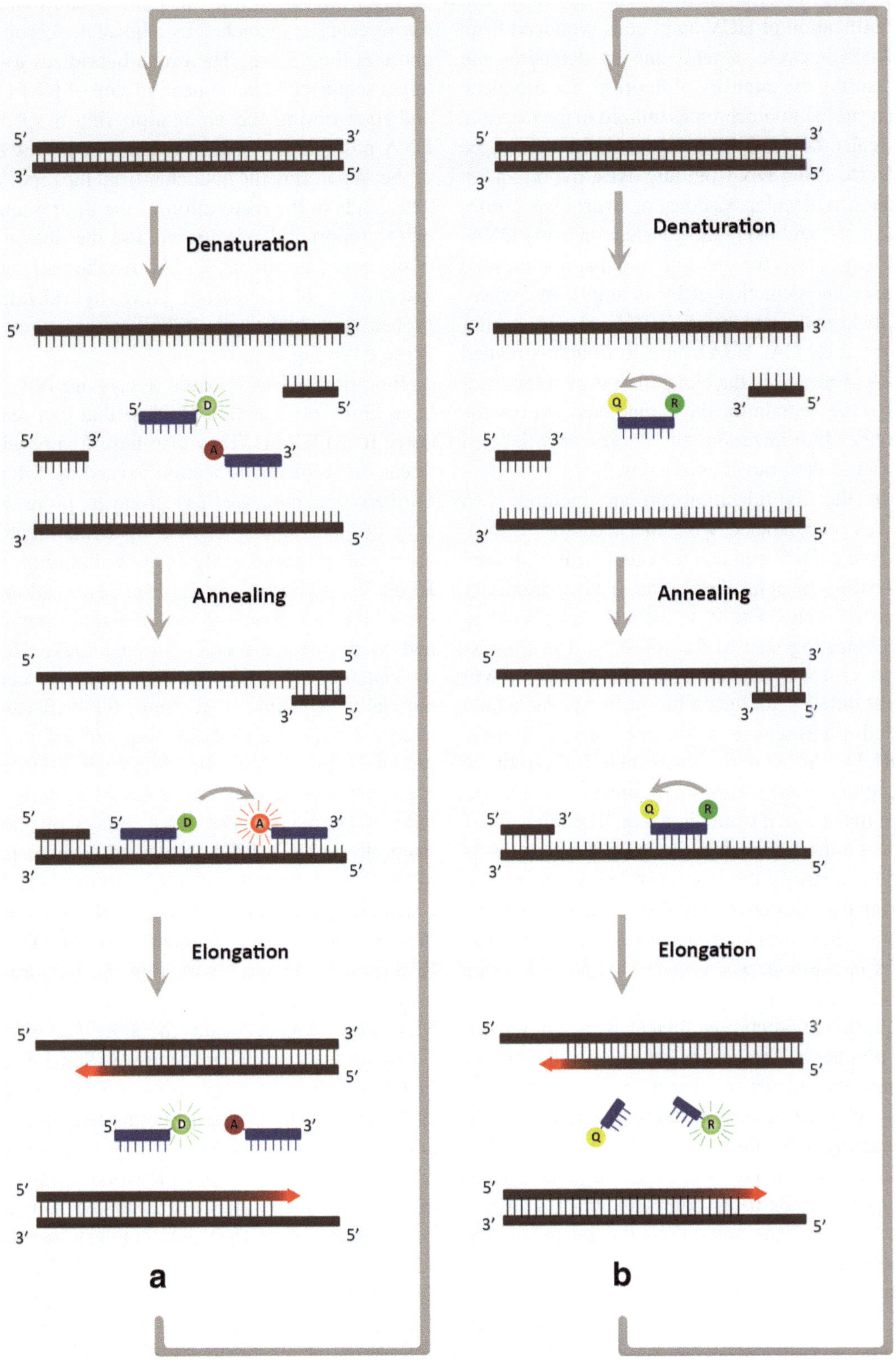
Denaturation
Annealing
Elongation
a
Denaturation
Annealing
Elongation
b

is then performed in different instruments. For the COBAS®Taqman assay, it is performed in either the COBAS®Taqman® Analyzer or the COBAS®Taqman® 48 Analyzer. For the Abbott RealTime™ assay, it is performed in the m2000rt™ system. In both assays sequences from the 5′UTR of the HCV RNA are amplified. Quantitative detection is performed via the hydrolysis probes method, where two different probes are used for the HCV RNA and IC amplicons. The fluorescence produced by the HCV RNA-specific probe is measured at a different wavelength from that at which the fluorescence of the IC-specific probe is measured. In order to calculate the initial amount of HCV RNA in the sample, the fluorescence measured above a certain critical threshold value for the HCV RNA is compared to that of a quantification standard(s). In the Abbott RealTime™ assay, quantification standards (QS) are amplified separately from the HCV RNA, and an internal control is added to the QS reactions as well. On the other hand in the COBAS Taqman® assay, the IC itself acts as the quantification standard [23, 26, 27]. In the Artus HCV QS-RGQ assay, HCV RNA extraction is performed in the instrument QIAsymphony SP/AS, while amplification and quantitative detection is performed in the Rotor-Gene Q real time PCR cycler. The assay amplifies a 240 bp region of the 5′UTR, and similar to the Abbott RealTime™ assay calculates the initial amount of HCV RNA in the sample relative to quantification standards amplified in separate reactions from that of the HCV RNA [28].

The COBAS AmpliPrep™/COBAS®Taqman® HCV assay has a linear range of quantification from 43 IU/mL to 6.9×10^7 IU/mL, with a LOD of 15 IU/mL. A clinical evaluation of the assay showed that it was able to detect HCV RNA concentrations down to 7.4 IU/mL with 100 % efficiency. It also showed that it had a specificity of 99 %, and linear quantification range ranging from 28 to 1.4×10^7 IU/mL [26]. Despite these good specifications, a study identified two problems in the assay. First, the assay was found to overestimate RNA levels in undiluted samples by about 0.6 logs, an over-estimation that increased with high viral load. The assay also underestimated RNA levels in 15 % of the test subjects infected with HCV genotype 2 and in 30 % of those infected with genotype 4, a problem that probably occurred due to a mismatch between the utilized probes or primers and the HCV RNA [23, 29]. Very recently, *Roche Molecular Systems Inc.* has issued a class 2 recall to the assay pertaining to the underestimation problem with genotype 4 [30]. However, this problem has been solved in the second version of the assay COBAS AmpliPrep™/COBAS®Taqman® HCV v2.0, which was recently launched in 2012.

With regard to the Abbott RealTime™ assay, a performance evaluation study showed that it has a specificity of 100 %, and a LOD of 12 IU/mL, which is the same value as the claimed LOD on the assay's package insert [31]. The Artus HCV QS-RGQ assay has a LOD of 36.2 IU/mL and a linear quantification range of 67.6 IU/mL up to 17,700,000 IU/mL. A recent study compared the performance of the assay with the COBAS AmpliPrep™/COBAS®Taqman® HCV assay, where linear regression analysis showed a good correlation between both tests, with the COBAS AmpliPrep™/COBAS®Taqman® HCV assay

Fig. 5.2 Schematic representation of amplicon detection in real time RT-PCR: (**a**) Detection by hybridization probes: The emission spectrum of the donor fluorochrome "D" overlaps with the excitation spectrum of the acceptor fluorochrome "A." This results in the excitation of the acceptor by FRET causing it to emit light at a longer wavelength than that of the donor which is then measured. (**b**) Detection by hydrolysis probes: DNA polymerases with double-strand-specific 5′exonuclease activities such as Taq polymerase and Tth polymerase are used in the assay to hydrolyze the bound probe. Once the probe is hydrolyzed, the quencher chromophore "Q" and the reporter fluorochrome "R" become separated, allowing the reporter to emit detectable fluorescence that is used to quantitatively detect the amount of target amplicons. *Modified from: Bustin SA. Absolute quantification of mRNA using real time reverse transcription polymerase chain reaction assays. J Mol Endocrinol. 2000;25:169–193 © Society for Endocrinology (2000). Reproduced by permission*

having a slightly better observed sensitivity than the Artus HCV QS-RGQ assay. The Artus assay was shown to detect higher levels of HCV RNA in HCV genotype 4 positive samples. Recently, the assay has obtained the European Conformity—In Vitro Diagnostic Medical Devices (CE-IVD) approval [28]. A list of the mentioned commercial real time RT-PCR-based molecular HCV assays with their linear quantification ranges is presented in Table 5.2.

Transcription-Mediated Amplification Assays

TMA-based assays provide a more sensitive alternative to RT-PCR for the qualitative detection of HCV RNA [4]. TMA is an isothermal process in which the desired region of viral RNA is reverse transcribed by a reverse transcriptase enzyme into cDNA using special primers containing T7 RNA polymerase promoter regions. The cDNA with the T7 promoter is then used as a template by T7 RNA polymerase to transcribe several copies of viral RNA, which re-enter the cycle to produce more copies of themselves [12, 13, 32]. Similar to commercial RT-PCR-based assays, the amplified region is included within the 5′UTR.

Versant®HCV RNA (Siemens Healthcare Diagnostics), Procleix HIV-1/HCV assay, and Procleix Ultrio (Gen-Probe and Novartis Diagnostics) are commercial TMA-based assays [4, 12]. The assays start by the extraction of HCV RNA using a chaotropic lysis buffer. The internal control is added in this step. The HCV RNA and the IC are then captured by 5′UTR specific probes immobilized on magnetic microparticles, which allow thorough washing of the sample. TMA starts by the hybridization of primers containing the T7 RNA polymerase promoter to their target sequence in the 5′UTR. Detection is carried out via a *Hybridization Protection Assay (HPA)* [33], where chemiluminescent amplicon-specific probes bind the HCV RNA and IC RNA amplicons. Chemiluminescence is then detected and the value of the signal-to-cut off ratio is then used to determine the test result [32, 34, 35].

TMA-based molecular HCV RNA assays have high analytical sensitivities and specificities almost reaching 100 % and LODs reaching less than 10 IU/mL. A multicenter evaluation of the Versant®HCV RNA assay showed that it can detect HCV RNA concentrations as low as 2.4 IU/mL with a specificity of 99.4 % [34]. The same assay was shown to be able to detect all HCV genotypes with near equal efficiency; in addition to being highly reproducible and robust in detecting HCV RNA from samples subjected to extreme conditions such as long-term storage, multiple freezing and thawing cycles, and presence of endogenous materials [32, 34, 36]. Similarly with the Procleix Ultrio assay, clinical evaluations showed that its LOD can reach an average of 4.6 IU/mL, with >95 % analytical sensitivity and >99.5 % specificity [35, 37].

Branched DNA Assays

These assays depend on signal amplification rather than target amplification, and are used to determine HCV viral load in serum or plasma. An example of a commercial bDNA HCV assay is the Versant HCV RNA 3.0 assay (Bayer Diagnostics, Emeryville, CA). The assay is performed in three steps: viral RNA *extraction*, *signal amplification*, and *quantification*. Extraction occurs by chemical lysis of HCV virions using a chaotropic buffer. The released RNA is then captured by specific synthetic oligonucleotide *capture probes* immobilized in welled plates. Signal amplification is achieved via a series of probe hybridizations resulting from the sequential addition of probes to the wells [7, 23, 38]. The first kind of probes added are the *target probes*, which bind the HCV RNA in a sandwich manner. Both the capture and target probes hybridize to the 5′UTR and core regions of the HCV genome. *Preamplifier probes* are then added which hybridize with the target probes. Finally, *amplifier probes* are added which hybridize with the preamplifier probes. This concludes the formation of the branched DNA complex and the signal amplification step. To quantify the amount of RNA, alkaline phosphatase-labeled probes are added to the wells and hybridize with the bDNA complex, followed by the addition of a chemiluminescent substrate. After incubation, the chemiluminescence produced by the reaction is used to quantify the amount of HCV RNA relative to a calibration curve constructed from chemiluminescence data of five standards [7, 23, 38].

Multicenter evaluation of the Versant HCV RNA 3.0 assay showed that the assay has a LOD of 615 IU/mL and a linear range of quantification of 615–7,690,000 IU/mL. The assay had a high analytical specificity of around 98 % and high reproducibility [10, 38]. Furthermore, due to the fact that HCV RNA is not amplified in this assay, the level of contamination is drastically reduced, which results in a much smaller number of false-positive results [7].

Laboratory Developed Tests (Home-Brewed Assays)

Instead of using expensive HCV commercial assays, home-brewed HCV assays are developed by some laboratories, especially in developing countries. In-house qualitative and quantitative assays are mostly based on conventional RT-PCR or real time RT-PCR technologies. Like in commercial assays, the 5′UTR, which contains sequences conserved among all HCV genotypes, is the preferred target for amplification. Table 5.3 lists some forward and reverse primers that have been used to amplify sequences within the HCV 5′UTR.

Genotyping Assays

The extensive genetic variability of HCV has lead to its classification into six major genotypes, and further into subtypes, and quasispecies. Epidemiologically, genotypes 1, 2, and 3 are spread worldwide, with genotypes 1 and 2 predominantly present in North America, Europe, and Japan, and genotype 3 in countries of south-east Asia like Pakistan and India [13, 44, 45]. Genotype 4 is mainly found in Northern and Central Africa and the Middle East, reaching its highest prevalence in Egypt, where more than 22 % of the population is infected with HCV. It is also recently becoming increasingly prevalent in European countries on the Mediterranean sea such as Italy, France, and Spain [2, 44, 46]. The prevalence of genotype 5 is almost exclusive to South Africa, while that of genotype 6 is predominant in south-east Asia in countries such as Vietnam and Indonesia [44, 47]. The duration and expected outcome of HCV treatment depends, in part, on the HCV genotype infecting the patient; a fact that made HCV genotyping an important step prior to the initiation of treatment. However, despite its importance, HCV genotyping is not done at all in certain countries due to the high costs of the test. Several genotyping technologies have been developed, the most important of which are *direct sequencing, DNA hybridization (line-probe assay), restriction fragment-length polymorphism (RFLP), multiplex real time RT-PCR, and primer-specific and mispair extension analysis (PSMEA).*

Many commercial genotyping assays rely on the presence of genotype-specific polymorphisms in the highly conserved 5′UTR of the HCV genome. Although relying on the sequence heterogenity in this region for HCV classification can cause problems in definitive genotype and subtype identification, as it has been proven that some genotype 6 variants share identical 5'UTR sequences with genotype 1a or 1b, it is still acceptable to rely on for HCV genotyping for the purposes of treatment response prediction and choosing the appropriate treatment regimen. According to Simmonds et al. [6], the results of HCV genotyping based on the analysis of the 5′-UTR nucleotide sequence showed 95 % concordance with those based on the analysis of the nucleotide sequence of the nonstructural protein 5B (NS5B) and Core/E1 regions of the genome, with the NS5B nucleotide sequence analysis being widely considered as the "gold standard" for HCV classification [6, 48, 49]. Failure to genotype an HCV isolate using commercial assays is rare (around 3 %), and is most probably due to either the presence of low viral levels below the assay's detection limit, the excessive mutations in the region analyzed, or both [4].

Direct Nucleic Acid Sequencing

Phylogenetic analysis of HCV nucleotide sequences is considered the reference method for

Table 5.3 Selected primers used for the amplification of regions within the 5′UTR of HCV RNA

Forward primers		Reverse primers		
Sequence (5′→3′)	Location[a]	Sequence (5′→3′)	Location[a]	Reference
GAAAGCGTCTAGCCATGGCGTTAGT	71–95	CTCGCAAGCACCCTATCAGG	292–311	[39, 40]
CTGTGAGGAACTACTGTCTT	45–64	GTGCTCATGGTGCACGGTCTACGAGACCTCC	319–349	[41]
TTCACGCAGAAAGCGTCTAG	63–82	CACTCGCAAGCACCCTATCAGGCA	290–313	[41]
GGCGACACTCCACCATAGATC	18–38	GGTGCACGGTCTACGAGACCT	321–341	[42]
CTGTGAGGAACTACTGTCTTC	45–65	CCCTATCAGGCAGTACCACAA	281–301	[42]
ACGCAGAAAGCGTCTAGCCATGGCGTTAGT	66–95	TCCCGGGGCACTCGCAAGCACCCTATCAGG	292–321	[43]

[a]location on H77 as identified by The Los Alamos HCV Sequence Database "QuickAlign" tool [39]

HCV genotyping or classification, with NS5B sequence analysis being considered as the gold standard [48]. This, however, is an expensive and time-consuming method of genotyping, which makes it impractical to follow in clinical investigations and limited its use to research settings [24, 49]. The TRUGENE®HCV assay (Siemens Healthcare Diagnostics) is a commercial genotyping assay for research use only based on the direct sequencing of a fragment from the 5′UTR via coupled amplification and sequencing technology (CLIP sequencing) [50]. In CLIP sequencing, the target nucleotide sequence is first amplified through several PCR cycles to provide a template for sequencing; then, the resultant amplicons are aliquoted into separate vessels containing fluorescently labeled primers and one of four dideoxynucleotides (ddNTPs) in pre-optimized concentrations. The amplicons are then further subjected to several PCR cycles, resulting in the production of ddNTP-terminated fragments that are then used to elucidate the investigated sequence via specialized equipment. The resultant sequence is then phylogenetically analyzed to determine the HCV genotype in question [51].

DNA Hybridization

Another way of identifying the HCV genotype can be achieved via the hybridization of genotype-specific probes to complementary regions on the HCV RNA containing genotype-specific polymorphisms. A commercial example for this method of genotyping is the VERSANT® HCV Genotype 2.0 Assay (LiPA), which is produced by Innogenetics and distributed by Siemens Healthcare Diagnostics, and is intended for research use only. In this assay, genotype-specific probes complementary to genotype-specific sequences in the 5′UTR and core regions of the viral RNA are immobilized in parallel lines on a nitrocellulose membrane. Biotinylated HCV RT-PCR amplicons of 5′UTR and core region fragments harboring sequences complementary to those probes are added onto the membrane where they would bind to their genotype-specific probes, followed by the addition of streptavidin-conjugated alkaline phosphatase. A chromogenic substrate is then added, and the genotype of the amplicon is determined by the formation of a colored precipitate in regions on the membrane containing the probes corresponding to the investigated genotype (genotype-specific colored band pattern). In an evaluation, the test was able to determine the genotypes of 96 % of the tested samples with a 99.4 % concordance with the direct sequencing (reference) method [52].

Restriction Fragment Length Polymorphism

The different genotype-specific polymorphisms result in different genotype-specific restriction sites which can be used for HCV genotyping. HCV DNA amplicons can be digested using certain restriction enzymes, and the sizes of the resulting fragments can be related to each genotype. Digestion should be done efficiently so that large undigested fragments don't interfere with the results and reduce the reliability of the assay. It is important to note that given the high rate of mutation of the HCV genome, the genotyping criteria of the RFLP assay must be continuously improved and updated to account for any changes in restriction sites due to the increasing heterogeneity of the virus [7, 53, 54].

Multiplex Real Time RT-PCR

Multiplex real time RT-PCR technology provides a faster and less contamination-prone way for HCV genotyping. The method involves the amplification of a specific region of the HCV genome via real time RT-PCR, where genotype-specific fluorescent probes complementary to genotype-specific polymorphic sites on that region are used to identify the HCV genotype. This can be done in separate reactions utilizing probes with the same fluorescent tag, or in one reaction tube utilizing probes with different fluorescent tags. Alternatively, a single probe can be used and genotyping can then be performed via melting curve analysis [55–59]. Commercially, a genotyping assay based on multiplex real time RT-PCR called RealTime HCV Genotype II (Abbott Laboratories) was developed. The assay is used to distinguish between the six major genotypes based on the 5′UTR, and the two genotype 1 subtypes *a* and *b* based on the NS5B region of the genome, using three reaction mixtures with probes tagged with three different reporter dyes [60]. The assay showed a high concordance of >95 % and 100 % with the line probe assay and restriction fragment mass polymorphism methods, respectively [61]. It has a detection limit >500 IU/mL; however, it was shown that even at this detection limit, it cannot detect minor genotypes in cases of mixed infection [61].

Primer Specific and Mispair Extension Analysis

In amplification reactions where mispair formation occurs during DNA synthesis, primer extension can occur normally especially if the utilized DNA polymerase lacks the 3′→5′ exonuclease proofreading capability. However, polymerases harboring this activity can to a great extent prevent primer extension when any mismatches are present. In a study conducted by Hu et al. [62], the ability of the enzyme *Pyrococcus furiosus (Pfu)* DNA polymerase to terminate primer extension in case of mispair formation due to its 3′→5′ exonuclease proofreading capability was effectively utilized for HCV genotyping [62]. The developed assay involves the amplification of regions in the 5′UTR containing genotype and subtype specific polymorphisms using the *pfu* DNA polymerase in a reaction vessel containing an incomplete set of dNTPs. If mispairing occurs at a polymorphic (type-specific) nucleotide on the PCR products of HCV RNA of a certain genotype/subtype adjacent to the 3′ end of the utilized primer due to the lack of the complementary dNTP in the reaction vessel, primer extension of the complementary strand would cease. On the other hand, it will proceed for PCR products of HCV RNA of different genotype(s)/subtype(s) that have dNTPs in the reaction vessel complementary to their polymorphic nucleotide of the same location. This will generate DNA fragments of different sizes which will give unique genotype/subtype specific band patterns on a DNA sequencing gel. The identification of genotype and subtype specific polymorphic regions can be controlled via the manipulation of the set of dNTPs utilized in the reaction and/or the use of different genotype specific primers. The assay's results showed 100 % concordance with those of RFLP analysis and direct nucleic acid sequencing genotyping methods. Furthermore, it was proven that PSMEA can detect low levels of mixed genotype HCV infections with high sensitivity.

Standard Reagents

The global use of molecular HCV assays and their established role in HCV diagnosis has made it a necessity to standardize these assays. This lead the World Health Organization (WHO) in 1997 to develop and produce the world's first international standard for HCV RNA nucleic acid amplification technology assays (denoted 96/790) to be used for the validation of HCV assays, and the calibration of their secondary standards and working reagents [23, 63]. This standard established a common unit of measure to be used in all molecular HCV assays, namely the *International Units per milliliter (IU/mL).* Establishing this international standard unit has allowed for the easy monitoring of the level of viremia in infected patients regardless of the assay used. The standard material 96/790 was produced by the dilution of a high titer isolate of HCV of genotype 1a in pooled human plasma. It was lyophilized and packed in vials to give a concentration of 10^5 IU/mL upon reconstitution. When the stocks of this material ran low, the WHO produced the second international standard 96/798 in 2003, which was produced from the same starting material and assigned the same potency of 10^5 IU/mL [64]. On the smaller scale, all molecular HCV assays include internal standard material (secondary standards) of known quantity. For quantitative assays, they include an external quantification panel quantified against the international standard.

When converting results of quantitative molecular HCV RNA assays from IU/mL into RNA copies/mL, no standard conversion factor exists. Instead, the conversion factor can vary anywhere from 1 to 5 depending on the assay used. Table 5.4 shows some of the conversion factors used with some common commercial assays [4, 65].

Table 5.4 IU/mL to RNA copies/mL conversion factors for commonly used molecular HCV RNA quantitative assays

Assay	Amplification technology	Conversion factor
Amplicor®HCV Monitor 2.0	RT-PCR	1 IU/mL = 0.9 copies/mL
COBAS Amplicor®HCV Monitor 2.0	RT-PCR	1 IU/mL = 2.7 copies/mL
SuperQuant™	RT-PCR	1 IU/mL = 3.4 copies/mL
LCx® HCV RNA	RT-PCR	1 IU/mL = 4.3 copies/mL
Versant® HCV RNA 3.0	bDNA	1 IU/mL = 5.2 copies/mL

Modified from references [4, 23]

Test Interpretation

In the diagnosis of HCV, a positive anti-HCV screening immunoassay means that the patient has been exposed to HCV. A negative result on the other hand can have more than one interpretation. First, if the tested individual belongs to a low-risk population, a negative anti-HCV screening assay is interpreted that he or she is free from infection [15]. If, however, the tested individual was immunocompromised and/or has an unexplained liver disease or is suspected to be in the early acute phase of infection, there is a good chance that the testing result is false-negative. In such case, a confirmatory molecular assay needs to be performed to confirm or refute the result of the screening immunoassay.

A positive molecular HCV assay confirms the presence of active HCV infection. A negative result, however, calls for repeating the test several weeks later to exclude the probability of transient aviremia. The biggest challenge facing molecular HCV assays in diagnosis is the differentiation between acute and chronic HCV infection. A positive molecular HCV assay result accompanied with a negative anti-HCV antibody screening test result may indicate that the patient is in the early acute phase of the infection; however, it can also mean that the anti-HCV assay result was false-negative, or that the patient is immunocompromised. A recent study by McGovern et al. suggests that HCV viral load fluctuations and levels of viremia should be used to distinguish between acute and chronic infections as part of the standard diagnostic criteria [7, 66]. Previous studies had shown that chronically infected patients have high HCV viral loads in their blood reaching >400,000 IU/mL in relatively stable levels with approximately 0.5 log fluctuations. On the other hand, they showed that the majority of acutely infected patients have low viral loads whose level fluctuated heavily until spontaneous viral clearance or viral persistence occurs. In McGovern et al., a cohort of acute HCV seroconverters were compared to a cohort of chronic HCV patients on the basis of viral load fluctuations and HCV RNA levels. The results showed that over 80 % of the acute seroconverters had low levels of viremia (<100,000 IU/mL) and viral load fluctuations, while only 13 % of the chronically infected patients had viremia levels below 100,000 IU/mL. These findings, however, need to be validated using larger cohorts of patients. The AASLD and EASL guidelines do not include viral load fluctuations and levels of viremia as standard parameters for differentiating between acute and chronic HCV infections. Based on these guidelines, differentiating between both cases is based on the clinical presentation of the patient, manifested in the presence/absence of disease symptoms, and whether there was a history of ALT elevation in the patient's blood or not, and the duration of this elevation [4, 14].

Before initiating treatment, the results of genotyping molecular HCV assays are necessary to direct the physician in choosing the optimal treatment duration for the patient. For patients infected with HCV genotypes 2 and 3, as it was aforementioned, the optimal treatment duration using peginterferon alpha in combination with ribavirin standard of care therapy is a maximum of 24 weeks, as for genotypes 4, 5, and 6, the optimal duration is a maximum of 48 weeks [4, 7, 19]. For genotype 1, the recommended optimal treatment duration using peginterferon alpha in combination with ribavirin therapy was a maximum of 48 weeks. However, with regard to the new triple therapy, the most recent

AASLD guidelines state that the optimal treatment duration for treatment-naïve patients taking the PI Boceprevir is between 24 and 44 weeks triple therapy, preceded by a 4 week "lead-in" treatment with peginterferon alpha and ribavirin therapy alone in order to improve treatment efficiency, while for those taking the PI Telaprevir, it is recommended to initiate treatment with a triple therapy regimen for 12 weeks, followed by 12–36 weeks of peginterferon alpha and ribavirin therapy alone [9].

In addition to directing the physician in choosing the optimal treatment duration for the patient, the results of quantitative and genotyping molecular HCV assays prior to treatment give an indication about the chances of treatment success. In general, patients infected with genotypes 2 or 3 and those having a starting viral load of <800,000 IU/mL have a better chance at treatment success than patients infected with genotypes 1, 4, 5, or 6 and those having a starting viral load of >800,000 IU/mL. With regard to peginterferon alpha and ribavirin therapy, patients infected with genotypes 2 and 3 have an 80 % chance of achieving SVR, while those infected with genotype 1 have only a 40–50 % chance [2, 7, 10, 19, 20]. With the new triple therapy however, the chances of treatment success with genotype 1 patients has risen to 60–80 % [9].

Just like there are virus-related factors associated with a higher likelihood of treatment success, there are also host-related factors such as female gender, young age (<40 years), and the favorable genotype of the interleukin (IL) 28B gene [67]. Three recent studies discovered a novel association between certain single nucleotide polymorphisms (SNPs) on the nucleotide sequence near the IL28B (or λ interferon 3) gene on chromosome 19 and the response to peginterferon alpha and ribavirin therapy in patients infected with HCV genotype 1 [67–70]. One of those SNPs is located at position rs12979860, where it was found that the presence of a cytosine nucleotide at this position is associated with a significantly higher chance of treatment success than the presence of a thymine nucleotide. Another example is the SNP located at position rs8099917, where a guanosine nucleotide present at this position is associated with better response to therapy than a thymine nucleotide [9, 67]. These SNPs are not only associated with a higher chance of success of peginterferon alpha and ribavirin therapy, recent clinical studies regarding triple therapy including PIs have shown that the IL28B genotype is also a predictor of the likelihood of success of the new therapy to HCV genotype 1 infection [9]. Thus far, the underlying mechanisms governing this association are not clear; however, the association is significant, and the AASLD has recommended that IL28B genotype testing may be considered if the HCV genotype 1 patient or his/her provider wish to acquire more information on the likelihood of response to therapy or the probable required duration of therapy [9, 67]. While so far this applies to genotype 1, more research needs to be done to investigate if the association is still valid for HCV infections of other genotypes. A recent study conducted by Asselah et al. [71] provides evidence that the same association between the rs12979860 SNP alleles and response to peginterferon alpha and ribavirin therapy observed in HCV genotype 1 infection is also present in genotype 4 infection [71].

After the initiation of therapy, quantitative molecular HCV assays continue to be performed at certain time intervals for purposes of treatment response monitoring and investigating the possibility of shortening the duration of therapy. A *rapid virological response (RVR)* is defined as the absence of HCV RNA from the patient's blood *4 weeks* after the initiation of therapy measured using a sensitive assay with a limit of detection (LOD) of 50 IU/mL. Achieving RVR predicts a high chance of achieving SVR, and allows limiting of the duration of therapy below the optimum [72]. *Early virological response (EVR)* is defined as a minimum 2 log decline or absence of HCV RNA from the patient's blood at *week 12* of therapy compared to its baseline at the start of treatment measured using a sensitive assay. Failing to achieve EVR is the most accurate predictor of the failure of achieving SVR, and may be an indication for the early stopping of therapy. An *end of treatment response (ETR)* is defined as the absence of HCV RNA from the patient's blood at the end of the course of therapy. It is not an accurate predictor of SVR; however, it must be achieved for SVR to occur. The reappearance of HCV RNA at any stage during the treatment before achieving ETR is called *virological breakthrough*, and its reappearance after ETR is called *virological relapse*. Patients who fail to achieve a minimum 2 log decrease in HCV RNA levels after week 24 of therapy are termed *null responders* [4].

Therapeutic decisions based on viral kinetics during peginterferon alpha and ribavirin therapy vary according to the HCV genotype infecting the patient. For patients infected with genotypes 2 and 3, clinical trials have shown that if RVR was achieved patients can benefit from shortening the treatment period from 24 weeks to 12–16 weeks; where the rate of achieving SVR at the shorter treatment period (62–94 %) is comparable to that at the optimal treatment period (70–95 %). However, patients treated for the shorter period exhibit a higher virological relapse rate (10–30 %) compared to those treated for the optimum duration (3–13 %); a problem that is efficiently solved by re-treatment with a standard 24 week course of therapy, where patients almost always achieve SVR [4, 73–76]. Hence, patients infected with HCV genotypes 2 and 3 and are intolerant to the optimum 24 weeks therapy may benefit from the discontinuation of treatment between weeks 12 and 16 of therapy given they achieve RVR. They should, however, be informed of the higher relapse rate associated with this discontinuation and the consequential requirement for re-treatment to achieve SVR [4]. If the patients infected with genotypes 2 and 3 did not achieve RVR, however, or have HIV coinfection, high viral load, liver cirrhosis, or immunosuppression, they must then be treated for 24 weeks, the optimum duration of therapy.

For patients infected with genotype 1 and 4 taking peginterferon and ribavirin combination therapy, clinical trials have shown that patients achieving RVR can be treated for 24 weeks instead of 48 with success [4]. Two clinical trials involving genotype 1 patients have demonstrated that the rate of achieving SVR among RVR patients treated for 24 weeks in the two trials was 89 %, a rate similar to that achieved by those treated for 48 weeks without achieving RVR [77, 78]. A similar trial for patients infected with genotype 4 demonstrated that the rate of achieving SVR among RVR patients treated for 24 weeks was 86 % [79]. Patients who fail to achieve RVR are tested again at week 12 of treatment for EVR. Two clinical studies have shown that 97–100 % of patients failing to achieve EVR also fail to achieve SVR and are labeled as nonresponders [80, 81]. Accordingly, if a patient fails to achieve a decline of at least 2 logs in viral load levels in response to treatment when tested for EVR, he or she may then discontinue treatment without limiting his/her chances of achieving SVR (according to the AASLD and EASL guidelines) [4, 14]. On the other hand, achieving EVR is not an accurate predictor for achieving SVR; however, achieving "complete" EVR (undetectable HCV RNA) is a better predictor of SVR than a 2 or more log decrease in viral load levels. Patients not achieving a complete EVR (≥2 log decrease of HCV RNA, with HCV RNA still detectable) must be retested at week 24; if HCV RNA is still detectable, then treatment must be stopped. If however HCV RNA was undetectable, an extension of peginterferon alpha and ribavirin therapy to 72 weeks must be considered [4].

As for the new triple therapy for genotype 1, treatment naïve patients taking the PI Boceprevir who are not suffering from cirrhosis may be considered to stop treatment at week 28 of therapy if they achieve undetectable viral levels (<10–15 IU/mL) at week 8 from the initiation of the lead-in therapy (i.e., RVR) and at week 24. Therapy must be stopped if viral load is >100 IU/mL at week 12 or if HCV RNA is detectable at week 24. For those taking Telaprevir and also not suffering from cirrhosis, treatment can be stopped at week 24 of therapy if undetectable viral levels were achieved at weeks 4 and 12. In case the viral load is >1,000 IU/mL at weeks 4 or 12 and/or if HCV RNA is detectable at week 24, therapy must be discontinued [9]. In Fig. 5.3, an algorithm depicting the role of HCV immunoassays and molecular assays in HCV diagnosis and management is presented.

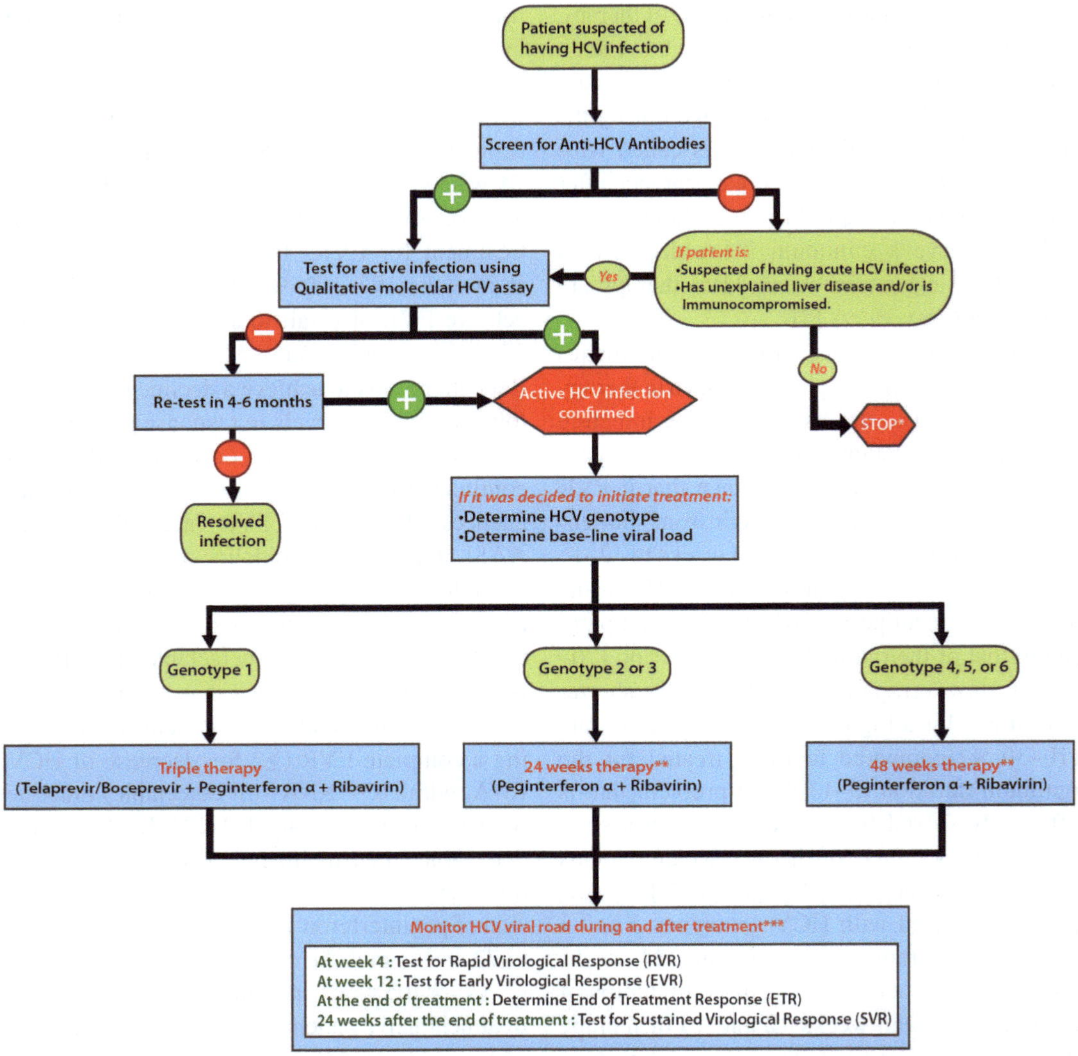

Fig. 5.3 Algorithm depicting the clinical applications of HCV immunoassays and molecular assays in HCV management: Immunoassays are needed for the initial screening of HCV infection. HCV qualitative molecular assays are needed as a supplemental test to anti-HCV antibody immunoassays to confirm the presence of active infection. Once the presence of active infection is confirmed, quantitative and genotyping molecular assays are performed prior to treatment to determine the best treatment route. During therapy, quantitative molecular assays are performed to monitor and adjust therapy. After the cessation of treatment, molecular assays are used to confirm HCV clearance. *In case of high-risk populations, patients may be prompted to repeat the anti-HCV antibody screening test in 1–3 months. **Optimum duration of therapy may be shortened based on the results of HCV viral load monitoring. ***Monitoring intervals during genotype 1 triple therapy are different from the usual intervals of peginterferon alpha and ribavirin combination therapy

How the Tests Have Changed Medical Practice

As evident from the most recent clinical practice guidelines of the AASLD and the EASL, molecular HCV assays are now a key player in HCV diagnosis and management [4, 9, 14]. In disease diagnosis, molecular HCV assays have now completely replaced the need for the recombinant immunoblot assay (RIBA) as a confirmatory test for the results of the EIA assays [4]. They can confirm the presence of active infection; even in immunocompromised patients where anti-HCV antibodies may not appear in the blood. Furthermore, since HCV RNA appears before anti-HCV antibodies in the blood, molecular assays have therefore allowed for the early detection of the virus in the acute phase of the disease, which greatly increases the chances of treatment success [7].

Prior to the treatment of HCV, molecular genotyping assays are necessary to direct the physician in choosing the optimum treatment regimen, and to predict the likelihood of treatment success. Furthermore, these assays have opened the door for the possibility of shortening the duration of therapy based on the patient's response to it, which is beneficial in limiting the exposure to the antiviral drugs leading to reduced drug side effects and cost savings.

Future Directions

HCV Nanodiagnostics

Over the past decade, several molecular nanodiagnostic assay prototypes have been developed. These prototypes are reported to be sensitive and generate results faster and at a fraction of the cost of the current amplification-based molecular assays [7, 82–84]. In this section, examples of such prototypes developed for detection of HCV will be discussed.

Assays Utilizing Gold Nanoparticles

When a bulk material is reduced in size to the nanoscale, it starts to exhibit unique optophysical properties different from those of the bulk material from which it was made, properties that can be easily manipulated by controlling the size, shape, and composition of the nanoscale material. Such unique properties and the ease of their manipulation have allowed the use of nanostructures in many promising biomedical applications, including in vitro molecular diagnostics.

Gold nanoparticles (AuNPs) are associated colloids typically in the size range of 0.8–250 nm and can be composed of pure gold, or of a gold shell surrounding a dielectric core made out of insulator material (e.g., silica). Such AuNPs having the core/shell structure are referred to as *nanoshells*, and have a size range of approximately 10–300 nm. AuNPs can be easily synthesized by the reduction of auric acid (H_3AuO_3) with sodium citrate (*citrate reduction method)*. They can be functionalized with biomolecules such as antibodies and oligonucleotides, an aspect that allows for their efficient use in molecular diagnostics [83, 85].

The popular use of AuNPs in nanodiagnostic assays can be attributed to their optical properties. When light strikes the surface of gold nanoparticles, its oscillating electric field component interacts with the free "conduction band" electrons of the gold atoms on the surface of the AuNPs causing them to oscillate about their atomic nuclei forming oscillating electric dipoles; such oscillations are called *surface plasmon oscillations*. Due to the spatial confinement of the free electrons in the particles, these oscillations will collectively have the same frequency as that of the incident light waves, a phenomenon called *surface Plasmon resonance*. This will result in increased absorption of the incident light, particularly at 520 nm, which is why colloidal AuNP solutions have an intense red color. However, when AuNPs aggregate, they interact by a phenomenon called *plasmon–plasmon interaction* which causes a red shift in their absorption spectrum, causing the color of the colloidal solution to turn to blue. This property of colloidal AuNP solutions has been utilized in several nanodiagnostic prototypes for the detection of nucleic acids [85, 86].

One example of utilizing the plasmon–plasmon interaction phenomenon of AuNPs in HCV RNA detection was developed by our research group, where unmodified AuNPs were used in a colorimetric qualitative assay to directly detect unamplified HCV RNA [87]. The assay depends on the fact that the surface of AuNPs prepared by the citrate reduction method is negatively charged using citrate groups coating it. These negative charges repel the AuNPs and the colloidal solution remains red. In presence of salt, however, the particles aggregate turning the color of the solution blue. This aggregation can be prevented by the addition of single stranded oligonucleotides, as they will adsorb on the surface of the AuNPs

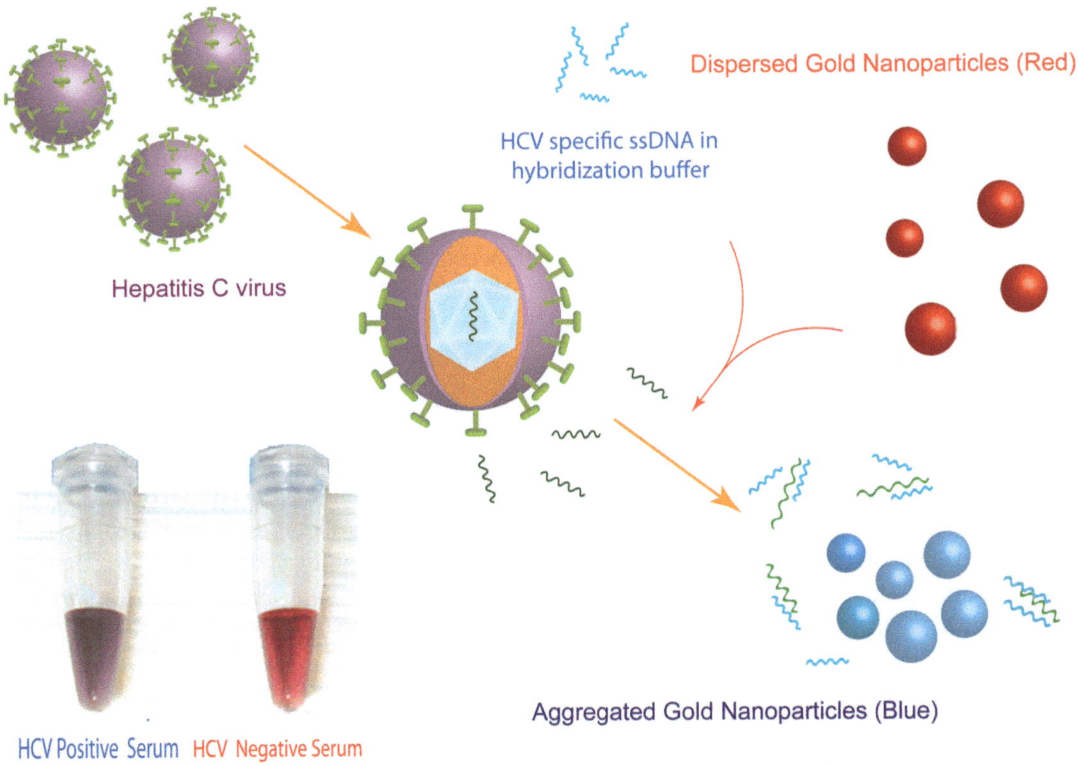

Fig. 5.4 Schematic representation of the HCV molecular nanodiagnostic assay. In the absence of HCV RNA, the single-stranded HCV oligotargeters remain bound to the AuNPs, thus maintaining their stability and the solution color remains *red*. If HCV RNA is present, the oligotargeters will hybridize with their complementary sequence on the HCV RNA leaving the AuNPs to aggregate in the presence of salt, and the color of the solution changes to *blue*

via electrostatic interaction exposing the sugar-phosphate backbone to the surrounding solution; this will maintain the repulsion forces between the AuNPs thus stabilizing them and the red color of the solution. In the developed assay, the role of the single stranded oligonucleotides is played by short oligonucleotide sequences (termed oligotargeters) complementary to a conserved region within the 5′UTR of HCV RNA. If a serum or plasma sample was HCV positive, the oligotargeters would hybridize with their complementary sequence on the HCV RNA, leaving the AuNPs to aggregate in presence of salt thus producing a blue color. On the other hand if the sample was HCV negative, the oligotargeters will remain adsorbed on the AuNPs, maintaining their stability and the red color of the solution. The assay was initially tested on 30 HCV RNA positive samples and 45 negative samples, and the results showed that it had a specificity of 88.9 % and sensitivity of 92 %. A schematic representation of the assay is presented in Fig. 5.4.

Another sensitive and selective assay was developed by Griffin et al. based on the same principle of plasmon–plasmon interactions except that the oligonucleotide sequences had a fluorescent tag that allowed the test to be quantitative [88]. When HCV RNA is absent from the tested sample, the fluorescent-labeled oligonucleotides would adsorb onto the AuNPs leading to the quenching of the fluorophore's fluorescence and the stabilization of AuNPs in the solution which remains red in color. Hence, the absence of HCV RNA is indicated by both the absence of fluorescence and the red color of the solution. On the other hand if HCV RNA was present in the sample, it will hybridize with the fluorescent tagged oligonucleotides sequestering them from the AuNPs, which will result in the restoration of the fluorophores' fluorescence and the aggregation of the AuNPs turning the solution to blue. The intensity of the emitted fluorescence is proportional to the amount of HCV RNA in the sample. The quenching of the fluorescence of the fluorophore tags occurs due to a phenomenon called *nanoparticle surface energy transfer (NSET)*, the efficiency of which depends on both the size of the AuNPs and the distance between the fluorophore and the nanoparticles.

Assays Utilizing Quantum Dots

Another kind of nanoparticles that can be used for in vitro molecular nanodiagnostics is quantum dots (QDs). QDs are fluorescent nanocrystals (2–10 nm) made of semiconductor material. They have a core/shell structure, where the material that forms the shell has a larger energy gap between its valence and conduction bands (i.e., band gap) than that of the core. The core material is usually made from elements of groups II and IV (e.g., CdSe) or III and V (e.g., InP), while an example of the higher band-gap material, the shell is made out of ZnS. The absorption and emission spectra of QDs, hence the color of their fluorescence, are a function of their size and composition, aspects which are both tunable. Like AuNPs, their surface can be easily functionalized with biomolecules [89].

QDs have unique optical properties that give them an advantage over commonly used fluorophores in several biological applications. First, they have wide absorption (excitation) spectra, which allows for the simultaneous excitation of QDs of different sizes using electromagnetic radiation of a single wavelength. Second, they have narrow, symmetrical emission spectra, which allow for their efficient use in multiplex simultaneous detection of cellular events or disease biomarkers. Finally, they have a long fluorescence lifetime, where they can emit light with a decay time of approximately 30–100 ns [90].

One example of an assay prototype utilizing QDs was developed by Gerion et al., where QD-conjugated DNA probes were used for the simultaneous detection of HCV and hepatitis B virus (HBV) on a microarray chip [7]. The assay involved first the hybridization of the HCV RNA or HBV DNA to immobilized capture probes on the microarray chip, followed by the addition of the QD-conjugated DNA probes, which would hybridize specifically to HCV RNA and/or HBV DNA. The assay can be used to detect single nucleotide polymorphisms with a true-to-false signal ratio higher than 10.

Summary

Hepatitis C virus molecular assays will have an increasing role in the management of HCV patients. More molecular assays may be developed for detection of viral and host factors that affect patient response to therapy. Inexpensive and sensitive nanoparticle-based assays that can directly detect unamplified HCV RNA may revolutionize HCV diagnosis. Proper management of treatment of HCV infected patients will require rapid detection of resistance against the medications used in order to adjust the treatment strategies. More studies are needed to develop and standardize the testing criteria for diagnosing acute HCV infections. This is important because the rate of response to therapy in the case of acute infection is significantly higher than that of chronic infection. Multianalyte microfluidic chips and other point-of-care devices will be developed for detection of blood-borne pathogen including HCV that will be mainly used by blood banks.

Acknowledgments Thanks to Mr. Tamer Samir and Ms. Lana Abdel-Hady for their help with the art work.

References

1. World Health Organization. Hepatitis. 2011. http://www.who.int/csr/disease/hepatitis/en/. Accessed 21 Aug 2011.
2. World Health Organization. Hepatitis C fact sheet N°164. 2011. http://www.who.int/mediacentre/factsheets/fs164/en/. Accessed 21 Aug 2011.
3. Centers for Disease Control and Prevention. Hepatitis C information for health professionals. 2011. http://www.cdc.gov/hepatitis/HCV/index.htm. Accessed 21 Aug 2011.

4. Ghany MG, Strader DB, Thomas DL, Seeff LB, American Association for the Study of Liver Diseases. Diagnosis, management, and treatment of hepatitis C: an update. Hepatology. 2009;49:1335–74.
5. Sharma SD. Hepatitis C, virus: molecular biology and current therapeutic options. Indian J Med Res. 2010;131:17–34.
6. Simmonds P, Bukh J, Combet C, et al. Consensus proposals for a unified system of nomenclature of hepatitis C virus genotypes. Hepatology. 2005;42:962–73.
7. Al Olaby RR, Azzazy HME. Hepatitis C virus RNA assasys: current and emerging technologies and their clinical applications. Expert Rev Mol Diagn. 2011;11:53–64.
8. Zeuzem S, Berg T, Moeller B, et al. Expert opinion on the treatment of patients with chronic hepatitis C. J Viral Hepat. 2009;16:75–90.
9. Ghany MG, Nelson DR, Strader DB, Thomas DL, Seeff LB, American Association for Study of Liver Diseases. An update on treatment of genotype 1 chronic hepatitis C virus infection: 2011 practice guideline by the American Association for Study of Liver Diseases. Hepatology. 2011;54:1433–44.
10. Scott JD, Gretch DR. Molecular diagnostics of hepatitis C virus infection: a systematic review. JAMA. 2007;297:724–32.
11. Alter MJ, Kuhnert WL, Finelli L, Centers for Disease Control and Prevention. Guidelines for laboratory testing and result reporting of antibody to hepatitis C virus. Centers for Disease Control and Prevention. MMWR Recomm Rep. 2003;52:1–16.
12. Chevaliez S, Pawlotsky JM. Hepatitis C virus serologic and virologic test and clinical diagnosis of HCV-related liver disease. Int J Med Sci. 2006;3:35–40.
13. Richter SS. Laboratory assays for diagnosis and management of hepatitis C virus infection. J Clin Microbiol. 2002;40:4407–12.
14. European Association for the Study of the Liver. EASL clinical practice guidelines: management of hepatitis C virus infection. J Hepatol. 2011;55:245–64.
15. National Institutes of Health Consensus Development Conference Panel. Management of hepatitis C. Hepatology. 1997;26:2S–10.
16. Mayo Medical Laboratories. Alternative approaches to the diagnosis of hepatitis C. http://www.mayomedicallaboratories.com/media/articles/algorithms/hcv-alt.pdf. Accessed 26 Mar 2011.
17. Esmat G, El Raziky M, El Kassas M, Hassany M, Gamil ME. The future for the treatment of genotype 4 chronic hepatitis C. Liver Int. 2012;32 Suppl 1:146–50.
18. Mayo Clinic. Hepatitis C treatments and drugs. 2011. http://www.mayoclinic.com/health/hepatitis-c/DS00097/DSECTION=treatments-and-drugs. Accessed 10 Sept 2011.
19. Hadziyannis SJ, Sette Jr H, Morgan TR, et al. Peginterferon-alpha2a and ribavirin combination therapy in chronic hepatitis C: a randomized study of treatment duration and ribavirin dose. Ann Intern Med. 2004;140:346–55.
20. Pawlotsky JM, Bouvier-Alias M, Hezode C, Darthuy F, Remire J, Dhumeaux D. Standardization of hepatitis C virus RNA quantification. Hepatology. 2000;32:654–9.
21. Hitzler WE, Runkel S. Routine HCV PCR screening of blood donations to identify early HCV infection in blood donors lacking antibodies to HCV. Transfusion. 2001;41:333–7.
22. Zou S, Dorsey KA, Notari EP, et al. Prevalence, incidence, and residual risk of human immunodeficiency virus and hepatitis C virus infections among United States blood donors since the introduction of nucleic acid testing. Transfusion. 2010;50:1495–504.
23. Le Guillou-Guillemette H, Lunel-Fabiani F. Detection and quantification of serum or plasma HCV RNA: mini review of commercially available assays. Methods Mol Biol. 2009;510:3–14.
24. Bukh J, Purcell RH, Miller RH. Importance of primer selection for the detection of hepatitis C virus RNA with the polymerase chain reaction assay. Proc Natl Acad Sci. 1992;89:187–91.
25. Bustin SA. Absolute quantification of mRNA using real-time reverse transcription polymerase chain reaction assays. J Mol Endocrinol. 2000;25:169–93.
26. Sarrazin C, Dragan A, Gartner BC, et al. Evaluation of an automated, highly sensitive, real-time PCR-based assay (COBAS Ampliprep™/COBAS TaqMan™) for quantification of HCV RNA. J Clin Virol. 2008;43:162–8.
27. Michelin BDA, Muller Z, Stelzl E, Marth E, Kessler HH. Evaluation of the Abbott RealTi*me* HCV assay for quantitative detection of hepatitis C virus RNA. J Clin Virol. 2007;38:96–100.
28. Paba P, Fabeni L, Perno CF, Ciotti M. Performance evaluation of the Artus hepatitis C virus QS-RGQ assay. J Virol Methods. 2012;179:77–80.
29. Chevaliez S, Bouvier-Alias M, Brillet R, Pawlotsky JM. Overestimation and underestimation of hepatitis C virus RNA levels in a widely used real-time polymerase chain reaction–based method. Hepatology. 2007;46:22–31.
30. Food and Drug Administration. Class 2 Recall COBAS® AmpliPrep/COBAS® TaqMan® HCV Test, CE-IVD. 2011. http://www.accessdata.fda.gov/scripts/cdrh/cfdocs/cfRes/res.cfm?ID=100296. Accessed 07 Sept 2011.
31. Chevaliez S, Bouvier-Alias M, Pawlotsky JM. Performance of the Abbott real-time PCR assay using m2000sp and m2000rt for hepatitis C virus RNA quantification. J Clin Microbiol. 2009;47:1726–32.
32. Sarrazin C. Highly sensitive hepatitis C virus RNA detection methods: molecular backgrounds and clinical significance. J Clin Virol. 2002;25:S23–9.
33. Dhingra K, Talpaz M, Riggs MG, et al. Hybridization protection assay: a rapid, sensitive, and specific method for detection of Philadelphia chromosome-positive leukemias. Blood. 1991;77:238–42.
34. Hendricks DA, Friesenhahn M, Tanimoto L, Goergen B, Dodge D, Comanor L. Multicenter evaluation of the VERSANT HCV RNA qualitative assay for detection

of hepatitis C virus RNA. J Clin Microbiol. 2003;41: 651–6.
35. McCormick MK, Dockter J, Linnen JM, Kolk D, Wu Y, Giachetti C. Evaluation of a new molecular assay for detection of human immunodeficiency virus type 1 RNA, hepatitis C virus RNA, and hepatitis B virus DNA. J Clin Virol. 2006;36:166–76.
36. Gorrin G, Friesenhahn M, Lin P, et al. Performance evaluation of the VERSANT HCV RNA qualitative assay by using transcription-mediated amplification. J Clin Microbiol. 2003;41:310–7.
37. Koppelman MH, Assal A, Chudy M, et al. Multicenter performance evaluation of a transcription-mediated amplification assay for screening of human immunodeficiency virus-1 RNA, hepatitis C virus RNA, and hepatitis B virus DNA in blood donations. Transfusion. 2005;45:1258–66.
38. Elbeik T, Surtihadi J, Destree M, et al. Multicenter evaluation of the performance characteristics of the Bayer VERSANT HCV RNA 3.0 Assay (bDNA). J Clin Microbiol. 2004;42:563–9.
39. Kuiken C, Yusim K, Boykin L, Richardson R. The Los Alamos HCV sequence database. Bioinformatics. 2005;21:379–84.
40. Murphy D, Willems B, Delage G. Use of the 5′ noncoding region for genotyping hepatitis C virus. J Infect Dis. 1994;169:473–5.
41. Verma V, Chakravarti A. Comparison of 50 noncoding-core with 50 noncoding regions of HCV by RT-PCR: importance and clinical implications. Curr Microbiol. 2008;57:206–11.
42. Shindo M, Di Bisceglie AM, Cheung L, et al. Decrease in serum hepatitis C viral RNA during alpha-interferon therapy for chronic hepatitis C. Ann Intern Med. 1991;115:700–4.
43. Roth WK, Lee JH, Rüster B, Zeuzem S. Comparison of two quantitative hepatitis C virus reverse transcriptase PCR assays. J Clin Microbiol. 1996;34:261–4.
44. World Health Organization. Hepatitis C. 2002. http://www.who.int/csr/disease/hepatitis/whocdscsrlyo2003/en/index2.html. Accessed 23 Jan 2012.
45. Attaullah S, Khan S, Ali I. Hepatitis C virus genotypes in Pakistan: a systemic review. Virol J. 2011; 8:433.
46. Khattab MA, Ferenci P, Hadziyannis SJ, et al. Management of hepatitis C virus genotype 4: recommendations of an international expert panel. J Hepatol. 2011;54:1250–62.
47. Chao DT, Abe K, Nguyen MH. Systematic review: epidemiology of hepatitis C genotype 6 and its management. Aliment Pharmacol Ther. 2011;34:286–96.
48. Podzorski RP. Molecular testing in the diagnosis and management of hepatitis C virus infection. Arch Pathol Lab Med. 2002;126:285–90.
49. Halfon P, Trimoulet P, Bourliere M, et al. Hepatitis C viral genotyping based on 5′ noncoding sequence analysis (Truegene). J Clin Microbiol. 2001;39:1771–3.
50. Ruano G, Kidd KK. Coupled amplification and sequencing of genomic DNA. Proc Natl Acad Sci USA. 1991;88(7):2815–9.
51. Ross RS, Viazov SO, Holtzer CD, et al. Genotyping of hepatitis C virus isolates using CLIP sequencing. J Clin Microbiol. 2000;38(10):3581–4.
52. Verbeeck J, Stanley MJ, Shieh J, et al. Evaluation of Versant hepatitis C virus genotype assay (LiPA) 2.0. J Clin Microbiol. 2008;46(6):1901–6.
53. Thiers V, Jaffredo F, Tuveri R, Chodan N, Brechot C. Development of a simple restriction fragment length polymorphism (RFLP) based assay for HCV genotyping and comparative analysis with genotyping and serotyping tests. J Virol Methods. 1997;65:9–17.
54. Yukimasa N, Yoshida K, Ohkushi H, et al. Hepatitis C virus genotyping by restriction fragment length polymorphism of polymerase chain reaction products generated with a HCV detection kit. Rinsho Byori. 2001;49:711–5.
55. Lindh M, Hannoun C. Genotyping of hepatitis C virus by Taqman real time PCR. J Clin Virol. 2005;34: 108–14.
56. Rolfe KJ, Alexander GJM, Wreghitt TG, Parmar S, Jalal H, Curran MD. A real-time Taqman method for hepatitis C virus genotyping. J Clin Virol. 2005;34: 115–21.
57. Bullock JC, Burns DE, Haverstick DM. Hepatitis C genotype determination by melting curve analysis with a single set of fluorescence energy transfer probes. Clin Chem. 2002;48:2147–54.
58. Schroter M, Zollner B, Schafer P, et al. Genotyping of hepatitis C virus types 1, 2, 3, and 4 by a one-step LightCycler method using three different pairs of hybridization probes. J Clin Microbiol. 2002;40:2046–50.
59. Fujigaki H, Takemura M, Takahashi K, et al. Genotyping of hepatitis C virus by melting curve analysis with SYBR Green I. Ann Clin Biochem. 2004;41:130–2.
60. Ciotti M, Marcuccilli F, Guenci T. A multicenter evaluation of the Abbott RealTime HCV Genotype II assay. J Virol Methods. 2010;167:205–7.
61. Sohn YH, Ko SY, Kim MH, Oh HB. Performance evaluation of the Abbott RealTi*me* HCV Genotype II for hepatitis C virus genotyping. Clin Chem Lab Med. 2010;48:469–74.
62. Hu YW, Balaskas E, Kessler G, et al. Primer specific and mispair extension analysis (PSMEA) as a simple approach to fast genotyping. Nucleic Acids Res. 1998;26:5013–5.
63. Saldanha J, Lelie N, Heath A. The WHO Collaborative Study Group. Establishment of the first international standard for nucleic acid amplification technology (NAT) assays for HCV RNA. Vox Sang. 1999;76:149–58.
64. Saldanha J, Heath A, Aberham C, et al. World Health Organization collaborative study to establish a replacement WHO international standard for hepatitis C virus RNA nucleic acid amplification technology assays. Vox Sang. 2005;88:202–4.
65. Highleyman L, Franciscus A. HCV diagnostic tools: HCV viral load tests. HCV Advocate. 2011. http://www.hcvadvocate.org/hepatitis/factsheets.asp. Accessed 6 Sept 2011.

66. McGovern BH, Birch CE, Bowen MJ, et al. Improving the diagnosis of acute hepatitis C virus infection with expanded viral load criteria. Clin Infect Dis. 2009;49:1051–60.
67. Ahlenstiel G, Booth DR, George J. IL28B in hepatitis C virus infection: translating pharmacogenomics into clinical practice. J Gastroenterol. 2010;45:903–10.
68. Ge D, Fellay J, Thompson AJ, et al. Genetic variation in IL28B predicts hepatitis C treatment-induced viral clearance. Nature. 2009;461:399–401.
69. Suppiah V, Moldovan M, Ahlenstiel G, et al. IL28B is associated with response to chronic hepatitis C interferon-alpha and ribavirin therapy. Nat Genet. 2009;41:1100–4.
70. Tanaka Y, Nishida N, Sugiyama M, et al. Genome-wide association of IL28B with response to pegylated interferon-alpha and ribavirin therapy for chronic hepatitis C. Nat Genet. 2009;41:1105–9.
71. Asselah T, De Muynck S, Broët P, et al. IL28B polymorphism is associated with treatment response in patients with genotype 4 chronic hepatitis C. J Hepatol. 2012;56(3):527–32.
72. Poordad F, Reddy KR, Martin P. Rapid virological response: a new milestone in the management of chronic hepatitis C. Clin Infect Dis. 2008;46:78–84.
73. Dalgard O, Bjoro K, Hellum KB, et al. Treatment with pegylated interferon and ribavarin in HCV infection with genotype 2 or 3 for 14 weeks: a pilot study. Hepatology. 2004;40:1260–5.
74. Mangia A, Santoro R, Minerva N, et al. Peginterferon alfa-2b and ribavirin for 12 vs. 24 weeks in HCV genotype 2 or 3. N Engl J Med. 2005;352:2609–17.
75. von Wagner M, Huber M, Berg T, et al. Peginterferon-alpha-2a (40KD) and ribavirin for 16 or 24 weeks in patients with genotype 2 or 3 chronic hepatitis C. Gastroenterology. 2005;129:522–7.
76. Yu ML, Dai CY, Huang JF, Hou NJ, Lee LP, Hsieh MY, et al. A randomized study of peginterferon and ribavirin for 16 versus 24 weeks in patients with genotype 2 chronic hepatitis C. Gut. 2007;56:553–9.
77. Jensen DM, Morgan TR, Marcellin P, et al. Early identification of HCV genotype 1 patients responding to 24 weeks peginterferon alpha-2a (40 kd)/ribavirin therapy. Hepatology. 2006;43:954–60.
78. Zeuzem S, Buti M, Ferenci P, et al. Efficacy of 24 weeks treatment with peginterferon alfa-2b plus ribavirin in patients with chronic hepatitis C infected with genotype 1 and low pretreatment viremia. J Hepatol. 2006;44:97–103.
79. Kamal SM, El Kamary SS, Shardell MD, et al. Pegylated interferon alpha-2b plus ribavirin in patients with genotype 4 chronic hepatitis C: the role of rapid and early virologic response. Hepatology. 2007;46:1732–40.
80. Fried MW, Shiffman ML, Reddy KR, et al. Peginterferon alfa-2a plus ribavirin for chronic hepatitis C virus infection. N Engl J Med. 2002;347:975–82.
81. Davis GL, Wong JB, McHutchison JG, Manns MP, Harvey J, Albrecht J. Early virologic response to treatment with peginterferon alfa-2b plus ribavirin in patients with chronic hepatitis C. Hepatology. 2003;38:645–52.
82. Azzazy HM, Mansour MM, Kazmierczak SC. Nanodiagnostics: a new frontier for clinical laboratory medicine. Clin Chem. 2006;52:1238–46.
83. Azzazy HM, Mansour MM. In vitro diagnostic prospects of nanoparticles. Clin Chim Acta. 2009;403:1–8.
84. Jain KK. Applications of nanobiotechnology in clinical diagnostics. Clin Chem. 2007;53:2002–9.
85. Radwan SH, Azzazy HM. Gold nanoparticles for molecular diagnostics. Expert Rev Mol Diagn. 2009;9:511–24.
86. Mansfield L. Nano-optics. In: Hornyak GL, Moore JJ, Tibbals HF, Dutta J, editors. Fundamentals of nanotechnology. Boca Raton, FL: CRC; 2009. p. 166–202.
87. Shawky SM, Bald D, Azzazy HM. Direct detection of unamplified hepatitis C virus RNA using unmodified gold nanoparticles. Clin Biochem. 2010;43:1163–8.
88. Griffin J, Singh AK, Senapati D, et al. Size- and distance-dependent nanoparticle surface-energy transfer (NSET) method for selective sensing of hepatitis C virus RNA. Chemistry. 2009;15:342–51.
89. Azzazy HM, Mansour MM, Kazmierczak SC. From diagnostics to therapy: prospects of quantum dots. Clin Biochem. 2007;40:917–27.
90. Jamieson T, Bakhshi R, Petrova D, Pocock R, Imani M, Seifalian AM. Biological applications of quantum dots. Biomaterials. 2007;28:4717–32.

Laboratory Testing for HIV Infection: Advances After 28 Years

6

Joseph Ntumbong Nkeze, Niel T. Constantine, and Richard Y. Zhao

Testing for HIV

Background

Following the identification of the human immunodeficiency virus (HIV) in the USA in 1984, the first test for HIV was licensed by the Food and Drug Administration (FDA) in 1985. This was an enzyme immunoassay (EIA) and was used mainly to ensure the safety of blood supply. People were deterred from using the blood bank just for learning about their HIV status and opinions were divided about the implication of a positive test result [1]. Counseling did not exist until 1987 when the United State Public Health Service (USPHS) issued guidelines making HIV testing and counseling a preventive strategy for those at high risk of infection. USPHS also recommended testing for those who were seeking treatment for other sexually transmitted diseases (STD) [2]. The first Western blot (WB) blood test kit was also licensed in 1987 and the first rapid test that provides results in as short as 10 min was licensed in 1992.

The recommendations for HIV testing were extended in 1993 to include in- and outpatients in hospitals, especially those in acute-care settings and emergency departments. Hospitals with HIV prevalence rates or an AIDS diagnostic rate of >1 % were encouraged to adopt voluntary counseling and testing for all patients aged 15–54 years [3]. In 1994, these guidelines for counseling and testing those at high risk stated specific prevention goals and strategies for each person (client-centered counseling) [4]. The first oral fluid test system was also licensed in 1994 and the test was subsequently granted a Clinical Laboratory Improvement Amendments (CLIA) waiver in 2004. In 1995, Zidovudine (AZT) was administered to HIV infected pregnant women and resulted in a significant reduction of vertical transmission. The USPHS then recommended that all pregnant women be counseled and encouraged to undergo voluntary testing for HIV [4, 5]. In 1996, the first HIV viral load (VL) test was approved and the first home and urine collection kits for HIV testing were introduced. In 2001, the USPHS recommendations were modified and are now part of routine prenatal care; the high

J.N. Nkeze, M.S.
Department of Pathology, University of Maryland School of Medicine, Baltimore, MD 21201, USA

N.T. Constantine, Ph.D., M.T. (A.S.C.P.)
Department of Pathology, University of Maryland School of Medicine, Baltimore, MD 21201, USA

Institute of Human Virology, University of Maryland School of Medicine, Baltimore, MD 21201, USA

R.Y. Zhao, Ph.D. (✉)
Department of Pathology, University of Maryland School of Medicine, Baltimore, MD 21201, USA

Department of Microbiology and Immunology, University of Maryland School of Medicine, Baltimore, MD 21201, USA
e-mail: rzhao@som.umaryland.edu

W.E. Highsmith Jr. (ed.), *Molecular Diagnostics: 12 Tests That Changed Everything*, Molecular and Translational Medicine, DOI 10.1007/978-1-4614-8127-0_6,

prevalence healthcare testing recommendations were extended to include clinical venues in both private and public sectors. HIV testing was targeted toward, and was the basis for, those in high risk settings [6, 7]. The OralQuick Advance Rapid HIV-1/2 Antibody Test that uses fingerstick blood or oral fluid was approved in 2002 and was granted a CLIA waiver in 2003 [8]. Knowledge gained from understanding the immunopathogenetic mechanisms of HIV infection, and the virus/host interaction in the past 30 years have been fundamental in the development and continuous improvement of diagnostic tests, which are able to detect either HIV-specific antibodies, antigens, or nucleic acids [9].

In 2003, the Centers for Disease Control and Prevention (CDC) introduced the initiative to advance HIV Prevention: *New Strategies for a Changing Epidemic*. The goal was to make HIV testing a routine part of medical care and also to further reduce prenatal transmission of HIV by the universal testing of all pregnant women and by using rapid tests during labor and delivery or postpartum if the mother's HIV status was unknown [10]. In March 2004, as result of a meeting with health consultants, a recommendation was made by the CDC to simplify the HIV screening process in order to make it more efficient, cost efficient, and to urge frequent diagnostic testing for patients with associated symptoms. A final recommendation on HIV testing in the healthcare setting was published in 2006 [11]. This recommendation came from a series of meetings with healthcare providers, HIV-infected individuals, and researchers. It recommended routine HIV screening for all adults, aged 13–64, and repeated screening at least annually for those at high risk. Screening should also be voluntary [11, 12]. The National Health Interview Survey recently reported that the number of people who said they have ever been tested for HIV since 2006 increased by 11.4 million, indicating an increasing adoption of this recommendation [13]. Finally, in the last few years, efforts have been extended to identify the large percentage of infected persons who do not know that they are HIV infected by offering testing to all persons admitted to emergency rooms.

Kinetics of HIV Virological and Serological Markers

Several HIV infection diagnostic markers from both the virus and the host appear at different times during the course of an infection. The kinetics and times of appearances are fairly consistent among different individuals and this must be taken into consideration when choosing an assay [9].

Early immunological and virological blood markers appear in the following order following infection: HIV RNA, HIV p24 antigen, and antibodies to HIV antigens [14]. Figure 6.1 shows the appearance of virological and serological markers following HIV-1 infection.

The viral RNA (viremia) is measurable in plasma as early as 8–12 days after infection and the number of viral copies in plasma increases exponentially to about one million copies of RNA/ml within a couple of months. Humoral and cell-mediated immune responses are then produced, are able to control HIV replication, and thus drastically reduce RNA copies to a constant lower level (set-point); at the same time, p24 antigen levels usually become undetectable because of complexing with antibody to HIV. In later stages of the infection, the RNA levels gradually increases over time reaching again high levels at the time of onset of AIDS-related symptoms [9]. The p24 antigen can be measured in blood a little later than viral RNA, usually as early as—17 days from infection. This is because the methods used for its detection are less sensitive than the nucleic acid-based amplification methods, which are used to detect viral RNA [15, 16]. Its concentration, however, remains high and the marker is detectable in blood for about a month and a half following its appearance [15]. The period before HIV-specific antibodies can be detected is known as the serological "window period." It is characterized by the absence of HIV-specific antibodies, detectable viremia (measurable RNA or p24 antigen), and variable CD4 lymphocyte levels. The detection of specific antibody to HIV signals the end of the window period and labels the individual as "seropositive" [9, 17]. The first HIV-specific antibodies to appear are IgM, usually within the first 3 weeks and peak between the 4th and 5th week (Fig. 6.1). The detection is,

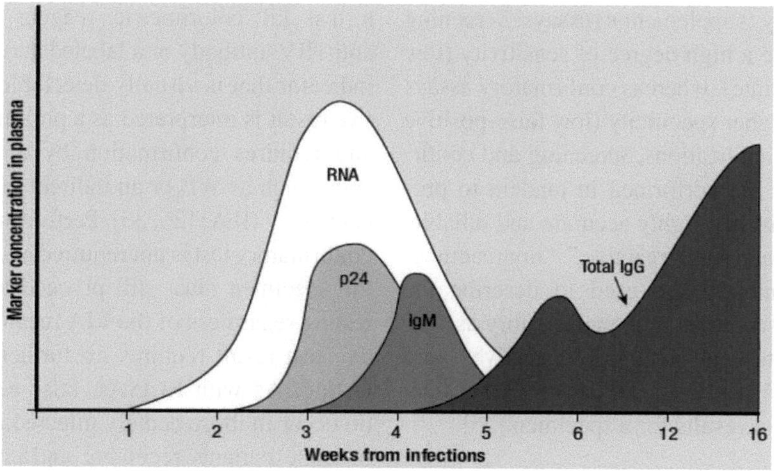

Fig. 6.1 Appearance of HIV-1 virological and serological markers during the first several weeks of infection. Note: total IgG antibody can be detected at about 3 weeks using third generation tests. Data from Butto et al. [9], the figure was adapted from a graphic courtesy of Federica Napolitani

however, strongly dependent on each individual's response [18, 19] and the specific test used. HIV-specific IgG antibodies usually appear at about 3–4 weeks after infection [15]. Anti-gp41 IgG antibodies have been detected as early as 13 days after infection using very sensitive noncommercial assays [20]. Anti-HIV IgG titers increase soon after their appearance, plateau at high levels between 3 and 6 months, and subsequently decrease as the immune system becomes less competent (e.g., when viral replication and p24 antigens increase at the time of AIDS). Some antibodies such as the IgG3 isotype directed against the p24 antigen [21, 22] may decrease after 10–12 weeks, giving this marker some utility as a means to predict "recent infection." Within 1–2 months after infection in most individuals, all HIV-specific antibodies are detectable regardless of the assay used [23]. Viremia usually decreases as the HIV antibodies appear. This is due to both a reduction in p24 and the formation of p24/anti-p24 antibody complexes. At the AIDS stage of the disease when the immune system is severely compromised, virus replication increases again to very high levels. Specific methods and approaches have been developed to detect infection both soon after infection, and long thereafter. These methods are discussed in detail below.

Serologic Testing: Methodology and Standard Reagents

Antibody-Based Diagnostic Tests

Detection of antibodies produced in response to HIV infection is the basis of most HIV screening tests. Such antibodies are nearly always detectable within 1–3 months following infection (depending on which test is selected) [7]. Various tests exist and they differ by testing principle, format, the type of specimen tested, test complexity, and how quickly the results are available. For example, whole blood, serum, plasma, oral fluid, finger-stick blood, urine, or immunoglobulin eluted from dried blood spots could all be the test matrix; the level of test complexity will determine where the test can be carried out, e.g., laboratory, point-of-care (POC) site, or home sample collection, and finally how quickly the results are available divide the tests into the conventional or rapid category [24]. Antibody detection tests are easy to perform and possess relatively high sensitivity and specificity. They are the choice of test technologies for the initial screening of people who are at high risk for HIV infection. These tests, however, are unable to detect acute infection; that is, during the window period before antibody is produced in an infected person. Antibody tests are generally classified as screening (initial tests) or confirmatory (supplemental) assays. Screening tests must have a high degree of sensitivity (low false-negative rate), whereas confirmatory assays must have a higher specificity (low false-positive rate). In most applications, screening and confirmatory assays are performed in tandem to produce results that are highly accurate and reliable. In general, the terms "reactive," "nonreactive," and "indeterminate" are used to describe the results of the screening and confirmatory assays, whereas the terms "positive," "negative," and "inconclusive" are used to describe the final interpretation of results for a specimen [25].

Blood-Based Rapid HIV Antibody Tests

Rapid HIV antibody tests have been widely used for years and most of them demonstrate sensitivities and specificities comparable to EIAs [12, 26–29]. They play an important role in HIV testing and access to testing in both clinical and nonclinical settings by overcoming some of the barriers of early diagnosis, thus improving linkage to care for those infected [30]. They are very useful in clinical settings such as public clinics, physicians offices, pregnancy clinics, and emergency rooms where rapid turnaround time for results is important. They are also most effective in cases of occupational exposure to provide results on the source patient so that the injured person can be treated in a clinically relevant time frame (usually within 2 h) [31]. Similarly, they are essential for detecting infection in a woman in labor whose HIV status is unknown; positive results would dictate the immediate institution of antiretroviral therapy to substantially reduce the risk of transmission to the newborn. Most assays are in a ready-to-use kit format that include all necessary reagents and require no specialized equipment [12]. Rapid HIV tests, similar to enzyme-linked immunosorbent assays (ELISAs), are screening tests and thus, the test results require confirmation if a reactive result is produced [30]. Currently FDA-approved rapid tests are listed in Table 6.1.

All rapid tests are interpreted visually, although some companies offer readers (e.g., Chembio, Medmira). HIV antigens fixed to the test membrane or contained in the test will bind to HIV antibodies if present in the specimen, and a test kit colorimetric reagent binds to the anti-HIV antibody or a labeled antigen creates an indicator that is visually detectable [30]. A reactive result is interpreted as a preliminary positive and requires confirmation by a more specific assay such as WB or an indirect immunofluorescent assay (IFA) [26, 33]. Performing an EIA as a confirmatory test is not required and if performed, the specimen must still proceed to WB or IFA testing regardless of the EIA result [34]. A negative test result requires no further confirmatory testing. As with ELISAs, false-negative results do occur in those acutely infected and also occur in some patients receiving antiretroviral (ARV) therapy with undetectable virus in whom antibody levels have waned below the sensitivity range of the test [6, 35].

The three most common formats of assays that can be used for whole blood tests are particle agglutination, immunoconcentration, and immunochromatography [12, 36]. Particle agglutination tests (not FDA licensed) require 10–60 min after the specimen containing antibodies is mixed with latex particles coated with HIV antigen; cross-linkage occurs and agglutination occurs. Immunoconcentration (flow through) devices use a solid-phase capture technology which involves immobilization of HIV antigens on a porous membrane. The specimen flows through the membrane and is absorbed into an absorbent pad. A dot or line visibly forms on the membrane after addition of a conjugate or color-producing reagent. This assay format usually requires several steps for the addition of specimen, wash buffers, conjugate (e.g., enzyme and substrate), or signal generating reagent (e.g., colloidal gold). They are performed in 5–15 min. Immunochromatographic (lateral flow) tests are the most recent development and incorporate both the antigen and signal reagent into the device. The specimen, followed by a buffer is applied to an absorbent pad where it binds to a conjugate (e.g., labeled antigen), and the complex migrates along a nitrocellulose strip and is captured by an immobilized antigen. A positive reaction results in a visual line on the membrane where the immobilized HIV antigen was applied. A procedural control line is usually applied to the

Table 6.1 FDA-approved rapid HIV immunoassays antibody screening tests [30–32]

Rapid HIV test	Specimen type	Sensitivity[a]	Specificity[a]	Time to result (min)	Window period for reading results	CLIA category
OraQuick ADVANCER Rapid HIV-1/2 Antibody Test http://www.orasure.com	Oral fluid Fingerstick and wholeblood Plasma	99.3 % 99.6 % 99.6 %	99.8 % 100 % 99.9 %	20–40 <10	20–40 min	Waived Moderate complexity
Uni-Gold Recombigen HIV http://www.unigoldhiv.com	Whole blood, fingerstick Serum and plasma	100 % 100 %	99.7 % 99.8 %	10–205	10–12 min	Waived
Reveal G-3 Rapid HIV-1 Antibody Test http://www.reveal-hiv.com	Serum Plasma	99.8 % 99.8 %	99.1 % 98.6 %	3–5	Immediately	Moderate complexity
MultiSpotHIV-1/HIV-2 Rapid Test http://www.biorad.com	Serum Plasma	100 % 100 %	99.9 % 99.9 %	10–15	Immediately or any time up to 24 h	Moderate complexity
Clearview HIV 1/2STAT-PAK http://www.invernessmedicalpd.com	Whole blood, fingerstick Serum and plasma	99.7 % 99.7 %	99.9 %% 99.9 %	5–20	15–20 min	Waived
Clearview COMPLETE HIV ½ http://www.invernessmedicalpd.com	Whole blood, fingerstick Serum and plasma	99.7 % 99.7 %	99.9 % 99.9 %	15–20	15–20 min	Waived
INSTI HIV-1 Antibody Test Kit http://www.biolytical.com	Whole blood, fingerstick, plasma	99.9 % 99.8 % 99.9 %	100 % 99.9 % 100 %	1	Immediately or anytime <5 min	Moderate complexity
DPP HIV 1/2 Assay http://www.chembio.com	Oral fluid Fingerstick Serum, plasma, and wholeblood	98.9 % 99.8 % 99.9 %	99.9 % 100 % 99.9 %	25 10 10	20–40 mins 10–25 mins 10–25 mins	Moderate complexity

[a]As determined during clinical trials

strip beyond the HIV-antigen line and acts as a means to show that the test procedure is accurate; in some manufacturer's devices, it indicates that a specimen has been added [37].

Rapid HIV assays could present some problems of sensitivity. Performance characteristics may be jeopardized when these tests are used in a venue different from a laboratory. For example, in a recent study performed on pregnant women in South Africa, three routinely used rapid HIV tests which performed well under laboratory conditions did not show the same performance when used in a clinical setting, giving a sensitivity of as low as 90.2 % [38]. Also, since the negative predictive value of these tests is low when compared to EIA, special precautions must be taken when using these tests in a population with high HIV prevalence and incidence. For example, in a recent study in Seattle in a population of MSM (men who have sex with men) with acute or recent infection, only 91 % of positive samples which had initially been tested with first- or second-generation EIA were positive with a rapid test [39]. In conclusion, rapid tests can be use for HIV diagnosis in both developing and developed countries and in most cases are as effective as ELISAs. However, there is still need for improvement in both its sensitivity and specificity.

Home Access HIV-1 Test System/Dried Blood Spots

One strategy for HIV testing was devised to encourage patients to get tested in a more confidential and convenient manner. Only one home sample collection kit is currently approved by the FDA: Home Access® HIV-1 (Home Access Health Corporation, Hoffman Estates, IL) [40]. This is an over-the-counter kit but is also available by mail. The patient collects the sample of blood from a fingerstick using a lancet that is provided, places it on the test card (dried blood spots), and mails it back to the company where it is tested. Pre and posttest counseling in the case of a negative result consist of a recorded message. For a positive result, a trained HIV counselor will conduct posttest counseling over the telephone. Testing is by an ELISA and IFA on fluid eluted from the dried blood card. The sensitivity and specificity of this strategy is claimed to approach 100 % [40, 41].

Antibody Testing with Fingerstick Blood and Oral Fluid Sample Types

Serological testing can also be performed on these sample types provided that the specific test has been validated for that specific specimen type. Three advantages of using these media are (1) collection of the sample is noninvasive, (2) the absence of needles increases the safety for the personnel collecting the sample [25], and (3) disposal of potentially infectious waste is minimized. Such tests are very applicable in resource limited regions where laboratory support is less available [24].

Oral Fluid

Most oral fluid-based assays collect oral fluid from patients that contain concentrated IgG antibodies for EIA and WB detection. Currently, there is one EIA and two rapid assays that can use oral fluid samples and are FDA licensed. Using the OraSure collection device (Epitope, Inc., Beaverton, OR), the oral fluid is collected by placing a cotton pad between the cheek and gum for about 2–5 min. A hypertonic solution in the pad will encourage transudation of oral mucosal transudate (the fluid portion from blood that moves through the capillaries at the tooth–gum margin) which is high in HIV-1 IgG. The pad is then transported to a laboratory in a preservative where an EIA and/or WB test can be performed. This EIA method has a sensitivity of 98–100 % and a specificity of 99–100 % [42–44]. HIV diagnosis from oral fluid has certain disadvantages, including the need for special collection devices for samples and that samples cannot be easily obtained from children [45]. The OraQuick rapid test that allows oral fluid for testing is described under the blood-based rapid test section (see Table 6.1).

Urine

Similar to the oral fluid tests, the urine-based test also relies on detection of anti-HIV antibodies. The Sentinel HIV-1 Urine Enzyme Immunoassay (Calpyte Biomedical Corporation, Alameda, CA) is a rapid EIA with a sensitivity of 99 % [46]. Compared to oral fluid, urine testing requires no special devices for sample collection [45]. One WB screening test (Cambridge Biotech HIV-1 Western Blot, Maxim Biomedical) has been approved for HIV-1 antibody detection in urine. The interpretative criteria for a reactive WB for urine require only the presence of a visible band at the gp160 region [47]. Being a screening urine WB assay, a serum WB is the mandated follow-up procedure. This is due to the low specificity of the urine test [6].

Vaginal Secretion and Seminal Fluid

Antibodies to HIV-1 and HIV-2 can be detected in both cervicovaginal secretions and seminal fluids. At present, no commercially available assay using vaginal secretions have been approved by FDA. However, rapid HIV EIA tests using seminal fluids are available to detect HIV antibodies with excellent sensitivity. An example is the Abbott recombinant HIV-1/HIV-2 third-generation immunoassay [48, 49]. Since HIV-1 and HIV-2 IgG can be detected in seminal fluid, an EIA for detection of these antibodies could be useful in rape situations where sero-status can guide the need for postexposure prophylaxis [50].

Confirmatory HIV Antibody Assays

Confirmatory assays for HIV greatly increase the specificity of detection when used in conjunction with screening assays. They are less sensitive (except the IFA), particularly for detection of seroconversion, but are more specific than screening assays. Confirmatory tests are more labor intensive, more prone to subjective interpretation, and more expensive than the screening assays. The primary goal of confirmatory testing is to ensure that individuals who test reactive by screening assays are not incorrectly identified as being infected with HIV (i.e., reducing false-positive screening test results). There are a number of tests that can be use to confirm HIV infection following a reactive initial screening test result.

EIAs

A second EIA or an EIA following a rapid test is the most commonly used method in developing countries to confirm infection (this is considered as an alternative confirmatory strategy to the routine screening test and WB or IFA testing algorithm) [51]. By using two EIAs or a rapid test/EIA in tandem, the predictive value of the combined result is near that of the routine testing algorithm. Because of viral gene heterogeneity, HIV-2 is not always detected in HIV-1 ELISA tests, but this problem has been resolved by the use of combined HIV-1/HIV-2 ELISA tests [52, 53]. The addition of HIV-1 subtype O antigens to the ELISA has allowed improved detection of this subtype of HIV-1 [54]. There are a number of reasons for false-positive and false-negative ELISA results. False-positive results can be due to technical error, cross-reacting antibodies, persons vaccinated for HIV, and several medical conditions [55]. Problems of cross-reacting antibodies have been minimized with the use of synthetic or recombinant HIV peptides in later generation tests. False-positive results may also occur in individuals participating in HIV vaccine trials [56]. Similarly, false-negative results can also occur for a variety of reasons. A nonreactive HIV ELISA result in a person at high risk of infection should always prompt consideration of the window period before seroconversion. Serological testing should be repeated on negative persons several weeks after a suspected infection [55].

There have been improvements in EIA methodologies such as the use of recombinant or synthetic peptide antigens instead of whole viral lysates (second generation) and also the use of double-antigen sandwich configurations (third-generation assays), all of which have led to increased sensitivity and specificity [57, 58]. Briefly, in a third-generation assay, recombinant HIV-1 and HIV-2 proteins and/or peptides, bound on the solid phase (bottom of a microplate, or a bead) will react with antibodies in the patient's serum. This is followed by a washing step to remove unbound constituents of the serum. The bound antibodies are detected through the

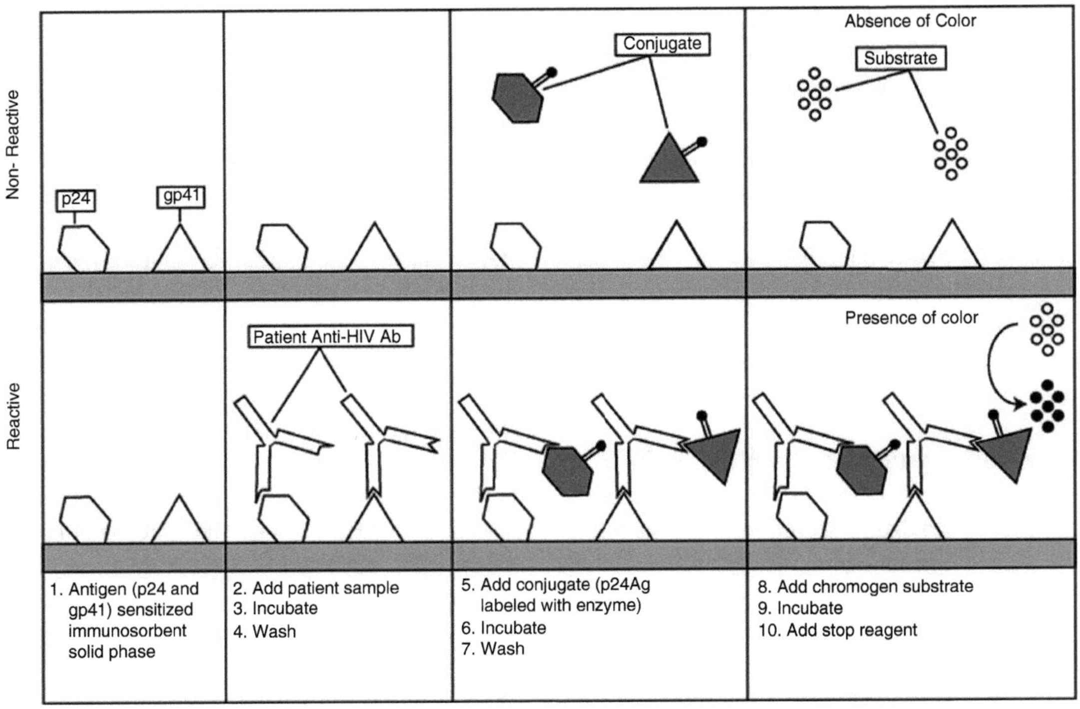

Fig. 6.2 Principle of a third-generation EIA [37]

addition of the same viral antigen conjugated with an enzyme molecule (antibody sandwiched between two antigens). Unbound conjugates are removed by another round of washing. The addition of a substrate of the coupled enzyme generates the development of a color whose optical density (OD) is read with a spectrophotometer. The OD of the color is proportional to the antibody activity in the serum. With the use of this "sandwich" format, higher sensitivity and specificity are ensured, since all potential classes of anti-HIV antibodies, including IgM, can be detected. A third-generation EIA reduces the "window period" to about 22 days after infection [14]. Current EIAs are estimated to be more than 99.9 % sensitive and an average specificity of 99.5–99.9 %. The use of these assays is mandatory when testing blood donations since any failure to identify a positive sample can have serious consequences for the transfused person and even the entire population [59].

Figure 6.2 shows an example of a third-generation EIA methodology.

Recently, fourth-generation EIA assays have been introduced which are able to reveal the presence of both the antibodies and the p24 major antigen of HIV. With this, the window period has been further reduced to almost the levels of HIV RNA detection [14, 60]. The definition of the window period therefore changes since its reduction is due to the early detection of HIV antigen and not antibodies as previously defined. Fourth generation assays detect HIV-1 p24 antigen 10–30 days earlier than the detection of antibody by Western blot and 5–7 days earlier than third-generation EIA [13]. The first fourth-generation assay approved by the FDA was the Abbott's ARCHITECT HIV Ag/Ab Combo assay (specificity of 99.20 % and sensitivity of 100 %) and most recently the Bio-Rad GS HIV Ag/Ab Combo EIA (specificity of 99.97 % and sensitivity of 100 %) [32]. Both assays can detect HIV p24 antigens, HIV-1 group M and O antibodies, and HIV-2 antibodies. They can also be used to detect acute infections, infection in pregnant women, as well as children as young as 2 years [13, 61, 62]. Currently, more fourth-generation EIA are pending FDA approval or under development from Ortho-Clinical Diagnostics and Siemens.

With more assays gaining approval and becoming available, becoming available, the CDC has moved forward with recommending a new testing algorithm that begins with these new fourth-generation assays. In a recent study, the Architect HIV Combo assay detected approximately 88 % of acutely infected individuals who had been missed by a third-generation ELISA test [63]. However, using a fourth-generation assay, there is a risk of a "second diagnostic window." This situation is rare but it can happen if there is both a drop in p24 antigen level and a delay in HIV-specific antibody development [13, 64].

Confirmatory Western Blot

The most common confirmatory assay for HIV antibody, the WB, is considered by many experts as the "gold standard" for HIV diagnostic testing. Briefly, in a WB, the virus is disrupted, and the individual proteins are separated by molecular weight via differential migration on a polyacrylamide gel and blotted onto a membrane support. HIV serum antibodies from the patient are allowed to bind to the proteins in the membrane support, and patterns of reactivity can be visibly read [25]. HIV-1 antigens detectable by WB can be divided into three groups: the env (envelope) glycoproteins (gp41, gp120, gp160), the gag or nuclear proteins (p17/18, p24/25, p40, p55), and the pol or endonuclease-polymerase proteins (p31/32, p66/68). Different groups have proposed different interpretation of the profiles. The Association of State and Territorial Public Health Laboratory Directors and the CDC have defined a positive HIV-1 WB as the presence of any two of the following bands: p24, gp41, or gp120–gp160 [65, 66]. If no band is present, the test is considered negative. If a single band is present or a combination of bands that do not meet the criteria for a positive result, the test is termed indeterminate. According to the WHO, a WB is positive if any two env bands are present [66]. A more restrictive recommendation is that from the American Red Cross which demands at least three bands, one from each group (i.e., one protein from gag, one from pol, and one from env) [67]. Figure 6.3 shows typical WB test results. More details and specific profiles have been published [37].

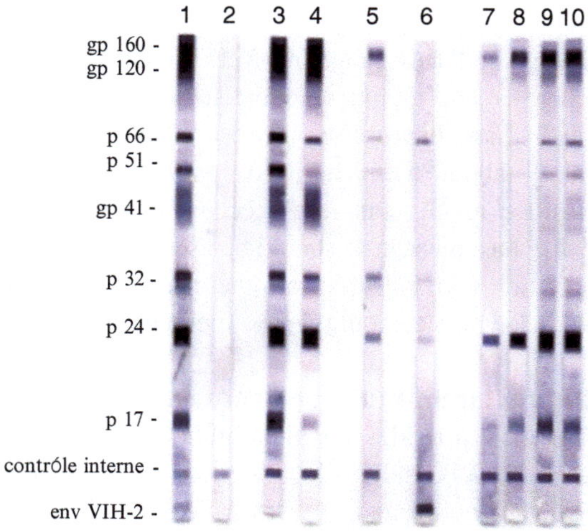

Fig. 6.3 Typical Western Blot results (HIV blot 2.2. Genelabs) [37]. Column 1: positive control; column 2: negative control; column 3–4: positive anti-HIV-1 serum; column 5: positive anti-HIV-1 serum group O; column 6: positive anti-HIV-2 serum; columns 7–10: sequential results from serum testing of a patient newly infected with HIV-1 over time (seroconversion panel)

As many as 10–20 % of WB results performed on sera with repeatedly reactive HIV-1 ELISA results are interpreted as indeterminate. This, however, depends on the population being tested [68]. Accessing the person's risk factor for HIV and repeating the WB test several weeks later is necessary to determine the significance of an indeterminate HIV-1 WB. If a positive result is not obtained after 6 months, the patient is usually considered not infected. The CDC guideline states that "a person whose Western blot test results continue to be consistently indeterminate for at least 6 months in the absence of any known risk factors, clinical symptoms or other findings may be considered to be negative for antibodies to HIV-1" [65]. If a recent HIV-1 infection is suspected, additional tests such as measurement of p24 antigen or HIV-1 nucleic acid tests may be useful. False-negative results may occur if the patient is infected with the rare HIV-1 serotype O and false-positive results have been reported in patients with hyperbilirubinemia, human leukocyte antigen (HLA) antibodies, other retroviruses, connective tissue disorders, and polyclonal antibodies [69, 70]. The sensitivity and specificity of the WB range between 96 and 100 % in most cases [71], unless there is early infection. The main disadvantage of a WB is its high price. There is also the unavoidable subjectivity when reading and interpreting the result and the uncertainty about the criteria of positivity. False-positive results can rarely occur with the WB [37]; thus, these tests should be used only in consultation with an expert or other provider who is knowledgeable about this test method.

Indirect Immunofluorescent Assay

The IFA provides an alternative confirmatory assay to WB, and one is approved as a screening test or a confirmatory test (Waldheim Pharmazeutika) [72]. This test is generally simple to perform, but the results are analyzed microscopically and require expertise for interpretation. In this assay, serum or plasma samples are incubated with T cells that have been infected with HIV and that express HIV antigens intracellularly and with uninfected T cells as a control. If a specimen contains antibodies against HIV antigens, the antibodies should bind to the infected T cells but not the control uninfected cells. Bound antibodies are then detected with an antihuman antibody conjugated to a fluorescent molecule such as fluorescein isothiocynate. The fluorescent molecule emits light when exposed to ultraviolet light. The degree and pattern of fluorescence determines whether a sample is infected with HIV [73]. The Fluorognost HIV-1 IFA (Waldheim Pharmazeutika GmbH, Vienna, Austria) is an FDA-approved confirmatory IFA for the detection of HIV-1 [73, 74]. Currently, there are no FDA-approved confirmatory IFA assays for HIV-2 infection [74]. Figure 6.4 illustrates appearance of an IFA positive test result.

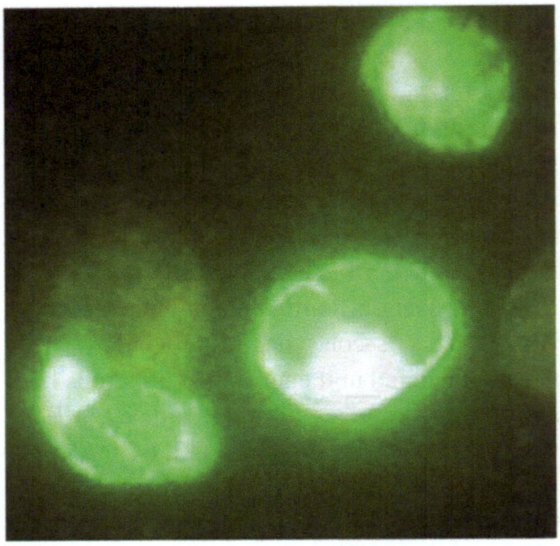

Fig. 6.4 Distinctive apple-green intracellular staining pattern in an HIV-1 positive specimen using the Fluorognost TM HIV-1 IFA. Data was adapted from a Sanochemia Leaflet [72], courtesy of Denis Underwood

Serologic Testing: Regulatory Issues

The regulation of HIV testing is primarily by the FDA except in situations where State laws also apply. Each test is restricted to the body fluid(s) that it was designed to analyze. Rapid HIV testing is usually performed in clinical laboratories that have an adequate Quality Assurance (QA) program where persons who use the test will receive and use the instructional materials provided with the tests. The FDA also requires that persons tested with rapid assays receive the "Subject Information" pamphlet provided with the test [75]. Rapid tests have been approved as waived tests or non-waived (moderately complex) (see Table 6.1) under CLIA. Classification depends on the sample type used or procedure used for testing [76, 77]. Waived tests use unprocessed specimens (whole blood, fingerstick blood, or oral fluid), are easy to use, and because their procedures are simple—have little risk for an incorrect result. Waived test can be performed at many clinical and nonclinical settings including community and outreach settings. The FDA restriction also includes that any facility planning to perform waived rapid tests must have a basic quality assurance (QA) plan with quality control (QC) that ensures that the test is carried out correctly, results are accurate, and errors are identified and corrected accordingly. Also, there are no federal requirements for personnel, quality assessment, or proficiency testing (PT), although the tests must comply with state and local regulations and laws. To perform only waived testing, an organization must obtain a certificate of waiver from the CLIA program and follow the manufacturer's instructions for the test procedure [78]. Rapid tests that use processed samples such as plasma and serum are classified as moderately complex non-waived tests under CLIA [76]. There is a requirement for QA, QC, PT, patient test management, personnel qualification, and inspections. Facilities that provide such testing must obtain a Certificate of Accreditation from an accreditation organization after it has been inspected for complying with a large number of requirements [76]. All confirmatory serological tests are classified as complex non-waived test under CLIA. The same requirements that apply to moderately complex tests also apply to complex tests. The main differences are in QC and personnel requirements.

The FDA assigns classes to medical devices in order to determine the type of premarketing submission/application required for them to be cleared for marketing. Manufacturers of HIV diagnostics assays are required to apply for a Premarket Approval application (PMA) from the FDA. A PMA is the process of scientific and regulatory review to evaluate the safety and effectiveness of Class III medical devices [79]. Apart from safety and effectiveness assurances, general and special controls also apply to Class III devices. General controls are the basic requirements of the Food, Drug and Cosmetic (FD&C) Act and they include: manufacturer registration with the FDA, good manufacturing techniques, proper branding and labeling, notification of the FDA prior to marketing the device, and general reporting procedures. An approved PMA is, in effect, a private license granting the applicant (or owner) permission to market the device.

Detection of Recent HIV Infection

Diagnosis of HIV infection during the acute phase of an infection has several important applications. First, the immune system can be better preserved; second, because viral loads are highest during acute infection, early intervention can minimize transmission to others, thereby limiting the spread of infection [80]. There are also advantages to know "when" a person has been infected; that is, whether they have had recent infection. Recent infection can be considered as the time when antibody levels are still rising (before they plateau at high levels); therefore, recent infection is between 3 and 6 months following infection. Most importantly, knowing how many persons in a population have recent infection allows the estimation of the incidence of HIV in that population. Incidence, in contrast to prevalence, is the rate of new infections. Thus, identifying recent infections (new infections) can be used to determine which populations should be targeted for interventions such as for education and vaccines. In addition, knowing the approximate time of HIV infection can be a beneficial tool for contact tracing so that contacts can be evaluated for infection and treatment. Conventional antibody assays are not able to differentiate between a recent infection and a chronic (established) infection. Thus, methods have been developed to identify a recent from established HIV infections. The tests have been given many names, including STARHS (serological testing algorithm for recent HIV seroconversion), TRI (tests for recent infection), S/LS (sensitive/less sensitive) tests, and detuned tests. These approaches must be used on persons who have already been confirmed to have antibodies to HIV [9]. There are generally two principles by which these TRI are based (1) antibody titer or (2) antibody avidity (191); one test examines antibody isotype.

The TRI assay first described was for antibody titer and was considered a detuning or S/LS test. By deliberately making a test less sensitive (LS) by changing test parameters, the result from an antibody positive person would change from positive to negative during the time interval when antibody levels had not reached their highest (plateau). So, if a sample were positive on the routine test (sensitive test, S) but negative on the less sensitive (LS) test, the person is considered as being recently infected. In a test with a similar principle, (BED-capture assay), the proportion of HIV-specific antibodies to the total IgG is used to differ recent from established HIV infection. In the second principle of a TRI, the approach is to identify recent infections by investigating the HIV-specific antibody avidity. It is known that antibody avidity to HIV antigens increases overtime during the first year of infection. Thus, low avidity HIV antibodies indicate a recent infection. These tests determine an avidity index (AI) (e.g., Abbott AxSYM commercial EIA) by determining how the antibodies respond to a chaotropic agent that dissociates weakly avid antibodies [81].

Test for recent infection are affected by a number of factors, primarily the HIV viral variability because immunodominant epitopes differ between the HIV-1 clades. It has been documented that these tests are indeed affected by viral variants. Another limitation is testing sera from individuals with AIDS or very low CD4 counts since these patients have low antibody titers and therefore would be classified as falsely recently infected (most experts believe there is a 5 % false positive rate because of AIDS [37]). Although not molecular assays, these TRI have influenced medical science in a positive manner, particularly for epidemiologic purposes.

How HIV Serologic Testing Has Changed Medical Practice

Early and accurate diagnosis and subsequent treatment can substantially slow down the advancement of the disease by keeping viral replication to a minimum (or eliminated). In this way, the immune system can be preserved and transmission to others can also be minimized or prevented if precautions are taken. The currently available HIV serological assays have made it possible for a rapid and accurate diagnosis especially at point-of-care facilities such as emergency rooms and are indispensable for occupational exposure cases and women in labor without a known HIV status. Safer blood and body tissue transplantation have also benefited following improvement in diagnostic techniques such the use of fourth-generation EIAs. With the wide range of new techniques currently available, choosing the appropriate method for identification and management will allow accurate information to be obtained regarding the patient's status for effective treatment [82].

Nucleic Acid-Based Tests for HIV

NAT Testing: Background

The advent of nucleic acid testing, and in particular, assessment of viral load (copy number of virions in blood) has revolutionized medical practice for HIV and Hepatitis C virus (HCV) infections. As better antiretroviral (ARV) drugs were developed, and with the application and use of highly active antiretroviral therapy (HARRT), cocktails of drugs targeting different points of the viral replication cycle, and monitoring of the viral load (VL) in patients rapidly became crucial in patient care and management [83, 84]. Rapid reduction in VL (0.7–3 logs) is typically observed in drug naïve patients within a few weeks after initiation of ARV therapy.

NAT Testing: Methodology and Standard Reagents

Viral nucleic acid (NA) detection and quantification may be achieved through laboratory techniques that either detect proviral cDNA in leukocytes or viral RNA in the cell-free compartment (plasma).

HIV proviral DNA assays allow the detection of cells that harbor quiescent provirus as well as cells with actively replicating virus [9]. This qualitative procedure is very sensitive and can detect between one and ten copies of HIV-1 proviral DNA per sample. Because of the extremely high sensitivity of this assay, small amounts of background "noise" in the environment or contamination during laboratory processing may result in amplification of products that can produce false-positive reactions [85]. Currently, the only recommended diagnostic use of this assay is for the detection of infection in infants born to mothers infected with HIV-1. The Roche HIV-1 Amplicor test, which is a qualitative PCR-based assay, can be used to detect HIV-1 DNA. Currently, there are no commercially available assays to quantify proviral DNA, which could potentially be useful in evaluating the efficacy of ARV therapies especially when the HIV-1 viral

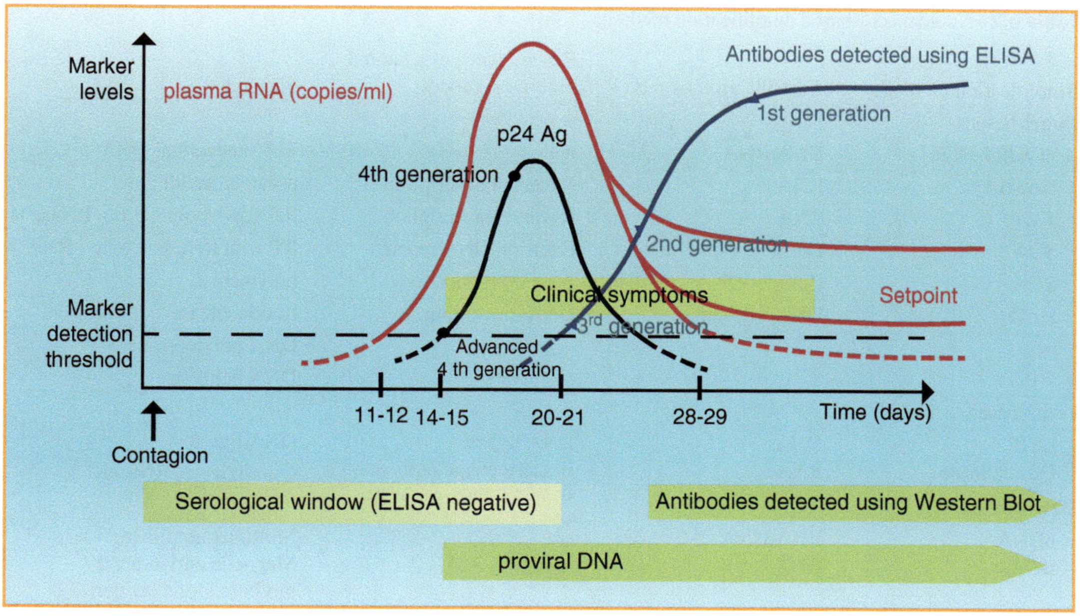

Fig. 6.5 Kinetics of viral markers during the early stages of infection and their diagnostic window periods [98]

RNA load is undetectable [86–88]. A number of research-based assays have been described for quantification of HIV-1 proviral DNA, but these assays are based on conventional PCR [89–92]. A limitation of some of these assays is that conventional PCR methods were used. As a result, the DNA copy numbers are calculated based on the final amplified gene products, which vary widely due to various factors affecting PCR. Several real-time PCR TaqMan-based protocols for quantification of HIV-1 proviral DNA have been reported [93–95], which provide a highly accurate and reproductive detection method for HIV-proviral DNA with a wide level of detection.

Quantification of HIV viral RNA has many advantages, e.g., used by clinicians to measure the baseline VL before initiation of ARV therapy, evaluate the efficacy of initial ARV therapy, predict drug resistance, and also to estimate the potential to develop AIDS-related opportunistic infections and diseases [83]. Nucleic acid tests (NAT), sometimes referred to nucleic acid amplification tests (NAAT), can also supplement antibody testing for the diagnosis of HIV infection in special situations such as in suspected acute infection, when antibodies are still undetectable and also in newborns of HIV-infected mothers in whom maternal antibodies are still present [9]. Plasma HIV RNA is usually measured in HIV infected individuals at baseline and thereafter. The level of VL measured at times about 1–2 months after infection is known as the "set point" and is positively correlated with the disease progression. Although HIV transmission through blood transfusion has decreased following the use of fourth generation screening assays, the application of NAT (in addition to using antibody testing) has further reduced the window period. It has been reported that, the risk of acquiring HIV through blood transfusion is reduced by approximately 50 % using NAT [96]. NAAT can detect HIV infection approximately 45 days earlier than first-generation EIAs, 32 days sooner than second-generation EIAs, 11 days sooner than third-generation EIAs, and 6 days sooner than fourth-generation EIAs [97, 98]. Figure 6.5 shows the kinetics of viral markers during the early stages of infection and a comparison of the window periods of various serological techniques with reference to NAAT.

Table 6.2 Nucleic acid-based amplification methods [106]

Amplification methods	Amplification targets	Resemblance of a natural biological process	Features
Target-based			
PCR/RT-PCR	DNA/RNA	n/a	Thermocycling, DNA
NASBA	RNA	Reverse transcription	polymerase/RT
TMA	RNA	Reverse transcription	RT, RNA polymerase, RNase H
SDA	DNA	Excision DNA repair	RT with RNase activity; RNA
RCA	Circular DNA	Plasmid replication	polymerase
HAD	DNA	DNA unwinding	Endonuclease
			DNA polymerase
			DNA helicase
Probe-based			
LCR	DNA	DNA ligase	DNA ligase
Qβ-replicase	RNA	Bacteriophage replication	Qβ-replicase, RNaseIII
Signal-based			
bDNA	RNA/DNA	n/a	Multimer amplifier
BCA	DNA	n/a	Magnetic enrichment; bio-barcodes detection

BCA bio-barcode assay, *bDNA* branched DNA, *HAD* helicase-dependent isothermal DNA amplification, *LCR* ligase chain reaction, *n/a* nonapplicable, *NASBA* nucleic acid sequence-based amplification, *PCR* polymerase chain reaction, *RCA* rolling circle amplification, *RNase* ribonuclease, *RT* reverse transcription, *SDA* strand displacement assay, *TMA* transcription-mediated assay

Determination of VL also provides vital information, especially to those individuals who are under ARV therapy. The minimal change in VL considered to be statistically significant (2 standard deviation) is a threefold, or 0.5 $\log_{10}$ copies/ml. Suppression of viral replication by ARV therapy to a level that is below the limits of detection (LOD) (below 40–75 copies/ml depending on the specific assay used) is the main objective of ARV therapy [99–102]. Standard HIV quantitative assays have a LOD of 400 copies/ml, whereas ultrasensitive assays may detect VL as low as 5–50 copies/ml. Also, some newer assays have a greater dynamic range than either the standard or ultrasensitive assay (e.g., 4.0×10 [1] to 1.0×10 [7] copies/ml) [25, 103, 104]. Therefore, assays that can detect <50 copies/ml are more useful than standard VL tests in predicting prolonged viral suppression and are recommended for monitoring patients who are receiving ARV therapy.

Three basic types of techniques are currently used to amplify HIV RNA for detection and quantification of VL (1) gene target-based amplification technology such as PCR or reverse transcription followed by PCR (RT-PCR) and TMA or NASBA. This type of method is designed to detect and amplify the target gene of interest; (2) signal-based amplification technique such as branched DNA (bDNA), which amplifies the signal rather than the gene target sequence; and (3) probe-based amplification techniques, e.g., ligase chain reaction (LCR) that relies on amplification of the probes that are homologous to a specific gene target [105].

The gene-based amplification technologies can be further divided into PCR-based or non-PCR-based methods. PCR is currently the best-known assay for the amplification of nucleic acid (NA). It is performed at various temperatures using a very specialized equipment known as the thermocycler. In contrast, most of the non-PCR methods take advantage of the natural NA amplification processes (Table 6.2). For example, the ligase chain reaction (LCR) mimics enzymatic ligation processes; nucleic acid sequence-based amplification (NASBA) mimics viral RNA reverse transcription and transcription; strand displacement assay (SDA) resembles the DNA excision repair process; and Qβ-replicase RNA amplification resembles bacteriophage replication. Another common feature of these non-PCR-based assays is that these assays can be carried out at constant temperature without thermocycling. The RT-PCR-based assays convert HIV RNA into DNA using an enzyme called reverse transcriptase (RT). This is followed by PCR, which increases the copy number of DNA for detection. The resultant DNA is then detected with a nucleic acid probe specific for a HIV-1 nucleic acid sequence that has been attached to an enzyme, or, the captured oligonucleotide (which is biotinylated) is detected using an avidin/enzyme agent. The enzyme–nucleic acid complex can react with another chemical and produce a color change, the intensity of which is used to quantify the DNA. The HIV-1 Amplicor Monitor Assay and the HIV-1 AmpliPrep TaqMan assay (Roche Molecular Diagnostics, Pleasanton, CA) are examples of target-based amplification assays. The difference between the HIV-1 Amplicor Monitor and AmpliPrep TaqMan assays are that the Monitor assay is based on the conventional PCR method and the TaqMan is a real-time PCR-based method. The real-time PCR is much more accurate and reproducible with a broader linear dynamic range than the conventional PCR method [107]. Other examples of target-based amplification assays include the Abbott *m2000* real-time PCR assay (Des Plaines, IL) and the Nuclisens HIV RNA QT (Organon-Teknika, Boxtel, The Netherlands) [108].

The bDNA assay, also known as the Versant HIV-1 RNA 3.0 assay or formally known as Quantiplex™, is one example of the signal amplification-based assays. HIV RNA is captured by complementary oligonucleotides called capture probes that are bound to the bottom of a plate. The hybridization probes are used to simultaneously bind the captured HIV RNA. Unlike the target-based assays, detection of the captured viral RNA is achieved by linkage of oligonucleotide-containing multi-amplifiers to the hybridization probes.

In the probe-based assays, the probes that are homologous to the target sequences are amplified. One of these assays is LCR [109, 110]. LCR is based on the principle that ligation of a DNA molecule is most efficient when the molecules are aligned in a head-to-tail fashion. Thus, typically two detection probes are specifically design to be complementary to a specific gene target sequence of interest. Once these probes are annealed to the gene target, addition of DNA ligase will join the two detecting molecules [111]. Repetition of hybridization, ligation, and denaturation will achieve probe-based amplification. The Abbott Laboratories (IL) markets HIV-1 LCx, which is based on LCR technology. Table 6.2 summaries the various types of nucleic acid-based amplification methods.

Although the sensitivity and specificity of these diagnostic tests are high (99 % and 98 %, respectively), they should be used in conjunction with serologic assays [112]. In addition, because most of these tests are designed to detect HIV-1 subtype B, they sometimes cannot detect other HIV strains and subtypes. Further improved real-time PCR-based assays have been introduced (Abbott Real Time HIV-1; Roche Amplicor TaqMan ver. 2.0) that are capable of detecting all subtypes of HIV group M and group O. The TaqScreen MPX from Roche is a NAT that has been approved by the FDA to simultaneously screen for HIV-1 group O and HIV-2. However, the current application of the test is for blood and tissue bank screening of samples from blood and organ donors. The TaqScreen MPX is not approved for clinical monitoring [113].

Despite being an indispensable clinical tool, VL testing still has some issues. It requires highly skilled personnel and the instruments are very expensive. Many developing countries cannot routinely use the currently available NAT assays [114, 115]. The increasing HIV viral variability can also have a serious impact on NAT sensitivity. Using these assays in geographic regions where multiple subtypes and CRFs (circulating recombinant forms) are present, can result in a failure to detect infection, since primers and probes used might not be the right ones to amplify nucleic acid of some HIV variants. A similar situation arises in countries where HIV-2 infection is endemic.

Other Viral Load Tests

An inexpensive HIV VL assay has been developed to measure viral reverse transcriptase (RT) activity (ExaVir Load Version 2; Cavidi AB, Uppsala, Sweden). The test is performed mostly manually and was designed primarily for resource-limited settings. The assay has a LOD of 400 copies/ml [116, 117]. However, it is not approved by the FDA for clinical use in the USA.

Detection of HIV-1 Non-B Subtypes

HIV-1 can be classified into group M (major), a rare group O (outlier), and a "new" group N (non-M, non-O) [118, 119]. Recently, a new HIV-1 group, which is designated as group P, has been reported [120]. Group M can be further divided into subtypes (A–D, F–H, J, and K) and circulating recombinant forms (CRFs) [119, 121]. The subtype B virus is at present the predominate subtype in the USA. Recent data however suggest increasing prevalence of HIV-1 non-B subtype in the USA. The clinical significance of emerging non-B viruses to HIV treatment and patient care is currently unknown. However, in the area of vaccine development, the extent of HIV diversity is an important consideration. Early candidate vaccines were developed based on the US HIV-1 B subtype type. However, non-B subtypes should also be included in future research and development of an effective vaccine against HIV [122]. This increase in HIV-1 non-B subtype is likely driven by global travel, immigration, commerce, tourism, and military deployment [123]. For example, in a study conducted from blood donors throughout the USA from 1997 to 2000, the prevalence of non-B subtypes was 2.3 % [124]. In a recent study conducted in the city of Baltimore and the State of Maryland, the non-B prevalence, which was determined using DNA sequencing analysis, was 13.2 % in a Maryland suburb of the Washington, DC area [125]. A similar high level of non-B HIV-1 subtypes in other part of the USA has also been reported [126, 127]. Therefore, new methods that are capable of detecting all of the non-B subtypes including circulating recombinant forms should be developed and used. Failure to detect or accurately quantify non-B HIV infection has been documented in some of the antibody and RNA-based assays [128–134].

p24 Antigen Measurements

Before the advent of viral RNA detection, quantification of HIV-1 in clinical specimens was based on gag (p24) protein detection or after in vitro cultivation of the virus [135]. p24 antigenemia can also be used to monitor disease progression. p24 antigen appears in blood approximately 1 week before antibodies are detected and can typically be detected in serum using EIA. Detecting p24 antigen by EIA is a relatively simple, inexpensive, and rapid method. However, the sensitivity is lower as compared to HIV RNA-based assays, but enhanced sensitivity have been reported by signal amplification [136–139]. Their specificity is high as long as a neutralization (confirmation) step is used [112]. These methods are commonly used in developing countries.

A real-time immuno-PCR (IPCR)-based assay, which uses HIV-p24 antigen as a marker for quantification of antigenemia, has been reported [140]. The real-time IPCR assay combines the p24 ELISA with real-time PCR amplification of the signal DNA molecules that are attached to the detecting antibody of p24. With the IPCR, the first protein is captured in the same way as in a typical ELISA, but the second antibody is conjugated with biotin that, through strong binding of biotin to streptavidin, links to biotinylated oligonucleotides. The protein level can then be quantified by amplifying the signal oligonucleotide linked to the antibody. The sensitivity level is in the range of femtograms (10^{-15} g/ml), which is at least 10^3 times more sensitive than a conventional ELISA assay [106]. Figure 6.6 shows a schematic representation of the IPCR assay in comparison with the conventional ELISA.

HIV Drug-Resistance Testing

The development of drug resistance in HIV-1 variants was first observed in patients treated with AZT. Viral isolates from such patients displayed phenotypic drug resistance in vitro, which later correlated with specific mutations in the reverse transcriptase (RT) gene [141].

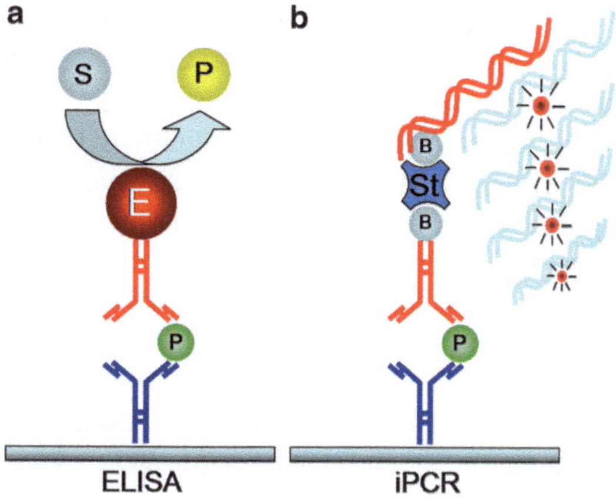

Fig. 6.6 Schematic presentation of immuno-PCR in comparison with ELISA. Comparison between ELISA (**a**) and immuno-PCR (**b**). *P* (*Green Circle*) p24 protein, *E* enzyme, *S* substrate, *P* (*yellow circle*) colored product, *B* biotin, *St* streptavidin: [106, 135]

Despite the approval of more nucleoside (NRTIs) and non-nucleoside RT inhibitors (NNRTIs) for treatment and also the introduction of double combination therapy, no long-term viral suppression was achieved. Following the introduction of protease (PR) inhibitors (PI) in 1996 and the use of a three drug regimen (two NRTIs with either a PI or an NNRTI), it was possible to achieve the basic requirement for sustaining successful antiretroviral treatment [142–145]. Keeping viral replication as low as possible is crucial in avoiding the emergence of resistant viral quasispecies carrying drug resistance-associated mutations. For most of the currently FDA approved RTI and PI, drug resistance-associated mutations in the RT and PR genes respectively have been reported. Factors such as poor adherence, malabsorption, other pharmacogenomic differences, or missing potency of the therapy regimen in the given patient (e.g., high VL and history of drug resistance) may result to insufficient drug level, allowing the virus to replicate in the presence of the drugs [141]. This might lead to the development of viral drug resistance.

The clinical significance of HIV-1 drug resistance has been well established. Treatment of patients with drugs to which their HIV-1 isolates are predicted to be resistant on the basis of genotypic or phenotypic assays will most likely result in no virological response (treatment failure). Alternatively, the use of drugs to which the virus is predicted to be susceptible enhances the likelihood of reestablishing virological control in patients in whom prior treatment regimens have failed [146]. The clinical utility of drug resistance testing as a guide to the selection of subsequent antiretroviral regimens for patients with virological failure of their current regimen have been demonstrated [147, 148]. Guidelines recommending drug resistance testing in managing failure of antiretroviral therapy has been proposed by several expert panels [149–151]. The current DHHS guidelines recommend that, if possible, treatment-experienced patients should receive a regimen containing two or three fully active drugs [152]. Following the increasing prevalence of resistance of HIV against antiretroviral therapeutic agents (mostly RTIs and PIs), there has been a rapid development of drug-resistance testing assays. The two main analytic approaches currently being use for the detection of HIV-1 drug-resistance are genotyping and phenotyping.

The genotyping detects mutations in the viral genes that encode protein targets for the RT or PR inhibitors. The presence or absence of specific mutations is predictive of antiretroviral activity [153]. Analysis is currently being done either by sequencing all relevant codons or by hybridization-based detection of mutations in selected codons mostly in the RT or PR genes. The Bayer (Visible Genetics) TRUGENE platform sequences the HIV-1 genes encoding RT (codon 40–247) and PR (codon 1–99). Prior to sequencing, RT-PCR is performed to amplify HIV-1 RNA target sequences in human plasma [135]. This qualitative assay is used in conjunction with clinical presentation, laboratory markers, and antiretroviral history.

HIV-1 phenotypic assays measure virological responsiveness in the presence of differing concentrations of ARV [153]; that is, it measures the ability of the patient's virus to grow in a cell culture in the presence of known concentrations of drugs [135]. Testing involves determining the IC_{50} (i.e., the median inhibitory concentration), which is defined as the drug concentration which inhibits viral replication by 50 %.

The ratio between the IC_{50} of the test virus and a reference (i.e., wild type) virus is known as the fold change. Clinical cutoff values are a correlative measure of virological response in treated patients and predict how viral resistance may affect future treatment response [153]. Two currently used phenotypic assays are Antivirogram (Virco, Durham, NC) and PhenoSense (Virologic, South San Francisco, CA).

Genotypic resistance assays have two major advantages over phenotypic assays. First, genotypic assays have a lower cost than phenotypic. Secondly, genotyping is more easily available in laboratories. In treatment-naïve patients, genotyping is the preferred method. They however come with certain disadvantages. These assays produce results in two or three categories, which incorrectly assume that HIV resistance is binary. Few ARV mutations express binary resistance (except the K103N mutation, which reduces susceptibility of NNRTIs, except Etravirine). The assays also vary in methodology and lack standardization [154]. Results, therefore, often have to be interpreted by experts. To maintain validity, genotypic algorithms must be continually updated with emerging data of viral isolates [155, 156].

Detection of drug resistance is predictive of treatment response and adds to knowledge obtained from drug history, VL measurements, or both [150, 153, 157]. Clinical studies have demonstrated that genotyping was superior to patient history alone in selecting affective regimens for treatment-experienced patients up to 1.5 years [158]. Genotyping assays have enabled physicians to select durable regimens without the use of active drug classes.

NAT Testing: Regulatory Issues

The FDA regulates HIV NAT. Some states also regulate testing. If the state under CLIA has stricter requirements, testing facilities in that state must follow the stricter state requirements. Just as the diagnostic confirmatory assays, all HIV NAT are classified as complex non-waived tests under the CLIA program. Therefore, the same requirements which were previously stated also apply here.

Similar to the HIV serologic assays, the NAT assays are classified by the FDA as Class III devices. However, the HIV drug-resistance genotyping assays such as the TRUEGENE HIV-1 Genotyping Kit and OpenGene DNA Sequencing System are classified as Class II devices [159]. Class II devices in addition to complying with the general controls also require a PMN or 510(k) prior to marketing. A 510(k) is a premarket submission made to FDA to demonstrate that the device to be marketed is at least as safe and effective (substantially equivalent) to a legally marketed device that is not subject to a PMA [160].

How NAT Methods for HIV Quantification Have Changed Medical Practice

Quantification of HIV VL and therapeutic responses is essential for the successful treatment and management of infected individuals following confirmation of infection with serologic assays. Quantitative techniques that provide accurate information about a patient's existing infection and immune status allow for physicians to make realistic prognosis and initiate or change therapy accordingly [82]. Following the design of better drugs targeting various parts of the viral life cycle, monitoring of the VL in patients using NAT techniques are crucial in patient care and management. Safer blood supply has been ensure with the use of NAT in blood transfusion medicine which has resulted to about a 50 % reduction in the risk of acquiring HIV following a blood transfusion [96]. NAAT has also been very useful in detecting acute HIV infection especially in situations that are undetectable even with fourth generation EIAs.

NAT Testing: Future Directions

Monitoring HIV Infection in Resource Limited Regions

HIV infection in resource limited areas remains a major cause of morbidity and mortality despite increasing availability of ARV therapies [161].

Quantification of HIV-1 viral RNA loads in plasma, although one of the most valuable clinical tools for initiation of therapy, evaluation of the efficacy of ARV, and predicting disease progression [162–164] are less available in resource-limited countries because of infrastructure and financial restraints. Plasma VL measurement, however, requires venous blood extraction, use of RNAase-free materials, freezers for storage, constant electricity supply to run the freezers, and also transport in a cold chain which makes it difficult to manage in resource-limited countries [162, 165]. Spotting and drying whole blood on a filter (dried blood spots) collected by lancet or fingerstick have proven to be highly economical and an effective alternative method for sample collection and storage. For example, the sample is easy to obtain, collection volume is small, no blood separation is required, and the samples can be transported at room temperature; thus, there is no need for cold-chain transportation [166]. In addition, the use of dried blood spot (DBS) or dried plasma spot (DPS) samples in VL determination appears to generate results that are less sensitive (approx. 2,000 copies/ml) than standard liquid plasma-based testing, but they nevertheless provide useful information in most of the clinical situations. Importantly, it has been demonstrated that HIV-1 RNA in DBS and DPS samples is stable over time under different conditions of temperature and humidity [164, 165, 167–172]. Therefore, DBS collections are valuable in resource-limited countries, but do not address the limitations associated with the testing process.

Individualized Molecular Genetic Testing for ARV Therapies

The genetic background of an individual has been shown to affect ARV therapies and the prognosis of HIV progression. For example, gene copy number of CCL3L1, a ligand of the CCR5 chemokine co-receptor or the CCL3L1–CCR5 genotypes, has been shown to be associated with each individual's susceptibility to HIV infection or with prognosis of HIV disease progression [173, 174]. However, no commercial genetic assay is currently available for such a determination. Certain variations in human leucocytes antigen (HLA) haplotypes such as HLA-B*5701 have also been reported to be associate with drug hypersensitivity to Abacavir (ABC) [175–177]. About 4–8 % of HIV patients treated with ABC (Ziagen) experience hypersensitivity that is characterized by rash, fever, gastrointestinal symptoms and can be life threatening [178]. Studies have shown that, screening for HLA-B*5701 before treatment with ABC and withholding ABC from persons who are positive for HLA-B*5701 appears to reduce the risk of an ABC hypersensitivity reaction [179, 180]. Current guidelines of the USDHHS recommend that patients be tested for HLA-B*5701 before ABC is initiated and that patients with HLA-B*5701 should not be given ABC. If HLA-B*5701 screening is not available, ABC may be used, with appropriate counseling and monitoring. It should be noted that ABC is FDA approved for anti-HIV therapy because studies have shown an improvement of CD4 T-lymphocyte counts and HIV VL on a 3-drug regimen of zidovudine (AZT), lamivudine (3TC), and ABC, in comparison with the 2-drug regimen of AZT and 3TC [181]. GlaxoSmithKline (GSK), manufacturer of ABC, has developed an approved genetic test for HLA-B*5701 [182].

Acknowledgments This work was supported in part by funding from the University of Maryland Medical Center and NIH-NINDS-R21-NS063880 (RZ).

References

1. Gebbie KM, Association of State and Territorial Health Officials (U.S.). Guide to public health practice--HTLV-III screening in the community: recommendations from a concensus conference convened by the association of state and territorial health officials, March 1–2, 1985. Atlanta, Georgia, Kristine Gebbie Presiding: ASTHO Foundation; 1985.
2. Centers for Disease Control (CDC). Public Health Service guidelines for counseling and antibody testing to prevent HIV infection and AIDS. MMWR Morb Mortal Wkly Rep. 1987;36:509–15.
3. Centers for Disease Control (CDC). Recommendations for HIV testing services for inpatients and outpatients in acute-care hospital settings. MMWR Morb Mortal Wkly Rep. 1993;42:1–10.
4. Centers for Disease Control (CDC). HIV counseling testing and referral: standards and guidelines.

Atlanta, GA: US Department of Health and Human Services, CDC; 1994.
5. Connor EM, Sperling RS, Gelber R, et al. Reduction of maternal-infant transmission of human immunodeficiency virus type 1 with zidovudine treatment. Pediatric AIDS Clinical Trials Group Protocol 076 Study Group. N Engl J Med. 1994;331:1173–80.
6. Centers for Disease Control (CDC). Revised guidelines for HIV counseling, testing, and referral and revised recommendations for HIV screening of pregnant women. MMWR Morb Mortal Wkly Rep. 2001;50:1–12.
7. Centers for Disease Control (CDC). Revised recommendations for HIV screening of pregnant women. MMWR Recomm Rep. 2001;50:63–85.
8. Kaiser Family Foundation. Global HIV/AIDS timeline: a timeline of key milestones. The Henry J Kaiser Family Foundation; 2010.
9. Butto S, Suligoi B, Fanales-Belasio E, Raimondo M. Laboratory diagnostics for HIV infection. Ann Ist Super Sanita. 2010;46:24–33.
10. Centers for Disease Control (CDC). Advancing HIV, prevention: new strategies for a changing epidemic—United States, 2003. MMWR Morb Mortal Wkly Rep. 2003;52:329–32.
11. Branson BM, Handsfield HH, Lampe MA, et al. Revised recommendations for HIV testing of adults, adolescents, and pregnant women in health-care settings. MMWR Recomm Rep. 2006;55:1–17. quiz CE1-4.
12. Branson BM. Piont of care rapid tests for HIV antibodies. J Lab Med. 2003;27:288–95.
13. Marone B. 30 years of HIV/AIDS: When will routine testing become reality? Clin Lab News. 2011;37: 1–4.
14. Weber B. Screening of HIV infection: role of molecular and immunological assays. Expert Rev Mol Diagn. 2006;6:399–411.
15. Fiebig EW, Wright DJ, Rawal BD, et al. Dynamics of HIV viremia and antibody seroconversion in plasma donors: implications for diagnosis and staging of primary HIV infection. AIDS. 2003;17:1871–9.
16. Kahn JO, Walker BD. Acute human immunodeficiency virus type 1 infection. N Engl J Med. 1998;339:33–9.
17. Steckelberg JM, Cockerill 3rd FR. Serologic testing for human immunodeficiency virus antibodies. Mayo Clin Proc. 1988;63:373–80.
18. Henrard DR, Daar E, Farzadegan H, et al. Virologic and immunologic characterization of symptomatic and asymptomatic primary HIV-1 infection. J Acquir Immune Defic Syndr Hum Retrovirol. 1995;9: 305–10.
19. Stramer SL, Glynn SA, Kleinman SH, et al. Detection of HIV-1 and HCV infections among antibody-negative blood donors by nucleic acid-amplification testing. N Engl J Med. 2004;351:760–8.
20. Tomaras GD, Yates NL, Liu P, et al. Initial B-cell responses to transmitted human immunodeficiency virus type 1: virion-binding immunoglobulin M (IgM) and IgG antibodies followed by plasma anti-gp41 antibodies with ineffective control of initial viremia. J Virol. 2008;82:12449–63.
21. Murphy G, Parry JV. Assays for the detection of recent infections with human immunodeficiency virus type 1. Euro Surveill. 2008;13. pii: 18966.
22. Wilson KM, Johnson EI, Croom HA, et al. Incidence immunoassay for distinguishing recent from established HIV-1 infection in therapy-naive populations. AIDS. 2004;18:2253–9.
23. Salahuddin SZ, Groopman JE, Markham PD, et al. HTLV-III in symptom-free seronegative persons. Lancet. 1984;2:1418–20.
24. DeSimone JA, Pomerantz RJ. New methods for the detection of HIV. Clin Lab Med. 2002;22:573–92.
25. New York Department of Health. Diagnostic, monitoring, and resistance laboratory testing for HIV. http://www.hivguidelines.org/wp-content/uploads/diagnostic-monitoring-and-resistance-laboratory-tests-for-hiv-posted-09-26-2011.pdf (2011). Accessed 12 Feb 2012.
26. Trinity Biotech. Uni-Gold™ Recombigen® HIV. Packgae Insert, 2004. http://www.fda.gov/downloads/BiologicsBloodVaccines/BloodBloodProducts/ApprovedProducts/PremarketApprovalsPMAs/UCM093428.pdf. Accessed 10 Mar 2012.
27. Health Research and Education Trust (HRET). Charts for comparing rapid HIV antibody screening tests. Health Research and Education Trust (HRET); 2005.
28. OraSure Technologies Inc. OraQuick advance rapid HIV-1/2 antibody test [package insert]. Bethlehem, PA: OraSure Technologies, Inc; 2004.
29. MedMira Laboratories Inc. Reveal rapid HIV-1 antibody test [package insert]. Halifax, Nova Scotia, Canada: MedMira Laboratories, Inc.; 2004.
30. Greenwald JL, Burstein GR, Pincus J, Branson B. A rapid review of rapid HIV antibody tests. Curr Infect Dis Rep. 2006;8:125–31.
31. Dechet A, Tokumoto J, Newstetter A, Teague R. The basics of HIV screening and testing. San Francisco, CA: Pacific AIDS Education and Training Center; 2009.
32. Food and Drug Administration. HIV diagnostic assays.http://www.fda.gov/BiologicsBloodVaccines/BloodBloodProducts/ApprovedProducts/LicensedProductsBLAs/BloodDonorScreening/InfectiousDisease/ucm080466.htm#HumanImmunodeficiencyVirusType1AntiHIV12Assay (2011). Accessed 20 Sept 2011.
33. Bio-Rad Laboratories. Multispot HIV-1/HIV-2 rapid test [package insert]. Redmond, WA: Bio-Rad Laboratories; 2004.
34. Centers for Disease Control (CDC). Quality assurance guidelines for testing using the OraQuick® Rapid HIV-1 antibody test. http://www.cdc.gov/hiv/rapid_testing/materials/QA-Guide.htm (2004). Accessed 10 Sept 2010.
35. O'Connell RJ, Merritt TM, Malia JA, et al. Performance of the OraQuick rapid antibody test for

diagnosis of human immunodeficiency virus type 1 infection in patients with various levels of exposure to highly active antiretroviral therapy. J Clin Microbiol. 2003;41:2153–5.
36. Respess RA, Rayfield MA, Dondero TJ. Laboratory testing and rapid HIV assays: applications for HIV surveillance in hard-to-reach populations. AIDS. 2001;15 Suppl 3:S49–59.
37. Constantine NT, Saville R, Dax E. Retroviral testing and quality assurance: essential for laboratory diagnosis. Ann Arbor, MI: Malloy Printers; 2005.
38. Black V, von Mollendorf CE, Moyes JA, Scott LE, Puren A, Stevens WS. Poor sensitivity of field rapid HIV testing: implications for mother-to-child transmission programme. BJOG. 2009;116:1805–8.
39. Stekler JD, Swenson PD, Coombs RW, et al. HIV testing in a high-incidence population: is antibody testing alone good enough? Clin Infect Dis. 2009;49: 444–53.
40. Brodie S, Sax P. Novel approaches to HIV antibody testing. AIDS Clin Care. 1997;9:1–5. 10.
41. Frank AP, Wandell MG, Headings MD, Conant MA, Woody GE, Michel C. Anonymous HIV testing using home collection and telemedicine counseling. A multicenter evaluation. Arch Intern Med. 1997; 157:309–14.
42. Gallo D, George JR, Fitchen JH, Goldstein AS, Hindahl MS. Evaluation of a system using oral mucosal transudate for HIV-1 antibody screening and confirmatory testing. OraSure HIV Clinical Trials Group. JAMA. 1997;277:254–8.
43. Emmons W. Accuracy of oral specimen testing for human immunodeficiency virus. Am J Med. 1997; 102:15–20.
44. Emmons WW, Paparello SF, Decker CF, Sheffield JM, Lowe-Bey FH. A modified ELISA and western blot accurately determine anti-human immunodeficiency virus type 1 antibodies in oral fluids obtained with a special collecting device. J Infect Dis. 1995; 171:1406–10.
45. Taye B, Woldeamanuel Y, Kebede E. Diagnostic detection of human immunodeficincy virus type-1 antibodies in urine, Jimma Hospital, south west Ethiopa. Ethiop Med J. 2006;44:363–8.
46. Urnovitz HB, Sturge JC, Gottfried TD. Increased sensitivity of HIV-1 antibody detection. Nat Med. 1997;3:1258.
47. Food and Drug Administration. CAMBRIDGE BIOTECH HIV-1 WESTERN BLOT KIT. http://www.fda.gov/downloads/BiologicsBloodVaccines/UCM167227.pdf (1998). Accessed 14 Feb 2012.
48. Belec L, Matta M, Payan C, Tevi-Benissan C, Meillet D, Pillot J. Detection of seminal antibodies to human immunodeficiency virus in vaginal secretions after sexual intercourse: possible means of preventing the risk of human immunodeficiency virus transmission in a rape victim. J Med Virol. 1995;45: 113–6.
49. Lauritzen E, Lindhardt B. Antibodies against human immunodeficiency virus (HIV) detected in human sera by immunoblotting. In: Bjerrum OJ, Heegaard NH. Handbook of immunoblotting of protein. CRC Press, Inc. Boca Raton, FL, 1989;(2):117–131.
50. Belec L, Gresenguet G, Dragon MA, Meillet D, Pillot J. Detection of antibodies to human immunodeficiency virus in vaginal secretions by immunoglobulin G antibody capture enzyme-linked immunosorbent assay: application to detection of seminal antibodies after sexual intercourse. J Clin Microbiol. 1994;32:1249–55.
51. Constantine NT, Kabat W, Zhao RY. Update on the laboratory diagnosis and monitoring of HIV infection. Cell Res. 2005;15:870–6.
52. George JR, Rayfield MA, Phillips S, et al. Efficacies of US Food and Drug Administration-licensed HIV-1-screening enzyme immunoassays for detecting antibodies to HIV-2. AIDS. 1990;4:321–6.
53. O'Brien TR, George JR, Holmberg SD. Human immunodeficiency virus type 2 infection in the United States. Epidemiology, diagnosis, and public health implications. JAMA. 1992;267:2775–9.
54. Bachmann P, Beyer J, Brust S, et al. Multicentre study for diagnostic evaluation of an assay for simultaneous detection of antibodies to HIV-1, HIV-2 and HIV-1 subtype 0 (HIV-0). Infection. 1995;23: 322–33.
55. Proffitt MR, Yen-Lieberman B. Laboratory diagnosis of human immunodeficiency virus infection. Infect Dis Clin North Am. 1993;7:203–19.
56. Sheon AR, Wagner L, McElrath MJ, et al. Preventing discrimination against volunteers in prophylactic HIV vaccine trials: lessons from a phase II trial. J Acquir Immune Defic Syndr Hum Retrovirol. 1998;19:519–26.
57. Bylund DJ, Ziegner UH, Hooper DG. Review of testing for human immunodeficiency virus. Clin Lab Med. 1992;12:305–33.
58. Gurtler L. Difficulties and strategies of HIV diagnosis. Lancet. 1996;348:176–9.
59. Fanales-Belasio E, Raimondo M, Suligoi B, Butto S. HIV virology and pathogenetic mechanisms of infection: a brief overview. Ann Ist Super Sanita. 2010;46:5–14.
60. Brust S, Duttmann H, Feldner J, Gurtler L, Thorstensson R, Simon F. Shortening of the diagnostic window with a new combined HIV p24 antigen and anti-HIV-1/2/O screening test. J Virol Methods. 2000;90:153–65.
61. Abbott Inc. Abbott's ARCHITECT HIV Ag/Ab Combo assay. http://www.fda.gov/downloads/BiologicsBloodVaccines/BloodBloodProducts/ApprovedProducts/LicensedProductsBLAs/BloodDonorScreening/InfectiousDisease/UCM216309.pdf (2011). Accessed 25 Sept 2011.
62. BIO-RAD. Bio-Rad GS HIV-1 Ag/Ab Combo EIA. http://www.fda.gov/downloads/BiologicsBloodVaccines/BloodBloodProducts/ApprovedProducts/PremarketApprovalsPMAs/UCM266211.pdf (2011). Accessed 25 Sept 2011.
63. Pandori MW, Hackett Jr J, Louie B, et al. Assessment of the ability of a fourth-generation immunoassay for human immunodeficiency virus (HIV) antibody

and p24 antigen to detect both acute and recent HIV infections in a high-risk setting. J Clin Microbiol. 2009;47:2639–42.
64. Meier T, Knoll E, Henkes M, Enders G, Braun R. Evidence for a diagnostic window in fourth generation assays for HIV. J Clin Virol. 2001;23:113–6.
65. Centers for Disease Control (CDC). Interpretation and use of the Western blot assay for serodiagnostic of human immunodeficiency virus type 1 infections. MMWR Morb Mortal Wkly Rep. 1989;38:1–7.
66. Tebourski F, Slim A, Elgaaied A. The significance of combining World Health Organization and Center for Disease Control criteria to resolve indeterminate human immunodeficiency virus type-1 western blot results. Diagn Microbiol Infect Dis. 2004;48:59–61.
67. O'Gorman MR, Weber D, Landis SE, Schoenbach VJ, Mittal M, Folds JD. Interpretive criteria of the western blot assay for serodiagnosis of human immunodeficiency virus type 1 infection. Arch Pathol Lab Med. 1991;115:26–30.
68. Celum CL, Coombs RW, Jones M, et al. Risk factors for repeatedly reactive HIV-1 EIA and indeterminate western blots. A population-based case–control study. Arch Intern Med. 1994;154:1129–37.
69. Jackson JB, Balfour Jr HH. Practical diagnostic testing for human immunodeficiency virus. Clin Microbiol Rev. 1988;1:124–38.
70. Jaffe HW, Schochetman G. Group O human immunodeficiency virus-1 infections. Infect Dis Clin North Am. 1998;12:39–46.
71. Centers for Disease Control (CDC). Update: serologic tests for HIV-1 antibody—United States, 1988 and 1989. MMWR Morb Mortal Wkly Rep. 1990;39:380–3.
72. SANOCHEMIA Pharmazeutika. Fluorognost TM HIV-1 IFA. http://www.fluorognost.com/ (1992). Accessed on 14 Feb 2012.
73. Zoon K. Use of Fluorognost HIV-1 immunofluorescent assay (IFA): Memo from US FDA Center for Biologics Evaluation and Research to all registered plasma and blood establishments. 1992.
74. Food and Drug Administration. Licensed/approved HIV, HTLV and hepatitis tests. http://www.fda.gov/cber/products/testkits.htm (2009). Accessed on 14 Feb 2012.
75. Armington K. Intergrating rapid HIV testing into fast-paced private setting. http://www.prn.org/images/pdfs/54_armington_kevin.pdf (2005). Accessed 12 Feb 2012.
76. Centers for Medicare and Medicaid Services (CMS). The clinical laboratory improvement amendments of 1988. Health Care Financ Rev 1989;10:141–6.
77. Centers for Disease Control (CDC). Quality assurance guidelines for testing using rapid HIV antibody tests waived under the clinical laboratory improvement amendments of 1988. CDC; 2007.
78. Centers for Disease Control (CDC). CLIA certificate of waiver fact sheet. http://www.cdc.gov/hiv/topics/testing/resources/factsheets/roltCLIA.htm (2007). Accessed 14 Feb 2012.
79. Food and Drug Administration. Device classification. http://www.fda.gov/MedicalDevices/DeviceRegulationandGuidance/Overview/ClassifyYourDevice/default.htm (2009). Accessed 28 Feb 2012.
80. Flanigan T, Tashima KT. Diagnosis of acute HIV infection: it's time to get moving! Ann Intern Med. 2001;134:75–7.
81. Suligoi B, Raimondo M, Fanales-Belasio E, Butto S. The epidemic of HIV infection and AIDS, promotion of testing, and innovative strategies. Ann Ist Super Sanita. 2010;46:15–23.
82. Darko A, Kabat W, Constantine N, Zhao R. Update on the Diagnosis and Monitoring of HIV-1 Infection. HIV AIDS. 2007;2:20–23.
83. Albrecht H, Hoffmann C, Degen O, et al. Highly active antiretroviral therapy significantly improves the prognosis of patients with HIV-associated progressive multifocal leukoencephalopathy. AIDS. 1998;12:1149–54.
84. de Mendoza C, Soriano V, Perez-Olmeda M, Rodes B, Casas E, Gonzalez-Lahoz J. Different outcomes in patients achieving complete or partial viral load suppression on antiretroviral therapy. J Hum Virol. 1999;2:344–9.
85. Louie M, Louie L, Simor AE. The role of DNA amplification technology in the diagnosis of infectious diseases. CMAJ. 2000;163:301–9.
86. Chun TW, Stuyver L, Mizell SB, et al. Presence of an inducible HIV-1 latent reservoir during highly active antiretroviral therapy. Proc Natl Acad Sci USA. 1997;94:13193–7.
87. Finzi D, Blankson J, Siliciano JD, et al. Latent infection of CD4+ T cells provides a mechanism for lifelong persistence of HIV-1, even in patients on effective combination therapy. Nat Med. 1999;5:512–7.
88. Finzi D, Hermankova M, Pierson T, et al. Identification of a reservoir for HIV-1 in patients on highly active antiretroviral therapy. Science. 1997; 278:1295–300.
89. Christopherson C, Kidane Y, Conway B, Krowka J, Sheppard H, Kwok S. PCR-Based assay to quantify human immunodeficiency virus type 1 DNA in peripheral blood mononuclear cells. J Clin Microbiol. 2000;38:630–4.
90. Bennett JM, Kaye S, Berry N, Tedder RS. A quantitative PCR method for the assay of HIV-1 provirus load in peripheral blood mononuclear cells. J Virol Methods. 1999;83:11–20.
91. Guenthner PC, Hart CE. Quantitative, competitive PCR assay for HIV-1 using a microplate-based detection system. Biotechniques. 1998;24:810–6.
92. Izopet J, Tamalet C, Pasquier C, et al. Quantification of HIV-1 proviral DNA by a standardized colorimetric PCR-based assay. J Med Virol. 1998; 54:54–9.
93. Desire N, Dehee A, Schneider V, et al. Quantification of human immunodeficiency virus type 1 proviral load by a TaqMan real-time PCR assay. J Clin Microbiol. 2001;39:1303–10.

94. Yun Z, Fredriksson E, Sonnerborg A. Quantification of human immunodeficiency virus type 1 proviral DNA by the TaqMan real-time PCR assay. J Clin Microbiol. 2002;40:3883–4.
95. Zhao Y, Yu M, Miller JW, et al. Quantification of human immunodeficiency virus type 1 proviral DNA by using TaqMan technology. J Clin Microbiol. 2002;40:675–8.
96. Pillonel J, Laperche S. Trends in risk of transfusion-transmitted viral infections (HIV, HCV, HBV) in France between 1992 and 2003 and impact of nucleic acid testing (NAT). Euro Surveill. 2005;10:5–8.
97. Patel P, Mackellar D, Simmons P, et al. Detecting acute human immunodeficiency virus infection using 3 different screening immunoassays and nucleic acid amplification testing for human immunodeficiency virus RNA, 2006–2008. Arch Intern Med. 2010;170:66–74.
98. Biomerieux. Diagnosis and moitoring HIV infection. Marcy l'Etoile, France: Biomerieux sa; 2006.
99. Hughes MD, Johnson VA, Hirsch MS, et al. Monitoring plasma HIV-1 RNA levels in addition to CD4+ lymphocyte count improves assessment of antiretroviral therapeutic response. ACTG 241 Protocol Virology Substudy Team. Ann Intern Med. 1997;126:929–38.
100. Murray JS, Elashoff MR, Iacono-Connors LC, Cvetkovich TA, Struble KA. The use of plasma HIV RNA as a study endpoint in efficacy trials of antiretroviral drugs. AIDS. 1999;13:797–804.
101. Marschner IC, Collier AC, Coombs RW, et al. Use of changes in plasma levels of human immunodeficiency virus type 1 RNA to assess the clinical benefit of antiretroviral therapy. J Infect Dis. 1998;177: 40–7.
102. Thiebaut R, Morlat P, Jacqmin-Gadda H, et al. Clinical progression of HIV-1 infection according to the viral response during the first year of antiretroviral treatment. Groupe d'Epidemiologie du SIDA en Aquitaine (GECSA). AIDS. 2000;14:971–8.
103. Yeghiazarian T, Zhao Y, Read SE, et al. Quantification of human immunodeficiency virus type 1 RNA levels in plasma by using small-volume-format branched-DNA assays. J Clin Microbiol. 1998;36:2096–8.
104. Shingadia DZY. Mesurement of plasma viral RNA load of human immunodeficiency virus type 1 (HIV-1). Am Med Lab Int J Infect Dis. 1997;2:4–5.
105. Bartlett J. Serologic tests for the diagnosis of HIV infection. http://www.uptodate.com (2003). Accessed on 10 Sept 2012.
106. Finan JE, Zhao RY. From molecular diagnostics to personalized testing. Pharmacogenomics. 2007;8: 85–99.
107. Iweala OI. HIV diagnostic tests: an overview. Contraception. 2004;70:141–7.
108. Abbott Inc. Abbott HIV-1 viral load test approved by FDA for use on new m2000TM molecular diagnostics instrument. http://www.abbott.com/global/url/pressRelease/en_US/60.5:5/Press_Release_0460.htm (2007). Accessed 10 Sept 2010.
109. Birkenmeyer L, Armstrong AS. Preliminary evaluation of the ligase chain reaction for specific detection of Neisseria gonorrhoeae. J Clin Microbiol. 1992; 30:3089–94.
110. Walker GT, Fraiser MS, Schram JL, Little MC, Nadeau JG, Malinowski DP. Strand displacement amplification – an isothermal, in vitro DNA amplification technique. Nucleic Acids Res. 1992;20:1691–6.
111. Benjamin Jr WH, Smith KR, Waites KB. Ligase chain reaction. Methods Mol Biol. 2003;226: 135–50.
112. Angela Caliendo. Techniques and interpretation of HIV-1 RNA quantitation. http://www.uptodate.com/contents/techniques-and-interpretation-of-hiv-1-rna-quantitation#H14118823 (2008). Accessed 15 April 2012.
113. Roche Molecular Diagnostics. Cobas® TaqScreen MPX Test. http://www.fda.gov/downloads/BiologicsBloodVaccines/BloodBloodProducts/ApprovedProducts/LicensedProductsBLAs/BloodDonorScreening/InfectiousDisease/UCM176443.pdf (2009). Accessed 14 Feb 2012.
114. Drosten C, Panning M, Drexler JF, et al. Ultrasensitive monitoring of HIV-1 viral load by a low-cost real-time reverse transcription-PCR assay with internal control for the 5′ long terminal repeat domain. Clin Chem. 2006;52:1258–66.
115. Fiscus SA, Cheng B, Crowe SM, et al. HIV-1 viral load assays for resource-limited settings. PLoS Med. 2006;3:e417.
116. Malmsten A, Shao XW, Aperia K, et al. HIV-1 viral load determination based on reverse transcriptase activity recovered from human plasma. J Med Virol. 2003;71:347–59.
117. Malmsten A, Shao XW, Sjodahl S, et al. Improved HIV-1 viral load determination based on reverse transcriptase activity recovered from human plasma. J Med Virol. 2005;76:291–6.
118. Foley B. An overview of the molecular phylogeny of lent viruses. Los Alamos, NM: Los Alamos National Laboratory; 2000.
119. Robertson DL, Anderson JP, Bradac JA, et al. HIV-1 nomenclature proposal. Science. 2000;288:55–6.
120. Plantier JC, Leoz M, Dickerson JE, et al. A new human immunodeficiency virus derived from gorillas. Nat Med. 2009;15:871–2.
121. Los Alamos National Laboratory. HIV sequence database. http://www.hiv.lanl.gov (July 2009). Accessed 14 Jan 2012.
122. Connor RI, Korber BT, Graham BS, et al. Immunological and virological analyses of persons infected by human immunodeficiency virus type 1 while participating in trials of recombinant gp120 subunit vaccines. J Virol. 1998;72:1552–76.
123. McCutchan FE. Global epidemiology of HIV. J Med Virol. 2006;78 Suppl 1:S7–12.
124. Delwart EL, Orton S, Parekh B, Dobbs T, Clark K, Busch MP. Two percent of HIV-positive U.S. blood donors are infected with non-subtype B strains. AIDS Res Hum Retroviruses. 2003;19:1065–70.

125. Carr J, Flynn C, Maheshwari V, Blattner W, Zhao R. Detection of HIV-1 non-B subtype in the city of Baltimore and state of Maryland. Molecular characterization of viral epidemics, Vol. 1. 6th conference on retroviruses and opportunistic infections, 2009.
126. Lin HH, Gaschen BK, Collie M, et al. Genetic characterization of diverse HIV-1 strains in an immigrant population living in New York City. J Acquir Immune Defic Syndr. 2006;41:399–404.
127. Brennan CA, Stramer SL, Holzmayer V, et al. Identification of human immunodeficiency virus type 1 non-B subtypes and antiretroviral drug-resistant strains in United States blood donors. Transfusion. 2009;49:125–33.
128. Emery S, Bodrug S, Richardson BA, et al. Evaluation of performance of the Gen-Probe human immunodeficiency virus type 1 viral load assay using primary subtype A, C, and D isolates from Kenya. J Clin Microbiol. 2000;38:2688–95.
129. Chew CB, Herring BL, Zheng F, et al. Comparison of three commercial assays for the quantification of HIV-1 RNA in plasma from individuals infected with different HIV-1 subtypes. J Clin Virol. 1999; 14:87–94.
130. Parekh B, Phillips S, Granade TC, Baggs J, Hu DJ, Respess R. Impact of HIV type 1 subtype variation on viral RNA quantitation. AIDS Res Hum Retroviruses. 1999;15:133–42.
131. Gobbers E, Fransen K, Oosterlaken T, et al. Reactivity and amplification efficiency of the NASBA HIV-1 RNA amplification system with regard to different HIV-1 subtypes. J Virol Methods. 1997;66:293–301.
132. Apetrei C, Loussert-Ajaka I, Descamps D, et al. Lack of screening test sensitivity during HIV-1 non-subtype B seroconversions. AIDS. 1996;10:F57–60.
133. Schable C, Zekeng L, Pau CP, et al. Sensitivity of United States HIV antibody tests for detection of HIV-1 group O infections. Lancet. 1994;344: 1333–4.
134. Phillips S, Granade TC, Pau CP, Candal D, Hu DJ, Parekh BS. Diagnosis of human immunodeficiency virus type 1 infection with different subtypes using rapid tests. Clin Diagn Lab Immunol. 2000;7: 698–9.
135. Zhang M, Versalovic J. HIV update. Diagnostic tests and markers of disease progression and response to therapy. Am J Clin Pathol. 2002;118(Suppl):S26–32.
136. Boni J, Opravil M, Tomasik Z, et al. Simple monitoring of antiretroviral therapy with a signal-amplification-boosted HIV-1 p24 antigen assay with heat-denatured plasma. AIDS. 1997;11:F47–52.
137. Nishanian P, Huskins KR, Stehn S, Detels R, Fahey JL. A simple method for improved assay demonstrates that HIV p24 antigen is present as immune complexes in most sera from HIV-infected individuals. J Infect Dis. 1990;162:21–8.
138. Schupbach J, Boni J. Quantitative and sensitive detection of immune-complexed and free HIV antigen after boiling of serum. J Virol Methods. 1993;43: 247–56.
139. Schupbach J, Flepp M, Pontelli D, Tomasik Z, Luthy R, Boni J. Heat-mediated immune complex dissociation and enzyme-linked immunosorbent assay signal amplification render p24 antigen detection in plasma as sensitive as HIV-1 RNA detection by polymerase chain reaction. AIDS. 1996;10:1085–90.
140. Barletta JM, Edelman DC, Constantine NT. Lowering the detection limits of HIV-1 viral load using real-time immuno-PCR for HIV-1 p24 antigen. Am J Clin Pathol. 2004;122:20–7.
141. Sturmer M, Berger A, Preiser W. HIV-1 genotyping: comparison of two commercially available assays. Expert Rev Mol Diagn. 2004;4:281–91.
142. Gulick RM, Mellors JW, Havlir D, et al. Treatment with indinavir, zidovudine, and lamivudine in adults with human immunodeficiency virus infection and prior antiretroviral therapy. N Engl J Med. 1997;337: 734–9.
143. Gulick RM, Mellors JW, Havlir D, et al. 3-Year suppression of HIV viremia with indinavir, zidovudine, and lamivudine. Ann Intern Med. 2000;133:35–9.
144. Hammer SM, Squires KE, Hughes MD, et al. A controlled trial of two nucleoside analogues plus indinavir in persons with human immunodeficiency virus infection and CD4 cell counts of 200 per cubic millimeter or less. AIDS Clinical Trials Group 320 Study Team. N Engl J Med. 1997;337:725–33.
145. Staszewski S, Morales-Ramirez J, Tashima KT, et al. Efavirenz plus zidovudine and lamivudine, efavirenz plus indinavir, and indinavir plus zidovudine and lamivudine in the treatment of HIV-1 infection in adults. Study 006 Team. N Engl J Med. 1999;341: 1865–73.
146. Kuritzkes DR, Grant RM, Feorino P, et al. Performance characteristics of the TRUGENE HIV-1 genotyping kit and the opengene DNA sequencing system. J Clin Microbiol. 2003;41: 1594–9.
147. Durant J, Clevenbergh P, Halfon P, et al. Drug-resistance genotyping in HIV-1 therapy: the VIRADAPT randomised controlled trial. Lancet. 1999;353:2195–9.
148. Tural C, Ruiz L, Holtzer C, et al. Clinical utility of HIV-1 genotyping and expert advice: the Havana trial. AIDS. 2002;16:209–18.
149. Panel on Antiretroviral Guidelines for Adults and Adolescents. Guidelines for the use of antiretroviral agents in HIV-1-infected adults and adolescents. http://www.aidsinfo.nih.gov/ContentFiles/AdultandAdolescentGL.pdf (27 Mar 2012). Accessed 15 April 2012.
150. Hirsch MS, Brun-Vezinet F, D'Aquila RT, et al. Antiretroviral drug resistance testing in adult HIV-1 infection: recommendations of an International AIDS Society-USA Panel. JAMA. 2000;283: 2417–26.
151. The EuroGuidelines Group for HIV Resistance. Clinical and laboratory guidelines for the use of

HIV-1 drug resistance testing as part of treatment management: recommendations for the European setting. The EuroGUidelines Group for HIV resistance. AIDS. 2001;15:309–20.
152. HHS panel on antiretroviral guidelines for adults and adolescents. Guidelines for the use of antiretroviral agents in HIV-1 infected adults and adolescents, Vol. 2011. Department of Health and Human Services; 2011. pp. 1–139.
153. MacArthur RD. Understanding HIV, phenotypic resistance testing: usefulness in managing treatment-experienced patients. AIDS Rev. 2009;11:223–30.
154. Perez-Elias MJ, Garcia-Arota I, Munoz V, et al. Phenotype or virtual phenotype for choosing antiretroviral therapy after failure: a prospective, randomized study. Antivir Ther. 2003;8:577–84.
155. King MS, Rode R, Cohen-Codar I, et al. Predictive genotypic algorithm for virologic response to lopinavir-ritonavir in protease inhibitor-experienced patients. Antimicrob Agents Chemother. 2007;51: 3067–74.
156. Sturmer M, Doerr HW, Staszewski S, Preiser W. Comparison of nine resistance interpretation systems for HIV-1 genotyping. Antivir Ther. 2003;8: 239–44.
157. Zolopa AR, Shafer RW, Warford A, et al. HIV-1 genotypic resistance patterns predict response to saquinavir-ritonavir therapy in patients in whom previous protease inhibitor therapy had failed. Ann Intern Med. 1999;131:813–21.
158. Haupts S, Ledergerber B, Boni J, et al. Impact of genotypic resistance testing on selection of salvage regimen in clinical practice. Antivir Ther. 2003;8: 443–54.
159. Food and Drug Administration. BK000038 Letter. http://www.fda.gov/BiologicsBloodVaccines/Blood BloodProducts/ApprovedProducts/Substantially Equivalent510kDeviceInformation/ucm088966.htm (2001). Accessed 28 Feb 2012.
160. FDA. Premarket notification (510k), 2010. Accessed 28 Feb 2012. http://www.fda.gov/MedicalDevices/DeviceRegulationandGuidance/HowtoMarketYour Device/PremarketSubmissions/PremarketNotification 510k/default.htm
161. Ghys PD, Zaba B, Prins M. Survival and mortality of people infected with HIV in low and middle income countries: results from the extended ALPHA network. AIDS. 2007;21 Suppl 6:S1–4.
162. Alvarez-Munoz MT, Zaragoza-Rodriguez S, Rojas-Montes O, et al. High correlation of human immunodeficiency virus type-1 viral load measured in dried-blood spot samples and in plasma under different storage conditions. Arch Med Res. 2005;36: 382–6.
163. Brambilla D, Jennings C, Aldrovandi G, et al. Multicenter evaluation of use of dried blood and plasma spot specimens in quantitative assays for human immunodeficiency virus RNA: measurement, precision, and RNA stability. J Clin Microbiol. 2003;41:1888–93.
164. Mwaba P, Cassol S, Nunn A, et al. Whole blood versus plasma spots for measurement of HIV-1 viral load in HIV-infected African patients. Lancet. 2003;362:2067–8.
165. Marconi A, Balestrieri M, Comastri G, et al. Evaluation of the Abbott Real-Time HIV-1 quantitative assay with dried blood spot specimens. Clin Microbiol Infect. 2009;15:93–7.
166. Lew J, Reichelderfer P, Fowler M, et al. Determinations of levels of human immunodeficiency virus type 1 RNA in plasma: reassessment of parameters affecting assay outcome. TUBE Meeting Workshop Attendees. Technology utilization for HIV-1 blood evaluation and standardization in pediatrics. J Clin Microbiol. 1998;36:1471–9.
167. Scott L. Dried blood spot (DBS) HIV viral load testing using the Abbott real-time HIV-1 assay, Fourth South African AIDS Conference, Durban, South Africa, 2009.
168. Katabira ET, Oelrichs RB. Scaling up antiretroviral treatment in resource-limited settings: successes and challenges. AIDS. 2007;21 Suppl 4:S5–10.
169. Ayele W, Schuurman R, Messele T, et al. Use of dried spots of whole blood, plasma, and mother's milk collected on filter paper for measurement of human immunodeficiency virus type 1 burden. J Clin Microbiol. 2007;45:891–6.
170. Fiscus SA, Brambilla D, Grosso L, Schock J, Cronin M. Quantitation of human immunodeficiency virus type 1 RNA in plasma by using blood dried on filter paper. J Clin Microbiol. 1998;36:258–60.
171. Kane CT, Ndiaye HD, Diallo S, et al. Quantitation of HIV-1 RNA in dried blood spots by the real-time NucliSENS EasyQ HIV-1 assay in Senegal. J Virol Methods. 2008;148:291–5.
172. Garrido C, Zahonero N, Corral A, Arredondo M, Soriano V, de Mendoza C. Correlation between human immunodeficiency virus type 1 (HIV-1) RNA measurements obtained with dried blood spots and those obtained with plasma by use of Nuclisens EasyQ HIV-1 and Abbott RealTime HIV load tests. J Clin Microbiol. 2009;47:1031–6.
173. Gonzalez E, Kulkarni H, Bolivar H, et al. The influence of CCL3L1 gene-containing segmental duplications on HIV-1/AIDS susceptibility. Science. 2005;307:1434–40.
174. Kulkarni H, Agan BK, Marconi VC, et al. CCL3L1-CCR5 genotype improves the assessment of AIDS risk in HIV-1-infected individuals. PLoS One. 2008;3:e3165.
175. Mallal S, Nolan D, Witt C, et al. Association between presence of HLA-B*5701, HLA-DR7, and HLA-DQ3 and hypersensitivity to HIV-1 reverse-transcriptase inhibitor abacavir. Lancet. 2002;359:727–32.
176. Hetherington S, Hughes AR, Mosteller M, et al. Genetic variations in HLA-B region and hypersensitivity reactions to abacavir. Lancet. 2002;359:1121–2.
177. Rauch A, Nolan D, Martin A, McKinnon E, Almeida C, Mallal S. Prospective genetic screening decreases

the incidence of abacavir hypersensitivity reactions in the Western Australian HIV cohort study. Clin Infect Dis. 2006;43:99–102.

178. Phillips E, Mallal S. Drug hypersensitivity in HIV. Curr Opin Allergy Clin Immunol. 2007;7:324–30.

179. Malla S, Phillips E, Carosi G, et al. PREDICT-1:a novel randomised prospective study to determine the clinical utility of HLA-B*5701 screening to reduce abacavir hypersensitivity in HIV-1 infected subjects (study CNA106030), Program and abstracts of the 4th international AIDS society conference on HIV pathogenesis. Treatment and prevention, Sidney, Australia, July 22–25, 2007.

180. Saag M, Balu R, Brachman P, et al. High sensitivity of HLA-B*5701 in whites and blacks in immunologically-confirmed cases of abacavir hypersensitiviity, Program and abstracts of the 4th international AIDS society conference on HIV pathogenesis. treatment and prevention, Sidney, Australia, July 22–25, 2007.

181. Fischl MAGS, Clumeck N, Peters B, Rubio R, Gould J, Boone G, West M, Spreen B, Lafon S. Ziagen (Abacavir, ABC, 1592) combines with 3TC and ZDV is highlly effective and durable through 48 weeks in HIV-1 infected antiretroviraal-therapy-naive subjects (CNA3003). 6th conference on Retroviruses and opportunistiic infections, Chicago, IL, January 31–February 4, 1999.

182. Nagle M. HIV therapy leads way in personalized medicine. http://www.drugresearcher.com/Emerging-targets/HIV-therapy-leads-way-in-personalised-medicine (Aug 2007). Accessed 10 Sept 2010.

Detection of Herpes Simplex Virus in Cerebrospinal Fluid Using Real-Time PCR

7

Thomas F. Smith, Mark J. Espy, and Matthew J. Binnicker

Background

Herpes simplex virus (HSV) is the most common, recognized cause of sporadic and severe encephalitis in the USA. The virus is estimated to account for at least 10–20 % of all viral encephalitis occurring in patients of all ages [30, 32, 57]. It is also important to underscore the worldwide impact of HSV infections in patients with superficial and systemic disease within every major organ system in both normal and immunocompromised hosts. Furthermore, this virus is usually the most frequent agent recovered in diagnostic laboratories from a variety of specimens using conventional (tube cell cultures) and rapid shell vial culture methods [18, 47]. Approximately 90 % of adults are seropositive for HSV, which is consistent with studies showing the detection of the viral genome in the trigeminal ganglia of 85–95 % of unselected autopsy cases [25]. Despite the high seroprevalence of HSV, the virus is rarely recovered from cerebrospinal fluid (CSF) specimens in viral culture, and this has been a major technical obstacle for the diagnosis of central nervous system (CNS) disease caused by this virus. Of 425 viral isolates recovered from CSF at the Mayo Clinic over a 12-year period (1984–1996), only 9 (2 %) were HSV [52].

The two genotypes of HSV (HSV-1, HSV-2) are members of the herpes virus family, along with varicella-zoster virus (VZV), human herpes viruses 6 and 7 (HHV-6 and HHV-7), cytomegalovirus (CMV), Epstein–Barr virus (EBV), and human herpes virus 8 [30, 57]. All herpes viruses are morphologically similar, although HSV types 1 and 2 are serologically and genetically unique based on a sequence homology of approximately 50 %. These double-stranded, linear DNA-containing viruses all produce latent infections in target host cells after primary infection and are generally reactivated by physical, metabolic changes, or altered immunosuppressive conditions [40].

Several target sequences of the HSV genome have been utilized by molecular assays designed to specifically detect signature nucleotides of the virus. These include several loci throughout the unique long (U_L) and unique short (U_S) regions of the 152-kb genome of HSV. Specific target regions include the thymidine kinase, DNA polymerase, DNA binding protein, and glycoprotein B and D genes [18, 19, 52].

Application of molecular methods, specifically polymerase chain reaction (PCR), for the detection of HSV DNA in CSF was a significant breakthrough that has changed the diagnostic focus and landscape of clinical virology laboratories worldwide [37].

T.F. Smith, Ph.D. • M.J. Espy, M.S.
M.J. Binnicker, Ph.D. (✉)
Division of Clinical Microbiology, Department of Laboratory Medicine and Pathology, Mayo Clinic, 200 First Street SW Hilton 4-54, Rochester, MN 55906, USA
e-mail: binnicker.matthew@mayo.edu

W.E. Highsmith Jr. (ed.), *Molecular Diagnostics: 12 Tests That Changed Everything*, Molecular and Translational Medicine, DOI 10.1007/978-1-4614-8127-0_7,

Over 20 years ago, Rowley et al. predicted the significance of these findings based on the sensitivity and specificity of their results [37]. Interestingly, a case report of HSV encephalitis using PCR technology to establish the laboratory diagnosis of this infection was published by Powell et al. in the same issue of the *Lancet* as the landmark publication of Rowley [34]. Subsequently, the growing implementation of PCR for the detection of HSV in CSF has confirmed the utility of this technology for diagnosing HSV CNS disease, rather than relying on invasive brain biopsy procedures and subsequent cell culture isolation for laboratory diagnosis of HSV infection [30, 37, 52]. In addition, several subsequent studies have corroborated the performance characteristics of molecular technology for the rapid and sensitive detection of HSV DNA in CSF [4, 14, 30, 39].

In this chapter, we review the expansive literature of the last two decades, which provides growing support for the routine use of molecular methods (e.g., PCR) for the detection of HSV DNA from CSF samples. In total, these studies have provided a data-driven alternative to the collection of temporal lobe brain biopsy specimens for inoculation of cell cultures. The detection of HSV DNA from CSF has served as a prototypic model assay for expansion of this technology to other pathogens and specimen types that are commonly encountered in clinical microbiology laboratories [19].

Clinical Applications

Before the laboratory diagnosis of HSV infections by molecular amplification technology, CNS disease caused by this virus was commonly diagnosed on clinical grounds. The presentation was often described as focal febrile encephalitis mainly involving the temporal lobes of the brain. Acute necrotizing encephalitis generally localizes in the orbitofrontal and temporal lobes with involvement of the cingulate and insular cortex; however, CNS disease caused by HSV in neonates tends to produce a more diffuse pathology [25]. Acute CNS onset is often accompanied by headache, altered mental status, focal neurological signs, and seizures [22, 27, 54, 57]. Without appropriate treatment, mortality may be as high as 70 % [22]. HSV type 1 has been predominantly associated with focal and severe necrotizing encephalitis, whereas type 2 has been predominant in infants, in patients with Mollaret's meningitis (benign recurrent aseptic meningitis), and in chronic atypical encephalitis presenting with headache and cognitive changes without focal neurological findings [1, 25].

Prior to molecular diagnostic methods, the diagnosis of HSV CNS disease was assessed by a typical clinical presentation combined with imaging techniques, abnormal cytologic findings, the presence of intrathecal antibodies to HSV, and growth of the virus in cell cultures from brain biopsy specimens. Magnetic resonance imaging provides the most sensitive imaging method for detecting early brain lesions; however, imaging techniques in general have not provided acceptable specificity for the routine laboratory diagnosis of CNS disease caused by HSV [3, 5, 22]. Detection of intrathecal antibodies (standardized by concomitant measurement of albumin) is not successful in the early acute phase of CNS disease caused by HSV; generally, these antibodies can only be reliably detected after 2–3 weeks into the clinical course [15].

Hematologic findings associated with HSV CNS disease typically have a profile of lymphocytic pleocytosis (10–200 cells/mm^3), normal glucose, and increased proteins (0.6–6 g/l) [25, 46]. Recovery of HSV from brain tissue has been considered the "gold standard" laboratory test for HSV CNS disease; however, the invasive surgical procedure is controversial and rarely used for this purpose [52].

PCR amplification of HSV DNA in CSF has been recognized for several years as the reference standard assay for the laboratory diagnosis of CNS disease associated with HSV infection. This molecular technology can detect HSV DNA in CSF specimens in approximately 95 % of cases [13]. False-negative results are most likely to occur early in the disease course (during the first 72 h), especially in patients with recurrent HSV CNS infections [2, 28]. Typically, HSV DNA is only detectable for approximately 10–14 days following the onset of clinical symptoms. Nevertheless, persistent DNA in CSF can be

Table 7.1 Percent of cerebrospinal fluid samples testing positive for herpes simplex virus type 1 or 2 by real-time PCR analysis or viral culture at Mayo Clinic, 2005–2011

		Number (%) CSF with result of			
	No. tested	Negative[a]	HSV-1	HSV-2	Indeterminate[b]
Viral culture	22,681	22,673 (99.9)	1 (0.004)	7 (0.03)	N.A.
Real-time PCR	86,262	83,833 (97.2)	604 (0.7)	1,721 (2.0)	104 (0.1)

[a]Number of CSF testing negative for HSV type 1 or 2 by viral culture or real-time PCR
[b]Positive for herpes simplex virus nucleic acid, but unable to distinguish between types 1 and 2
CSF cerebrospinal fluid, *HSV-1* herpes simplex virus type 1, *HSV-2* herpes simplex virus type 2, *N.A.* not applicable

present in immunosuppressed patients and those with chronic underlying diseases [41].

PCR testing is sensitive, specific, and importantly, the diagnostic results can be available within a day following receipt of the specimen into the laboratory. Importantly, a past study performed in our laboratory tested 500 specimens (288 genital, 192 dermal, and 20 ocular) by real-time PCR and compared the results with routine cell culture for the identification of HSV. We found that PCR was 23.1 % more sensitive compared to cell culture for the routine laboratory detection of non-CNS clinical specimens [18]. We have used PCR for the diagnosis of both CNS (since 1992) and mucocutaneous HSV infections (since 2000). Interestingly, a review of all CSF samples submitted to our laboratory for viral culture (n=22,681) and/or HSV PCR (n=86,262) between 2005 and 2011 showed a higher overall percent positive rate by PCR (2.8 %) compared to viral culture (0.04 %). Furthermore, the implementation of PCR at our institution has increased the detection of HSV-2 CNS disease by nearly 100-fold compared to viral culture over the past 6 years (2.0 % versus 0.03 %) (Table 7.1). Due to these and other data, PCR has been recognized as the gold standard laboratory test for the diagnosis of all HSV infections for several years [16, 18, 19, 53].

Methodology

In this section, we will discuss a variety of methods used by clinical laboratories to facilitate the detection of HSV DNA in CSF. A critical pre-analytical step for PCR assays is nucleic acid extraction. Proper extraction should isolate and concentrate the nucleic acid while providing a product free of inhibitors. Extraction of clinical specimens can be carried out by either manual or automated methods.

A number of commercial manufacturers have developed manual extraction kits for use in the clinical laboratory. These kits vary as to method, cost, and time for extraction. This variability allows the clinical laboratory the flexibility to choose the kit that best suits its needs. The reagents used in manual extraction kits are non-corrosive and safe to use by the clinical laboratory, and they are also generally inexpensive and easy to use. The limitations to manual extraction kits are that these methods often require multiple manipulations, which can increase the potential for contamination of target DNA to other specimens. Further, manual extraction is a laborious, time-consuming process, which requires extensive training of laboratory personnel to achieve consistency and ensure reproducible results.

To overcome many of these limitations, automated extraction instruments have been developed and manufactured by a number of different companies. Similar to manual extraction methods, automated systems vary in method, cost, and time required for extraction. Additionally, they can also vary as to specimen capacity and size of the instrument (footprint). Studies indicate that automated extraction is equivalent, and in some instances superior, to manual methods [17]. Automated extraction systems are designed to process large numbers of samples in a consistent manner and keep sample manipulation to a minimum, reducing the potential for cross contamination of samples. Automated systems are typically walkaway, and do not require constant attention, resulting in recovery of nucleic acids which is consistent and reproducible. Potential drawbacks to the use of automated systems include cost (both for the instrument and the disposables required by the instrument) and space requirements needed to accommodate the footprint of the instrument. Certain companies (e.g., Roche Applied Sciences, Qiagen) have manufactured smaller versions of their automated extractors. While these smaller versions extract fewer samples, they are also less expensive and have a smaller footprint than the parent instrument.

Our current practice at the Mayo Clinic is to extract all CSF samples using the Roche MagNA Pure (Roche Diagnostics, Indianapolis, IN) using a total nucleic acid extraction kit (Roche). While this extraction method works well for the majority of CSF specimens, we also encounter CSF specimens with inadequate sample volume (e.g., <200 μl). For these low volume CSF specimens, the sample is diluted to a total volume of 200 μl with media followed by MagNA Pure extraction. Recently, we compared processing low volume CSF specimens by our current method (MagNA Pure extraction of diluted CSF) to an experimental protocol whereby 50 μl of CSF is heated at 100 °C for 5 min followed by direct PCR analysis for HSV DNA. This study demonstrated that the heating method yielded sensitive detection of HSV in low volume CSF specimens and showed superior performance characteristics compared to extracting DNA by the MagNA Pure from diluted CSF [60].

Detection Technologies and Platforms

Real-time PCR detection of HSV DNA in CSF is based on a combination of probes and real-time PCR instruments. There are a variety of detection technologies that have been developed, with each demonstrating certain advantages and limitations.

SYBR Green

SYBR Green is an asymmetrical cyanine dye which is used as a nucleic acid stain. It preferentially binds to double-stranded DNA and is used to detect the accumulation of any double-stranded DNA product. While SYBR Green provides for sensitive detection of target nucleic acid, it is not specific and, therefore, is not routinely used in the clinical diagnostic laboratory. Because of the lack of specificity, SYBR Green is mainly used in screening assays and in the early stages of development of real-time PCR tests.

5′ Nuclease (TaqMan) Probes

5′ nuclease probes, which are commonly referred to as TaqMan probes, were the first real-time fluorescent probes developed. The probe itself is a short oligonucleotide sequence that contains a 5′ fluorescent dye and a 3′ quenching dye. To generate a fluorescent signal, the probe must first bind to a complementary target strand of DNA at 60 °C. Second, Taq polymerase must cleave the 5′ end of the probe separating the fluorescent dye from the quenching dye, allowing generation of a detectable signal. Typically, TaqMan probes are used to detect a single target; however, differentiation of a single nucleotide polymorphism from the wild-type sequence is possible using this technology. This requires the use of a second probe with a sequence complementary to the polymorphism and a fluorescent dye with a different emission spectrum than that of the wild-type probe [19].

Eclipse Probes

Eclipse probes are similar to TaqMan probes in that both are labeled with a fluorescent dye and a quenching molecule. However, they differ in the orientation of the probe and quencher molecules with the fluorescent dye being attached to the 3′ end and the quencher on the 5′ end in eclipse probes. A minor groove-binding molecule (MGB) is also incorporated at the 5′ end next to the quencher molecule. The MGB molecule stabilizes the binding between the probe and target molecule and blocks probe hydrolysis. Since the Eclipse probe is not destroyed it is available for further analysis such as confirming the amplified product by its specific melting temperature [50].

Molecular Beacons

Molecular beacons are similar to TaqMan probes in that they have a fluorescent dye on the 5′ end and a quencher dye on the 3′ end of the probe, but they are designed not to be cleaved by the 5′ nuclease activity of Taq polymerase. A region at each end of the molecular beacon probe is complementary to itself, and at low temperatures, the ends anneal creating a hairpin structure. This hairpin structure brings the two dyes in close proximity, quenching the fluorescence from the reporter dye. The probe has a central region which is complementary to the target DNA. At high temperatures the probe and target become single stranded. As the temperature is lowered, the central complementary region of the probe binds to the target nucleic acid. This binding causes the hairpin structure to open, thereby separating the fluorescent dye from the quenching dye and allowing detection of a light signal from the reporter dye. As with TaqMan probes, molecular beacons typically detect a single target; however, by using multiple beacon probes with different reporter dyes single nucleotide polymorphisms can be detected [19].

Scorpion Probes

Scorpion probes have a hairpin structure similar to molecular beacons with a reporter dye on the 5′ end; however, unlike molecular beacons, the quencher dye is directly linked to the 5′ end of a PCR primer via a blocker molecule. This allows the scorpion probe to serve simultaneously as a PCR primer and probe. During PCR, the primer is extended and the complementary target strand is synthesized. The hairpin loop unfolds and the probe hybridizes to the newly synthesized target sequence. The reporter dye is no longer in proximity to the quencher dye generating a fluorescent signal. Because the primer and probe are incorporated as a single molecule, generation of a fluorescent signal is essentially instantaneous providing stronger signals and shorter reaction times [8].

FRET Hybridization Probes

FRET hybridization probes are two DNA probes designed to anneal in close proximity to each other (e.g., within several base pairs). The first probe has a fluorescent dye attached to its 3′ end and the second probe has an acceptor dye attached to its 5′ end. As both probes anneal to their target sequence, fluorescence from the 3′ dye is absorbed by the acceptor dye on the 5′ end of the second probe. The second dye is excited and emits light at a third wavelength, which serves as the detection signal. The 3′ end of the second probe is phosphorylated so that it can't be used as a primer by Taq polymerase during PCR amplification. FRET hybridization probes allow melting curve analysis of the amplification product. A single nucleotide polymorphism in the target DNA under a FRET hybridization probe will generate a signal, but the melting curve will display a lower melting temperature than that of the wild-type control. This allows for differentiation of HSV types 1 and 2, due to minor base pair differences in the region of the DNA targeted by the probes. FRET hybridization probes and molecular beacons are recycled in each round of the PCR cycle. This is in contrast to TaqMan probes which are destroyed with each round of PCR amplification [19]. Several examples of real-time PCR assays designed to detect HSV in CSF samples are listed in Table 7.2.

Real-Time PCR Instruments

Real-time PCR instruments perform two critical functions (1) they amplify nucleic acids and (2) detect signal generated by target-specific probes. The usual considerations for choosing a real-time instrument include cost (instrument, disposables), footprint, maintenance, and service. Other considerations can include the volume of samples tested, turnaround time, software (result

Table 7.2 Examples of real-time PCR assays developed for the detection of HSV types 1 and 2 in cerebrospinal fluid

Target	Probe technology	Platform	Sensitivity/specificity (%)	Reference
DNA polymerase	TaqMan	Roche LC	91/95	[26]
DNA polymerase	FRET	Roche LC	100/100	[23]
Glycoprotein G	Eclipse	ABI HT9700	100/100	[50]
Glycoprotein G	SYBR Green	Roche LC	91/84	[20]

LC LightCycler, *FRET* fluorescence energy transfer

analysis), and probe detection formats. All real-time instruments support all or some of the dyes used for TaqMan probes and molecular beacons; however, only the Roche LightCycler supports FRET hybridization probe detection with melting curve analysis. Real-time instruments can be divided into high and low capacity instruments. High capacity instruments can amplify up to 96 specimens at one time and are particularly useful for laboratories that test large numbers of specimens. A significant drawback to high capacity instruments is that they often have slower thermocycling parameters compared to lower capacity instruments due to the use of solid-phase material (heating block principle) for heat conductance. Low capacity instruments test fewer samples, but typically yield faster thermocycling (compared to high throughput platforms), which may give the clinical laboratory greater flexibility for real-time PCR testing. Some instruments use specialized reaction vessels (e.g., Cepheid SmartCycler, Roche LightCycler, and FOCUS integrated cycler). These vessels aid in rapid heat transfer and provide more rapid thermocycling. In addition, several manufacturers have developed analyte-specific reagents (ASRs), which can be used in conjunction with their real-time PCR instruments (Cepheid, FOCUS, Roche Diagnostics). The commercial availability of these reagents for use with the manufacturer's real-time PCR instruments makes it considerably easier for clinical laboratories to adapt real-time PCR platforms into their workflow. This has allowed for real-time PCR technology to be rapidly evaluated and implemented for the detection of HSV in clinical samples, including CSF.

Standard Reagents

The use of standard reagents (FDA-approved assays) helps to ensure continuity and consistency among clinical laboratories by decreasing variability in testing protocols and reagents used. Unfortunately, FDA-approved assays for detecting HSV DNA in CSF specimens do not currently exist. While ASR reagents are commercially available (Roche Diagnostics, Cepheid, FOCUS Diagnostics) and have demonstrated excellent sensitivity, they are manufactured by different companies and vary as to target, type of probe, and detection platform. Laboratories that use the same ASR reagents can benchmark results with each other; however, accurate comparison of results between laboratories using different ASR reagents is not possible, as the results can vary significantly depending on the target and detection platform that is utilized.

Regulatory Challenges

As noted in the sections above, the vast majority of molecular tests for the detection and typing of HSV from clinical samples often use ASR reagents and are categorized as laboratory developed tests (LDTs). These assays utilize a diverse array of target genes, amplification platforms, and detection technologies [4, 16, 20]. Laboratory developed tests require clinical laboratories to complete independent validation studies to demonstrate that the performance characteristics of the assay are acceptable prior to implementing the assay for routine testing. In May 2010, EraGen Bioscience (Madison, WI) received FDA clearance for their MultiCode® HSV 1&2 kit. This was the first FDA-cleared, molecular PCR test for the qualitative detection and typing of HSV 1 and 2. This represented a significant advance in the diagnosis of HSV infection by providing a FDA-cleared, rapid (<4 h turnaround time), and sensitive molecular approach. However, the EraGen MultiCode HSV assay was only cleared for testing vaginal lesion swab specimens from symptomatic female patients. Importantly, the device is not FDA cleared for use with CSF samples or clinical specimens other than vaginal lesions. Therefore, clinical laboratories that test CSF are currently required to validate the assay as an FDA-modified test, or LDT. To this point, Selvaraju et al. performed an evaluation of the EraGen MultiCode assay using CSF samples to determine the performance characteristics of the assay for this sample type. This group found the sensitivity and specificity of the EraGen assay to be 100 % (25/25) and 100 % (43/43), respectively, using CSF samples that were known to be positive ($n=25$) or negative ($n=43$) for HSV type 1 or 2. In addition, they demonstrated that the analytical sensitivity of the assay was approximately 10^1 copies/reaction [44].

In March 2011, Becton Dickinson (BD; Franklin Lakes, NJ) was the second to receive FDA clearance for their BD ProbeTec™ HSV Q^x assay, which uses strand displacement amplification (SDA) technology. This was the first fully automated HSV molecular assay to be FDA cleared, meaning that clinical laboratories could potentially increase throughput and decrease the turnaround time of results. However, the BD ProbeTec HSV test was FDA cleared for only clinician-collected, external anogenital specimens. Therefore, similar to the EraGen HSV test, clinical laboratories using the BD assay for CSF testing are required to complete extensive validation studies to demonstrate the accuracy of this assay on any non-FDA-cleared sample types.

The lack of FDA-cleared assays for a particular analyte poses a unique set of challenges to clinical laboratories, especially for (1) sample types that are difficult to obtain and (2) disorders or infections that are relatively rare. This is especially true for the development and validation of molecular tests for the detection of HSV in CSF. The Clinical Laboratory Improvement Amendments (CLIA) of 1988 require that laboratories performing FDA-modified tests, or LDTs, validate the following performance characteristics prior to implementing the test (1) accuracy, (2) precision, (3) reference range, (4) reportable range, (5) analytical sensitivity, and (6) analytical specificity [11]. These validation requirements, which are enforced by the Centers for Medicare & Medicaid Services (CMS) and reviewed by accrediting agencies, such as the College of American Pathologists (CAP) and the New York State (NYS) Department of Health, can be challenging for clinical laboratories to complete. The CAP Molecular Pathology Checklist states that laboratories should complete validation studies "with an adequate number and representative (reasonable) distribution of samples for each type of specimen expected for the assay" [9]. Furthermore, CAP requires that "the results of each validation study are compared to another valid assay, such as comparison to another test method or specimen exchange with a laboratory performing the same type of test" [10]. While meeting these requirements is essential to ensuring the accuracy of any test, it can be very challenging for clinical labs to validate HSV PCR tests using CSF samples due to the (1) the lack of a standardized reference method, (2) the difficulty in obtaining CSF specimens, and (3) the low prevalence of positive CSF samples [57].

The NYS Department of Health also provides validation guidelines for clinical labs developing nucleic acid amplification tests (NAATs). These guidelines recommend the incorporation of positive and negative lysis/extraction controls into the assay, as well as an inhibition control to ensure that patient samples are free of amplification inhibitors. If an inhibition control is not incorporated into the assay, the laboratory should test ~500 samples to verify that inhibition is occurring in <1 % of each validated specimen type (NYS Micro NAAT Checklist). This may be challenging for some laboratories to accomplish, especially small clinical laboratories that receive low numbers of CSF samples. For the verification of accuracy, the NYS guidance document recommends that laboratories include at least 30 positive and 10 negative samples for each specimen type and conduct "a randomized, blinded validation study where the assay results are compared to those of a gold standard or FDA-approved assay, or results of spiked clinical samples are compared to predicted results based on spiking values" [49]. This presents obvious challenges for the validation of HSV PCR assays on CSF, as the gold standard diagnostic method for HSV CNS disease has historically involved a temporal lobe brain biopsy (a procedure that is rarely performed); furthermore, FDA-cleared HSV molecular assays for CSF samples do not exist. Therefore, clinical laboratories have typically addressed these requirements by testing a mixture of clinical and spiked CSF samples that are known to be positive for HSV nucleic acid by an alternative PCR assay. Due to the regulatory challenges associated with validating LDTs, clinical laboratorians need to work closely with their partners in industry to develop and verify FDA-cleared assays for the detection of HSV in CSF samples.

Test Interpretation

In the context of a clinically compatible syndrome, the detection of HSV nucleic acid in CSF should be considered a critical laboratory result that prompts immediate communication to the healthcare provider. This is based on the extremely reliable performance of PCR for the detection of HSV in CSF, with past studies showing that the sensitivity and specificity of PCR exceed 90 % in patients with biopsy-proven disease [55, 58]. However, there are important caveats to the interpretation of HSV PCR testing that should be considered, including the possibility for false-negative and false-positive results.

Despite the high sensitivity of molecular amplification methods, cases of PCR-negative herpes simplex encephalitis (HSE) have been described [35, 55]. In a 2002 report by Weil et al. [55], the authors describe three patients with initial PCR-negative results who later had positive PCR findings for HSV-1 on a subsequent CSF sample. It is possible that the HSV viral load in CSF is below the limit of detection for PCR during the early stage of disease. Furthermore, there are some data indicating that the HSV viral load may increase during the first several days following the administration of antiviral therapy [36, 55]. Therefore, it has been suggested that for patients with presumed HSE that are negative by PCR on initial testing, a second lumbar puncture (collected 2–7 days later for PCR testing) should be considered to reduce the potential for false-negative results [55, 61].

A second important consideration is how to interpret a positive HSV PCR result in the absence of a clinically compatible disease. In 2008, Plentz et al. [33] reported on a study in which 1,387 CSF samples collected from 1,218 patients were tested for up to five different herpes viruses by PCR. Among the 1,218 patients tested, 30 (2.5 %) were positive for HSV-1/2 nucleic acid. Interestingly, a review of the clinical histories demonstrated that 25 of these patients presented with typical symptoms of HSV CNS disease, while five patients had an atypical presentation. Furthermore, the authors noted that among the five patients with a positive result and an atypical clinical manifestation, each of them had a HSV viral load that was very low (e.g., <1,000 copies/ml CSF). Whether these results reflect (1) active disease, (2) subclinical infection, or (3) false-positive results due to PCR contamination is difficult to determine. To this point, the authors concluded that the detection of low levels of HSV nucleic acid in the CSF requires a critical evaluation of the laboratory and clinical findings to accurately interpret the significance of the results.

In recent years, the role of quantitative HSV PCR has been assessed to determine its potential role in monitoring the effects of antiviral therapy, as well as potentially establishing a patient's prognosis. Ziyaeyan et al. [61] analyzed CSF samples collected from 236 patients with suspected HSE, of which 22 (9.3 %) had positive results. The HSV viral loads ranged from 2.5×10^2 to 1.7×10^6 copies/ml (median $= 4.8 \times 10^4$ copies/ml). Interestingly, ten patients had sequential CSF samples available for testing, which showed a significant ($p = 0.047$) decline in viral load between the first and second samples after the initiation of antiviral therapy. Several other important observations were made in this report, including (1) the higher the initial viral load, the longer the PCR remained positive for HSV nucleic acid following the initiation of treatment, and (2) a duration of antiviral therapy of at least 8 days was required to revert a positive patient to PCR negative.

In a similar study, Schloss et al. [41] evaluated a quantitative PCR assay using 92 CSF samples collected from 29 patients with HSE. Testing revealed that the initial CSF samples showed viral loads between 2×10^2 and 4.2×10^6 copies/ml (median = 1.9×10^5 copies/ml). A review of patient outcomes demonstrated that there was no correlation between the initial HSV CSF viral load and the prognosis. However, HSV nucleic acid was still detectable after 20 days of treatment in three patients, and the persistence of elevated viral loads in the CSF correlated with poor patient outcome. The authors concluded that quantification of HSV in CSF does not appear to be useful as a prognostic marker for HSE; however, it was suggested that care providers consider repeating a lumbar puncture prior to discontinuing antiviral therapy in patients with HSE. The persistence of HSV nucleic acid in CSF for long periods of time (e.g., ≥20 days) may suggest more severe disease and, potentially, support the extension of antiviral treatment [31, 41].

How the Test Has Changed Medical Practice

The seminal findings and astute predictions by Rowley et al. in 1990 provided direction to clinical laboratorians and their industry partners regarding the translational potential of molecular testing, especially for detection of viruses that may not replicate well in cell culture (e.g., HSV from CSF) [37]. A key element related to the importance of molecular testing for HSV DNA in CSF was the ability to enhance the management of patients with CNS disease due to this viral infection. Past studies have shown that patients with HSV CNS disease who are treated with acyclovir have reduced mortality (19–28 %) compared to a mortality of 50–54 % in individuals treated with vidarabine [59]. Importantly, the effectiveness of acyclovir treatments depends on the early and specific detection of HSV DNA [6, 56]. The implementation of real-time PCR has led to a significant increase in the detection of HSV in CSF samples, with a retrospective study performed at our institution showing a nearly 100-fold increase in the detection of HSV-2 by PCR compared to viral culture (Table 7.1).

Certainly, the molecular detection of human immunodeficiency virus (HIV) and the hepatitis viruses (e.g., hepatitis B and C viruses) were prototypic, industry developed assays that clearly demonstrated the utility by rapid detection and quantitation of viral pathogens for the management of patients with these infections. Similarly, conventional diagnostic methods including imaging techniques, serology, and cell culture detection of HSV infection in CSF were replaced by conventional PCR (initial gel electrophoresis followed by Southern blot resolution of targeted nucleic acids). These cumbersome techniques have now been replaced by real-time, automated instruments that provide rapid, sensitive, and specific laboratory results in the clinical laboratory. Many diagnostic laboratories have since extended real-time applications of molecular testing for the rapid detection of signature nucleotide targets for a wide variety of pathogenic microorganisms [18, 19]. Specimens submitted for the diagnosis of HSV from all anatomical sites accounted for over 70 % of the total viruses detected at the Mayo Clinic [47, 48]. Due to the impact of real-time PCR, several clinical virology laboratories in the USA have converted from the use of cell culture isolation to real-time molecular techniques for the detection of viral pathogens.

Because of the routine collection of CSF from patients with CNS disease, molecular testing for HSV DNA has been integrated into the standard operating procedures of many clinical laboratories. Rationale for this decision has been driven by data showing that PCR allows for a rapid and sensitive diagnosis in patients with CNS infection caused by HSV-1/2 [27, 54, 57].

Molecular amplification of target HSV DNA from CSF has clearly become the standard diagnostic technology for the clinical laboratory [42].

Future Directions

The implementation of real-time PCR for the diagnosis of HSV CNS disease has made an extraordinary impact on reducing the morbidity and mortality associated with this infection. However, given the nonspecific clinical presentation of viral encephalitis and the urgency to make a diagnosis, future studies should be aimed at improving our ability to detect and identify the causative agent in an even more timely fashion. In recent years, an area of significant interest has been the development of multiplex assays [7, 12, 21, 29] that are able to detect a number of different viral pathogens, including HSV, in a single reaction [24, 38, 43, 45].

In a recent study, Shi et al. [45] evaluated a PCR microarray designed to simultaneously detect HSV types 1 and 2, VZV, EBV, CMV, and HHV-6A/B in CSF specimens ($n=290$) collected from children presenting with clinical suspicion for viral encephalitis. The results of the PCR microarray assay were compared to those of individual TaqMan-based real-time PCR assays. The results showed that the analytical sensitivity of the PCR microarray was approximately ten copies/reaction, with a clinical sensitivity and specificity of 91.7 % (11/12) and 100 % (278/278), respectively. Interestingly, one of the CSF samples showed evidence of a double infection with HSV-2 and CMV, which was supported by sequencing studies. Furthermore, the PCR microarray could provide results for seven herpes viruses in as few as 4 h. In a similar study, Sankuntaw et al. [38] developed a multiplex real-time PCR assay for the detection of HSV-1, HSV-2, VZV, EBV, and CMV in clinical CSF samples. The analytical sensitivity of the multiplex PCR assay was determined to be one copy/reaction for HSV-1 and VZV and ten copies/reaction for HSV-2, EBV, and CMV. Testing of 62 clinical CSF samples showed that 39 (62.9 %) were positive for one ($n=21$ CSF) or multiple viruses ($n=18$). The clinical sensitivity of the multiplex PCR ranged from 75 % for EBV to 100 % for HSV-1 and VZV. These reports suggest that multiplex assays may provide a promising alternative to single analyte tests for the diagnosis of viral CNS disease, especially when the clinical and radiographic presentation is not specific for a particular viral agent.

An area where clinical laboratories must continue to improve is decreasing the turnaround time for providing results of HSV CSF testing. Although many real-time PCR systems can provide results in as few as 4 h following receipt of the sample in the testing laboratory, new technologies are emerging that allow for extraction and amplification of certain analytes in fewer than 60 min [51]. These systems utilize microfluidics, which increases the surface area and significantly reduces the PCR cycling times and the volume of sample required for testing. Several commercial manufacturers, including BioFire Inc. (Salt Lake City, UT) and Focus Diagnostics (Cypress, CA), have developed microfluidics-based PCR assays that allow for nucleic acid extraction and target amplification in as little as 30 min. This technology could be readily applied to the detection of HSV in CSF samples, with a significant reduction in turnaround time potentially translating into improved patient outcomes.

Perhaps the most pressing future need related to HSV diagnostics is the availability of FDA-cleared assays for the detection of HSV nucleic acid in CSF samples. The lack of a FDA-cleared assay for CSF has forced clinical laboratories to develop and implement LDTs, which generally demonstrate excellent performance but are not standardized and, in some situations, may not have been properly validated. In the near future, clinical laboratorians should work closely with their partners in industry to develop and validate molecular assays that can be cleared by the FDA for detection of HSV in CSF samples. This will help ensure that clinical laboratories are using standardized and approved methods for the diagnosis of this potentially life-threatening disease.

References

1. Afonso N, Gunasena S, Galla K, Podzorski R, Chandrasekar P, Alangaden G. Appropriate use of polymerase chain reaction for detection of herpes simplex virus 2 in cerebrospinal fluid of patients at an inner-city hospital. Diagn Microbiol Infect Dis. 2007;57:309–13.
2. Akyldz BN, Gumus H, Kumandas S, Coskun A, Karakukucu M, Yklmaz A. Diffusion-weighted magnetic resonance is better than polymerase chain reaction for early diagnosis of herpes simplex encephalitis: a case report. Pediatr Emerg Care. 2008;24:377–9.
3. Al-Shekhlee A, Kocharian N, Suarez JJ. Re-evaluating the diagnostic methods in herpes simplex encephalitis. Herpes. 2006;13:17–9.
4. Aslanzadeh J, Osmon DR, Wilhelm MP, Espy MJ, Smith TF. A prospective study of the polymerase chain reaction for detection of herpes simplex virus in cerebrospinal fluid submitted to the clinical virology laboratory. Mol Cell Probes. 1992;6:367–73.
5. Avkan Oguz V, Yapar N, Sezak N, Alp Cavus S, Kuruuzum Z, Sayiner A, Ada E, Cakir N, Yuce A. Two cases of herpes encephalitis with normal cerebrospinal fluid findings. Mikrobiyol Bul. 2006;40:93–8.
6. Bell DJ, Suckling R, Rothburn MM, Blanchard T, Stoeter D, Michael B, Cooke RP, Kneen R, Solomon T. Management of suspected herpes simplex virus encephalitis in adults in a U.K. teaching hospital. Clin Med. 2009;9:231–5.
7. Bergallo M, Costa C, Margio S, Sidoti F, Terlizzi ME, Cavallo R. Development of a multiplex polymerase chain reaction for detection and typing of major human herpes viruses in cerebrospinal fluid. Can J Microbiol. 2007;53:1117–22.
8. Broude NE. Molecular beacons and other hairpin probes. In: Fuchs J, Podda M, editors. Encylclopedia of diagnostic genomics and proteomics. London, England: Informa Healthcare; 2005. p. 846–50.
9. CAP. Validation studies-specimen types, vol. MOL.31015; 2011.
10. CAP. Validation study comparison, vol. MOL.31130; 2011.
11. Department of Health and Human Services. Clinical laboratory improvement amendments of 1988: final rule. Fed Regist. 1992;57(40):7001–7186. 42 CFR part 493.1253.
12. Chesky M, Scalco R, Failace L, Read S, Jobim LF. Polymerase chain reaction for the laboratory diagnosis of aseptic meningitis and encephalitis. Arq Neuropsiquiatr. 2000;58:836–42.
13. Davis L. Diagnosis and treatment of acute encephalitis. Neurologist. 2000;6:145–59.
14. DeBiasi RL, Kleinschmidt-DeMasters BK, Weinberg A, Tyler KL. Use of PCR for the diagnosis of herpes virus infections of the central nervous system. J Clin Virol. 2002;25 Suppl 1:S5–11.
15. Domingues RB, Lakeman FD, Pannuti CS, Fink MC, Tsanaclis AM. Advantage of polymerase chain reaction in the diagnosis of herpes simplex encephalitis: presentation of 5 atypical cases. Scand J Infect Dis. 1997;29:229–31.
16. Espy MJ, Ross TK, Teo R, Svien KA, Wold AD, Uhl JR, Smith TF. Evaluation of LightCycler PCR for implementation of laboratory diagnosis of herpes simplex virus infections. J Clin Microbiol. 2000;38:3116–8.
17. Espy MJ, Rys PN, Wold AD, Uhl JR, Sloan LM, Jenkins GD, Ilstrup DM, Cockerill 3rd FR, Patel R, Rosenblatt JE, Smith TF. Detection of herpes simplex virus DNA in genital and dermal specimens by LightCycler PCR after extraction using the IsoQuick, MagNA Pure, and BioRobot 9604 methods. J Clin Microbiol. 2001;39:2233–6.
18. Espy MJ, Uhl JR, Mitchell PS, Thorvilson JN, Svien KA, Wold AD, Smith TF. Diagnosis of herpes simplex virus infections in the clinical laboratory by LightCycler PCR. J Clin Microbiol. 2000;38:795–9.
19. Espy MJ, Uhl JR, Sloan LM, Buckwalter SP, Jones MF, Vetter EA, Yao JD, Wengenack NL, Rosenblatt JE, Cockerill 3rd FR, Smith TF. Real-time PCR in clinical microbiology: applications for routine laboratory testing. Clin Microbiol Rev. 2006;19:165–256.
20. Franzen-Rohl E, Tiveljung-Lindell A, Grillner L, Aurelius E. Increased detection rate in diagnosis of herpes simplex virus type 2 meningitis by real-time PCR using cerebrospinal fluid samples. J Clin Microbiol. 2007;45:2516–20.
21. Frias C, Matas L, Ferre X, Millan M, Marti S, Hernandez A, Ausina V. Usefulness of adding multiplex nested-polymerase chain reaction assay of cerebrospinal fluid samples to routine diagnostic testing for herpes virus encephalitis. Eur J Clin Microbiol Infect Dis. 2001;20:670–2.
22. Harrison NA, MacDonald BK, Scott G, Kapoor R. Atypical herpes type 2 encephalitis associated with normal MRI imaging. J Neurol Neurosurg Psychiatry. 2003;74:974–6.
23. Issa NC, Espy MJ, Uhl JR, Smith TF. Sequencing and resolution of amplified herpes simplex virus DNA with intermediate melting curves as genotype 1 or 2 by LightCycler PCR assay. J Clin Microbiol. 2005; 43:1843–5.
24. Jaaskelainen AJ, Piiparinen H, Lappalainen M, Vaheri A. Improved multiplex-PCR and microarray for herpesvirus detection from CSF. J Clin Virol. 2008; 42:172–5.
25. Kennedy PG, Chaudhuri A. Herpes simplex encephalitis. J Neurol Neurosurg Psychiatry. 2002;73:237–8.
26. Kessler HH, Muhlbauer G, Rinner B, Stelzl E, Berger A, Dorr HW, Santner B, Marth E, Rabenau H. Detection of Herpes simplex virus DNA by real-time PCR. J Clin Microbiol. 2000;38:2638–42.

27. Kimberlin D. Herpes simplex virus, meningitis and encephalitis in neonates. Herpes. 2004;11 Suppl 2: 65A–76.
28. Kohira I, Ninomiya Y. A case of recurrent aseptic meningitis (Mollaret meningitis) with back pain in which was detected the DNA of herpes simplex virus type 2 in cerebrospinal fluid. Rinsho Shinkeigaku. 2002;42:24–6.
29. Koskiniemi M, Rantalaiho T, Piiparinen H, von Bonsdorff CH, Farkkila M, Jarvinen A, Kinnunen E, Koskiniemi S, Mannonen L, Muttilainen M, Linnavuori K, Porras J, Puolakkainen M, Raiha K, Salonen EM, Ukkonen P, Vaheri A, Valtonen V. Infections of the central nervous system of suspected viral origin: a collaborative study from Finland. J Neurovirol. 2001;7:400–8.
30. Lakeman FD, Whitley RJ. Diagnosis of herpes simplex encephalitis: application of polymerase chain reaction to cerebrospinal fluid from brain-biopsied patients and correlation with disease. National Institute of Allergy and Infectious Diseases Collaborative Antiviral Study Group. J Infect Dis. 1995;171:857–63.
31. Mejias A, Bustos R, Ardura MI, Ramirez C, Sanchez PJ. Persistence of herpes simplex virus DNA in cerebrospinal fluid of neonates with herpes simplex virus encephalitis. J Perinatol. 2009;29:290–6.
32. Olson LC, Buescher EL, Artenstein MS, Parkman PD. Herpesvirus infections of the human central nervous system. N Engl J Med. 1967;277:1271–7.
33. Plentz A, Jilg W, Kochanowski B, Ibach B, Knoll A. Detection of herpesvirus DNA in cerebrospinal fluid and correlation with clinical symptoms. Infection. 2008;36:158–62.
34. Powell KF, Anderson NE, Frith RW, Croxson MC. Non-invasive diagnosis of herpes simplex encephalitis. Lancet. 1990;335:357–8.
35. Puchhammer-Stockl E, Presterl E, Croy C, Aberle S, Popow-Kraupp T, Kundi M, Hofmann H, Wenninger U, Godl I. Screening for possible failure of herpes simplex virus PCR in cerebrospinal fluid for the diagnosis of herpes simplex encephalitis. J Med Virol. 2001;64:531–6.
36. Roos KL. Pearls and pitfalls in the diagnosis and management of central nervous system infectious diseases. Semin Neurol. 1998;18:185–96.
37. Rowley AH, Whitley RJ, Lakeman FD, Wolinsky SM. Rapid detection of herpes-simplex-virus DNA in cerebrospinal fluid of patients with herpes simplex encephalitis. Lancet. 1990;335:440–1.
38. Sankuntaw N, Sukprasert S, Engchanil C, Kaewkes W, Chantratita W, Pairoj V, Lulitanond V. Single tube multiplex real-time PCR for the rapid detection of herpes virus infections of the central nervous system. Mol Cell Probes. 2011;25:114–20.
39. Sauerbrei A, Wutzler P. Laboratory diagnosis of central nervous system infections caused by herpesviruses. J Clin Virol. 2002;25 Suppl 1:S45–51.
40. Schiffer JT, Corey L. Herpes simplex virus. In: Mandell GL, Bennett JE, Dalin R, editors. Principles and practices of infectious diseases. 7th ed. Philadelphia, PA: Churchill Livingston; 2010. p. 1443–962.
41. Schloss L, Falk KI, Skoog E, Brytting M, Linde A, Aurelius E. Monitoring of herpes simplex virus DNA types 1 and 2 viral load in cerebrospinal fluid by real-time PCR in patients with herpes simplex encephalitis. J Med Virol. 2009;81:1432–7.
42. Schmutzhard E. Viral infections of the CNS with special emphasis on herpes simplex infections. J Neurol. 2001;248:469–77.
43. Scott LJ, Gunson RN, Carman WF, Winter AJ. A new multiplex real-time PCR test for HSV1/2 and syphilis: an evaluation of its impact in the laboratory and clinical setting. Sex Transm Infect. 2010;86:537–9.
44. Selvaraju SB, Wurst M, Horvat RT, Selvarangan R. Evaluation of three analyte-specific reagents for detection and typing of herpes simplex virus in cerebrospinal fluid. Diagn Microbiol Infect Dis. 2009;63: 286–91.
45. Shi J, Wu Y, Cai M, Shang S. Rapid diagnosis of herpetic encephalitis in children by PCR-microarray technology for simultaneous detection of seven human herpes viruses. Eur J Pediatr. 2010;169:421–5.
46. Simko JP, Caliendo AM, Hogle K, Versalovic J. Differences in laboratory findings for cerebrospinal fluid specimens obtained from patients with meningitis or encephalitis due to herpes simplex virus (HSV) documented by detection of HSV DNA. Clin Infect Dis. 2002;35:414–9.
47. Smith TF, Espy MJ, Jones MF. Molecular virology: current and future trends. In: Persing DH, Tenover FC, Versalovic J, Tang YW, Unger ER, Relman DA, White TJ, editors. Molecular microbiology diagnostic principles and practices. Washington, DC: ASM Press; 2004. p. 543–8.
48. Smith TF, Espy MJ, Wold AD. Develpment, implementation, and optimization of lightcycler PCR assays for detection of herpes simplex virus and varicella-zoster virus from clinical specimens. In: Reischl U, Wittwer C, Cockerill F, editors. Rapid cycle real-time PCR methods and applications. Berlin, Germany: Springer; 2002. p. 189–200.
49. State of New York. Department of Health. Approval of microbiology nucleic acid amplification assays. Microbiology Molecular Checklist; 2011. p. 1–11.
50. Stevenson J, Hymas W, Hillyard D. Effect of sequence polymorphisms on performance of two real-time PCR assays for detection of herpes simplex virus. J Clin Microbiol. 2005;43:2391–8.
51. Sun Y, Dhumpa R, Bang DD, Hogberg J, Handberg K, Wolff A. A lab-on-a-chip device for rapid identification of avian influenza viral RNA by solid-phase PCR. Lab Chip. 2011;11:1457–63.
52. Tang YW, Mitchell PS, Espy MJ, Smith TF, Persing DH. Molecular diagnosis of herpes simplex virus infections in the central nervous system. J Clin Microbiol. 1999;37:2127–36.
53. Tang YW, Rys PN, Rutledge BJ, Mitchell PS, Smith TF, Persing DH. Comparative evaluation of colorimetric microtiter plate systems for detection of herpes simplex virus in cerebrospinal fluid. J Clin Microbiol. 1998;36:2714–7.
54. Tyler KL. Update on herpes simplex encephalitis. Rev Neurol Dis. 2004;1:169–78.

55. Weil AA, Glaser CA, Amad Z, Forghani B. Patients with suspected herpes simplex encephalitis: rethinking an initial negative polymerase chain reaction result. Clin Infect Dis. 2002;34:1154–7.
56. Whitley R, Arvin A, Prober C, Burchett S, Corey L, Powell D, Plotkin S, Starr S, Alford C, Connor J, et al. A controlled trial comparing vidarabine with acyclovir in neonatal herpes simplex virus infection. Infectious Diseases Collaborative Antiviral Study Group. N Engl J Med. 1991;324:444–9.
57. Whitley RJ. Herpes simplex encephalitis: adolescents and adults. Antiviral Res. 2006;71:141–8.
58. Whitley RJ. Herpes simplex viruses. In: Scheld WM, Whitley RJ, Durack DT, editors. Infections of the central nervous system. 2nd ed. Philadelphia, PA: Lippincott-Raven; 1997. p. 73–89.
59. Whitley RJ, Gnann Jr JW. Acyclovir: a decade later. N Engl J Med. 1992;327:782–9.
60. Wright PA, Espy MJ, Irish C, Smith TF, Pritt BS. Evaluation of a sample-conserving heat processing method for low volume csf specimens submitted for HSV PCR. Clinical virology symposium meeting, Daytona Beach, FL; 2010.
61. Ziyaeyan M, Alborzi A, Borhani Haghighi A, Jamalidoust M, Moeini M, Pourabbas B. Diagnosis and quantitative detection of HSV DNA in samples from patients with suspected herpes simplex encephalitis. Braz J Infect Dis. 2011;15:211–4.

Toward a Safer Blood Supply: The Impact of Molecular Testing

8

Niel T. Constantine, Patricia A. Wright, Ahmed Saleh, and Anna DeMarinis

Background on the Test

Introduction

Blood banks in the USA strive to have the safest blood supply in the world. To accomplish this, testing for infectious diseases is federally mandated through strict regulatory measures and is continuously monitored for effectiveness and accuracy. Extraordinary quality assurance oversight is omnipresent and monitored by several government and nongovernmental organizations including the Food and Drug Administration (FDA), American Association of Blood Banks (AABB), and various state health authorities.

Infectious disease testing technologies perpetually evolve to offer improvement and are instituted, sometimes even before licensing by the FDA, when they offer better safety for the blood supply. In addition, testing strategies have improved for better efficiency, such as multiplexing to detect multiple agents simultaneously. Further, testing algorithms that include serologic and molecular technologies are perpetually being changed to provide better test indices (e.g., sensitivity and specificity). Testing for additional agents (e.g., Trypanosoma, West Nile Virus) has been added to the testing menu and inclusion of others (e.g., Babesia, Leishmania) is being considered. Finally, the identification of prions in blood, although important, cannot be considered at present because there is currently no suitable test available for screening blood.

Currently, blood banks are mandated to test for human immunodeficiency virus types 1 and 2 (HIV-1/HIV-2), hepatitis B virus (HBV), hepatitis C virus (HCV), human T-cell lymphotropic virus types I and II (HTLV-I/HTLV-II), *Treponema pallidum* (syphilis), *Trypanosoma cruzi* (Chagas Disease), and West Nile Virus (WNV). Some use serologic testing only, while others are tested by only molecular assays, and some by combinations of serologic and molecular methods. Although all blood banks must test for all agents, the choice of methods and strategies (e.g., pooling) varies among the

N.T. Constantine, Ph.D., M.T. (A.S.C.P.) (✉)
Department of Pathology and Institute of Human Virology, University of Maryland School of Medicine, Baltimore, MD, USA
e-mail: nconstantine@ihv.umaryland.edu

P.A. Wright, B.A., M.T.(A.S.C.P.)S.B.B.
Signature Healthcare-Brockton Hospital, Brockton, MA, USA

A. Saleh, Ph.D.
Department of Pathology and Institute of Human Virology, University of Maryland School of Medicine, Baltimore, MD, USA

Faculty of Science, Zoology Department, Cairo University, Cairo, Egypt

A. DeMarinis, M.A., M.T.(A.S.C.P.)S.B.B., C.Q.A.(A.S.Q.)
The DeMarinis Group, LLC, North Attleborough, MA, USA

W.E. Highsmith Jr. (ed.), *Molecular Diagnostics: 12 Tests That Changed Everything*, Molecular and Translational Medicine, DOI 10.1007/978-1-4614-8127-0_8,

organizations (e.g., American Red Cross [ARC], American Blood Centers [ABC], and others [e.g., New York Blood Center, Houston Blood Center, etc.]).

In this chapter, we aim to present a summary of infectious disease testing in USA blood banks, concentrating on the molecular assays that have revolutionized the testing arena and contributed to enhancing the safety of the blood supply. To set the stage and to describe the strategies used by blood banks, we include a brief background on the infectious agents, their risk to the blood supply, and what technologies are available for each. Subsequently, we concentrate on the molecular methods including their applications, usefulness, limitations, interpretation of results, and the basics of their methods; details on the molecular methodologies can be found in other chapters. Finally, we provide some information on the costs of these tests, the regulatory aspects that form the framework for ensuring blood safety, and the impact of molecular testing on changing medical practice in the blood bank. Although background is presented for all required testing in USA blood banks, the emphasis is on molecular assays and how they have unequivocally contributed to making the blood supply safer.

Importance of Screening the Blood Supply for Infectious Agents

There are nearly 16 million whole blood donations per year in the USA [1]. This includes about seven million from the ARC, and the rest from the ABC and major blood centers throughout the USA. All of the agents mentioned above can be transmitted effectively through plasma and blood transfusions, although some can only be transmitted through the transfusion of cellular components (e.g., HTLV). Some are much more prevalent, while others may be prevalent only in certain geographic areas (e.g., *Trypanosoma cruzi* in infected blood is highest in the southern USA). Importantly, blood components (typically 2–3 including red blood cells, platelet concentrates, and fresh frozen plasma) from a single infected donor can be used for transfusion to multiple recipients, thereby resulting in infection of a number of persons receiving one or more components from that same donor. The risk of infection by any particular agent varies and is dependent on the viral load of the agent and the amount of blood transfused [2]. Nevertheless, the risk of transfusion-transmitted infection is high, and detection, sequestration, and ultimately, elimination of infected units are of essential importance. Although all risks cannot currently be eliminated for any agent, they are minimized to the degree that the tests allow. The current risks are dependent somewhat on the prevalence of the infectious agent present (see section "Clinical Significance"), and the population tested; that is, a higher risk donor population has a higher chance of containing infectious units that are in the window or eclipse period (see Fig. 8.1). Transfusion-transmitted infections result not only in morbidity and mortality, but also in potential lawsuits. Finally, newer technologies have the potential to further reduce the eclipse period [5, 6] (see Future Directions section), but these research techniques require further development.

Infectious Agents for Which Screening is Required

Blood donation (and the subsequent transfusion of the donated blood) is a complex process that may follow one of several pathways. A single unit of whole blood can be collected from an individual and subsequently processed through simple centrifugation into components such as red blood cells (RBC), platelet concentrates (PC), and fresh frozen plasma (FFP; frozen immediately after centrifugation). Alternatively, a donor may choose to donate one or more units of whole blood for his own use during, for example, a planned surgical procedure (autologous donation). In addition, in-process centrifugation of a single donor (direct centrifugation while the blood is being withdrawn; a process called apheresis) can be used for larger collections of red blood cells, white blood cells, and platelets. Furthermore, large-volume plasma-only collections (source plasma) can be

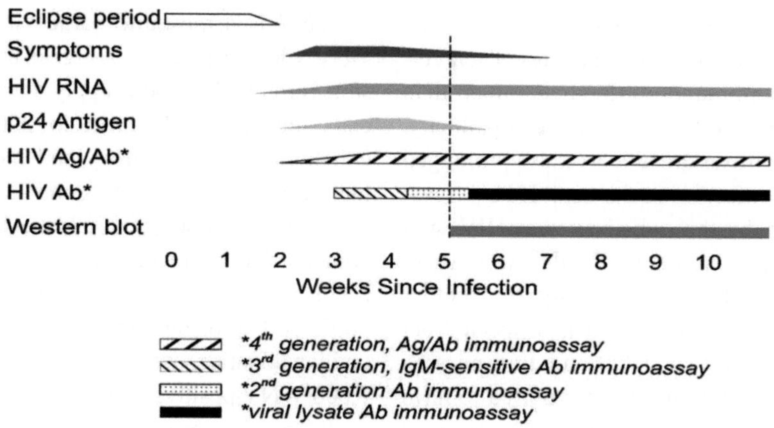

Fig. 8.1 Kinetics of the appearance of viral and serologic markers for HIV [3, 4] ([4] with permission from Elsevier)

taken from individual donors for subsequent fractionation through chemical methods into many products such as immune serum globulin and albumin. These types of blood donor collections have somewhat different regulatory requirements, vis-à-vis infectious disease testing. This chapter will focus on the testing of traditional whole blood donations used only for processing into components. However, for interested readers, a brief summary of the differences in the testing required for autologous, apheresis, and source plasma donations is found in the Regulatory Issues section.

The agents of major threat to the blood supply are blood-borne pathogens that are primarily viruses, but also include spirochetes (*Treponema or T. pallidum*), and protozoa (*Trypanosoma or T. cruzi*). Each causes a disease that can result in substantial morbidity and mortality. Each agent, the condition it causes, and the general methods of detection are described briefly below.

HIV is a ribonucleic acid (RNA) virus that is transmitted through blood, vertically from mother to child, and sexually; included are HIV-1 and HIV-2 types, both of which cause acquired immunodeficiency syndrome (AIDS). HIV-1 is present globally and consists of a variety of subtypes (clades). Although HIV-2 is less prevalent in the USA (about 200 cases identified), its identification has become more important because the treatment selection must be altered since it is less responsive to first-line HIV therapy [7]. Of particular importance is the understanding of the kinetics of markers that can be used for detecting HIV infection (see Fig. 8.1).

HBV infection causes liver inflammation and can lead to chronic hepatitis and hepatocellular carcinoma. The deoxyribonucleic acid (DNA) virus can be transmitted easily through blood transfusion, and it is estimated that in the past, 30 % of multi-transfused recipients could be at risk for contracting HBV [8]. The tests used to identify current and previous infection with HBV consist of testing for hepatitis B core antibody (anti-HBc) to detect recent and established infection after antigen has disappeared, and hepatitis B surface antigen (HBsAg) to detect early or chronic (carrier) infection.

HCV, previously known as non-A, non-B hepatitis, has become a major concern among diagnosticians and those trying to protect the blood supply. It is the most common cause of viral hepatitis in the USA. The RNA virus is prevalent throughout the world, with the highest rates occurring in Egypt [9], and high rates (up to 70 %) in intravenous drug users (IVDU) in the USA [10]. Infection results in acute hepatitis and chronic hepatitis (in 40–70 %) and may progress to hepatocellular carcinoma. In the USA, the threat of infectious units is substantial, but has been minimized by the institution of serologic and molecular methods for testing blood donors.

HTLV types I and II cause infections that can lead to leukemia or a variety of neurologic diseases.

Each is a single-stranded RNA-type C virus that has tropism for human T lymphocytes. Their cellular effect is immunoproliferative rather than causing an immunodeficiency via cytopathicity. Both of these viruses are able to cause prolonged asymptomatic infection in the host. HTLV transmission occurs by the same routes as HIV, specifically sexual, parenteral, IVDUs who share contaminated needles, and vertically from mother to child; perinatal transmission is suspected but remains unproven. In addition, transmission through breastfeeding has been reported to have a risk of 18–30 % [11]. Transfusion is the most efficient mode of HTLV transmission, with seroconversion occurring in about 27 % of recipients following exposure to contaminated cellular products, although this seroconversion rate is less than that of HIV, HCV, and HBV [12]. Currently, the testing of blood units for HTLV-I and HTLV-II is mandated in the USA and these screening programs have successfully lowered the risk of transfusion-related transmission. HTLV-I-infected blood may be an efficient means of disease production and has been linked to the development of tropic spastic paraparesis (TSP) occurring 1 month to 3 years after transfusion. Infection can also lead to Adult T-cell Leukemia (ATL), an aggressive disease associated with the proliferation of T lymphocytes. HTLV-II infection has been described in a patient having "hairy cell" leukemia and may be associated with Large Granular Lymphocyte (LGL) leukemia. However, presently the agent is not conclusively linked to any specific disease. HTLV-II is much more common in IVDUs than is HTLV-I, but a clear association with disease state or medical condition has not been found.

Syphilis is caused by the spirochete *T. pallidum*, a sexually transmitted disease that can result in latent infection and subsequent neurological disease. Theoretically, the organism has the potential to be transmitted through the blood supply, although there have been no documented transfusion-transmitted syphilis cases since 1968 [13]. This organism cannot survive beyond 72 h in donated blood stored at 1–6 °C. This would make platelets, concentrates (routinely stored at room temperature) the only component capable of transmitting infection.

WNV is a mosquito-borne virus that causes West Nile encephalitis, a disease that is transmissible through the blood supply. Public health officials recognized this risk in 2002. The FDA collaborated with industry and blood collection facilities to develop new donor screening tests, and in the summer of 2003, the FDA approved clinical trials for these new tests and blood banks began screening the blood supply. By July 1, 2003, 100 % of military donations and 95 % of civilian donations were screened, resulting in over 1,000 WNV-positive donations being identified.

T. cruzi is a protozoan parasite found primarily in Central and South America, but it has been estimated that more than 300,000 individuals are infected in the USA [14]. Infection by *T. cruzi* causes Chagas disease, a condition that may be self-limiting with complete resolution but typically establishes a lifelong infection that can lead to cardiomyopathy and congestive heart failure; it may also cause megaviscera. Although it is transmitted by a vector, human-to-human transmission occurs through blood and organ transfusion, and vertically from mother to child [15–18]. As many as 45,000 cases of cardiomyopathy and up to 300 new congenital infections may occur per year in the USA [14, 19]. Many cases are asymptomatic, where there are no signs or symptoms; this presents a particular challenge to blood donations [20].

Evolution of Infectious Disease Testing in the Blood Bank

With the discovery in 1965 of the "Australia antigen" by Blumberg et al. [21], a test to detect the presence of HBV exposure in blood donors could be conceived. This antigen, later renamed HBsAg, was the basis for donor hepatitis testing, which began in 1969. At that time, HBV was the most significant transfusion-transmitted disease. Also at that time, many blood donors were not volunteers; they were paid for their blood. The lack of a reliable test and the use of paid donors resulted in a very high risk that a transfusion recipient would contract HBV. Data from the National Institutes of Health (NIH) showed that a multiply transfused recipient had a

30 % risk of contracting posttransfusion hepatitis [8]. In 1970, the NIH Blood Bank simultaneously adopted an all-volunteer donor system and introduced a first-generation assay to screen for HBsAg. The outcome of this dual intervention was dramatic; posttransfusion hepatitis rates fell to a new baseline level of approximately 10 %. By the mid-1970s, once the national blood donor pool became a voluntary one and more sensitive testing for HBV exposure became routine, the incidence of posttransfusion hepatitis B dropped to 0.3–0.9 % [22]. The "first-generation" HBsAg testing employed agar gel-based immunodiffusion, followed by the second-generation testing that used counter-immunoelectrophoresis (CIE). Beginning in 1972, the methods of choice were the third-generation assays of reverse passive hemagglutination (RPHA) and radioimmunoassay (RIA). Subsequently, the development of enzyme immunoassays (EIA) was a major breakthrough in infectious disease testing, including the testing of blood donors because the method was easy to perform and sensitive.

Serologic assays for HIV, HTLV-I/II, and HCV were established for use in the USA in 1985, 1997, and 1998, respectively. Once a virus was identified, screening tests for antibody to the virus (e.g., anti-HIV, anti-HTLV-I/II, or anti-HCV) were developed rapidly. As new tests were developed and approved, an FDA requirement quickly followed that routine donor screening include nucleic acid tests/testing (NAT), in addition to the serologic methods then in use.

Syphilis testing was first instituted for blood donor screening in the 1950s using the rapid plasma reagin (RPR) test and currently uses an automated testing method with confirmation using a serologic EIA test for total antibody and a test for reagin. No cases of transfusion-transmitted syphilis have been recorded since 1968 [13].

Testing for *T. cruzi* was instituted in 2007, with the test being an EIA to qualitatively detect antibodies to *T. cruzi*; confirmation testing is performed by radioimmunoprecipitation assay (RIPA). Although it is possible to transmit *T. cruzi* through blood transfusion, the ARC has not, to date, identified any recipients infected by blood transfusions from donors who subsequently tested as confirmed positive.

WNV testing was instituted in 2003 as a NAT only test. Since donor screening was implemented, there have been nine cases of transfusion transmission; all were due to very low viral loads below the detectable level. To further reduce the risk of such transmissions in areas where WNV is endemic or cases of WNV infection have been identified, testing has recently switched from testing in small pools to testing individual units.

As these test methods for screening and confirmation were being established and implemented, it was well recognized that there was a possibility that an infected blood donor could be missed by these tests if the donor was in an early stage of infection (a false-negative test), where seropositivity was below the lower limit of the test's ability to detect the antibody or the antigen of interest. This "window of infectivity" is different for the many viruses of interest, but it exists for all of them. The thrust of research that followed was to develop test methods that could detect these very low levels of target viruses. NAT for viral RNA/DNA detection was found to address that problem effectively.

Clinical Significance

Prevalence and Incidence of Infectious Diseases in Blood Donors

HIV

The prevalence of HIV infection in blood donors and the risk of receiving an infected unit are shown in Table 8.1. An analysis of a decade of results (1999–2008) after NAT was introduced revealed that 32 HIV RNA-positive/antibody-negative donors were detected in 66 million donations collected and screened in that decade. These infections translate to 1 in 2,060,000 donations that were screened for HIV. A follow-up for 22 of the NAT HIV positive showed that 16 seroconverted within a 15-day median. A further follow-up of 12 of these donors, who continued with the study, became antibody-confirmed positive within a median of 21 days [25].

Table 8.1 Prevalence rates and risk of infections for HIV, HBsAg, HCV, syphilis, and HTLV in blood donors

Agent	Positive rate (%) 2000–2001 [23]	Number of pos., 2000–2001 [23]	Risk of Infections from negative blood, 1999–2006 [24]
HIV	0.0011	30	1:2,135,000
HBsAg	0.0012	33	1:205,000–488,000
HCV	0.0013	35	1:1,935,000
Syphilis	0.0037	100	[a]
HTLV	0.0002	5	1:3,000,000
Any one confirmed	0.0080	216	[a]

Adapted from Zou [23] and Stramer [24]
[a]Not indicated

HBV

The prevalence rate for HBV infection and the risk of receiving an infectious unit from blood donors are shown in Table 8.1. In 2011, a study by Stramer et al. [26] reported using a triplex NAT test for HCV, HBV, and HIV and compared the results of HBV detection by the routine HBsAg and anti-HBc serology assays (PRISM ChLIA, a chemiluminescence immunoassay, Abbott Diagnostics, Abbott Park, IL). The PROCLEIX® ULTRIO® assay and the PROCLEIX®TIGRIS System automated platform (Gen-Probe and Novartis) were used since 2008 in three of five ARC National Testing Laboratories for this comparison. A minipool (MP) of 16 samples (84 %) or individual samples (16 %) were screened by the NAT. The study included 3,694,858 donations from 2,137,275 donors. The ULTRIO® triplex assay was able to distinguish 9 HBV DNA-positive donors before seroconversion (1 in 410,540), 7 of which were false positives due to previous HBV vaccinations, as compared with 426 positive by both NAT and serologic analysis (1 in 8,673). These only had a brief acute phase of infection that is not proved to be transmitted by blood transfusion. The author concluded that the cost of such assays is not justified based on this low number of detections of HBV and their medical significance.

Nevertheless, since 2009, the ARC has adopted this triplex NAT, using an MP of 16 donations (MP-NAT) for the detection of HCV, HBV, and HIV. The screening results of the triplex screening versus the HBsAg and anti-HBc to identify the HBV-infected donors for one full year (June 2009 to end of June 2010) were recently examined by Stramer et al. [27]. Out of 6.5 million donations screened, 699 were confirmed HBV-infected. MP-NAT detected only 477 (68 %) while 697 (99 %) showed reactivity to one or more by serologic testing. The prevalence of NAT-positive, seronegative donors (two donors) was 1 per 3.23 million. Among NAT reactive donors, two (0.4 %) had negative serology (representing early infection) and ten (2.1 %) were HBsAg-confirmed positive and anti-HBc nonreactive.

HCV

In 1999, NAT for HIV and HCV was first introduced for the screening of blood donated through the ARC centers all over the USA. Data compiled for the period of 1999–2008 were analyzed to examine the effect of NAT for the safety of blood donation screening [25]. NAT testing revealed 244 HCV RNA positives that were antibody-negative donors in 66 million donations. These infections account for 1 in 270,000 screened for HCV. The current risk of transfusion-transmitted HCV is 1:1,390,000 [28].

HTLV

It is estimated that 15–20 million individuals have HTLV infection [29]. Within adult populations, the prevalence rates vary depending on risk groups and geographic location, but range from very low to as high as 37 % in some areas of Japan. ATL and HTLV-associated myelopathy (HAM)/TSP most frequently occur in southern Japan, which also coincides with a high prevalence of virus carriers. The incidence of seropositive donors increases with age, and the virus has a high prevalence in families when the mother is seropositive. In Europe and North America, the virus has been mainly detected in intravenous drug users (IVDUs) and specific immigrant populations.

In the USA, the prevalence of HTLV-I and HTLV–II ranges from 0.025 % in asymptomatic blood donors and 3 % in blood transfusion recipients to 7–49 % in IVDUs and commercial sex workers. In the USA, the risk of contracting HTLV from receiving contaminated donor blood is estimated to be less than 1 in 2,000,000 units [28], but the risk of seroconverting after transfusion of HTLV-1-contaminated blood ranges from 40 to 60 % [29]. Among first-time donors, HTLV-I/II prevalence has decreased from 10 per 10,000 in 2000 to 5 per 10,000 in 2009 [30]. The estimated risk of collecting blood during the infectious window period for repeat blood donors is about 1 in 3,000,000 (Table 8.1).

WNV

National blood donor screening for WNV started in June 2003, after the documentation of WNV transfusion-associated transmission (TAT) in 2002. Blood donations were screened with investigational NAT in MP formats, and blood collection agencies reported screening results to state and local public health authorities. During 2003–2005, 1,425 presumptive viremic donors were reported to the Centers for Disease Control and Prevention (CDC) from 41 states. Of 36 investigations of suspected WNV TAT in 2003, six cases were documented. Estimated viremia levels were available for donations implicated in four TAT cases. National blood screening for WNV identified and removed these potentially infectious blood donations in 2003 through 2005. Despite the success of screening in 2003, some residual WNV TAT risk remained due to donations containing very low levels of virus. Screening algorithms employing selected individual donation testing were designed to address this residual risk and were fully implemented in 2004 and 2005 [31].

T. pallidum

No cases of transfusion-transmitted syphilis have been recorded since 1968 [13].

T. cruzi

The CDC estimates that there are more than 300,000 *T. cruzi*-infected persons in the USA; the majority is unaware of their infection. Data from the testing of allogeneic blood donors for *T. cruzi* during 2007–2009 (nearly three million donations from over one million donors) showed the prevalence rates of confirmed donors to be 0.01 % per donation tested and 0.026 % per blood donor were repeatedly reactive; 89 of those were confirmed by RIPA, yielding an overall seroprevalence of 1 per 33,039 donations and 1 per 13,292 donors; the national seroprevalence of *T. cruzi* in USA blood donors was estimated to be 1 in 27,500 donations screened [32, 33]. One of 200 donors born in Central or South America and 1 of 800 donors born in Mexico were confirmed positive by RIPA. In the USA, it was found that the highest prevalence from donors was in California followed by Las Vegas, Nevada, and parts of Texas. It was concluded by the authors that blood donors or transfusions, although recognizing that autochthonous infection occurred in the USA, do not substantially contribute to the burden of *T. cruzi* infections in the USA.

Table 8.1 illustrates the prevalence rates in blood donors and the risk of infections from negative blood.

Methodology and Interpretation

Serologic Testing

HIV

HIV serologic screening tests vary among facilities, but all must use FDA-licensed tests, and all donors are tested. Most blood banks use an EIA that detects HIV-1, HIV-2, and HIV-1 group O to maximize chances of detecting all HIV infections. Moreover, they can choose between third- or fourth-generation assays. The former is an indirect detection format where antibody is detected with the use of an anti-immunoglobulin conjugate, while the latter uses an antigen sandwich format that offers detection of IgG and IgM antibodies [3]. They all offer high throughput, simplicity, and are fully automated so thousands of samples can be tested daily; they usually possess front-end processors of blood, including barcoding and robotic apparatuses that add samples and all reagents. Other types of immunoassays are available, including fluorometric immunoassays (FIAs) or ChLIA that use fluorescence or luminescence, respectively, as the signal rather than a colorimetric readout. The configurations of these assays have been described [3]. Reactive results are repeated to minimize technical errors, and repeatedly reactive samples are further tested by a confirmatory (supplemental) assay such as the HIV-1 Western blot (WB) or HIV indirect immunofluorescent assay (IFA). The confirmatory test is used to counsel the donor. HIV-2 confirmation is not performed because no supplemental tests for HIV-2 are licensed; however, a rapid FDA-licensed test can be used for HIV-1 and HIV-2 differentiation. Repeatedly reactive samples by the screening test result in deferral of the donor and quarantine of the blood donation. More specifically, donors are deferred who are NAT nonreactive (or if NAT was not performed) and who were repeatedly reactive by a screening test for HIV-1 or HIV-2 or HIV-1/2 antibody, with an HIV-1 WB or IFA that was indeterminate, unreadable, negative, or was not performed. Performance of an investigational HIV-2 supplemental test (if available) is optional.

In addition to the use of serologic assays to identify most donors who are infected, NAT (see below) has been added to detect acute HIV and HCV infection (before antibody is produced). As shown in Fig. 8.1, NAT can detect HIV infection 1–2 weeks before seroconversion, but both serologic and molecular assays are used in combination to detect most HIV infections except during the eclipse period. In response to recommendations or guidelines by CDC and the Clinical Laboratory Standards Institute (CLSI) recently [34], algorithms are being considered that will specifically identify HIV-1 or HIV-2 infection. Although blood banks have not yet revised their algorithms to differentiate HIV-1 from HIV-2, this may be considered in the future. At present, the serologic screening assays detect antibodies to both HIV-1 and HIV-2 (although they do not differentiate the viral types), while some of the molecular assays used in the blood banks detect only HIV-1. Because the screening serologic assays detect infection by both viruses, the blood supply can be kept relatively safe from both viruses (except during very early infection).

The serologic screening tests detect antibodies from about 3 weeks after infection throughout established infection; however, with treatment or during the late stages of AIDS, antibody levels decrease and serologic tests can become negative [35]. Newer fourth-generation serologic tests additionally detect HIV-1 p24 antigen in an effort to decrease the serologic window period [3], but these are not currently performed in blood banks because of the use of NAT, which has a higher sensitivity for early infection than does p24 antigen testing. Viral RNA can be detected at about 11 days postinfection, while p24 antigen is detected at about day 17, and antibody at day 21 (Fig. 8.1). However, no technique can detect infection during the eclipse period (time zero to about 11 days) where even NAT cannot detect infection; this period varies, most likely due to host factors, the size of the inoculum, as well as the sensitivity of the test, and has been estimated to have a range of 6–12 days [36, 37]. While the sensitivity and specificity of EIA methods are very high, the risk of false-negative results due to early infection and the risk of false-positive results due to autoimmune conditions or other infectious agents (or unknown reasons) in screening blood donors were identified as significant issues. HIV infection rates have decreased among blood donors and the window period has been shortened from about 45 days in the early 1990s [38] to about 11 days at present (with molecular tests). Similarly, the window period for HCV has declined to about 10 days [23].

HBV

The ARC currently tests for HBsAg and Anti-HBc using the fully automated PRISM ChLIA (Abbott); some blood banks may use a colorimetric EIA. Samples that are HBsAg reactive are repeated and then confirmed using a neutralization assay to rule out false-positive HBsAg reactions. Anti-HBc appears in the serum of individuals infected with HBV 1–4 weeks after the appearance of HBsAg, and at the onset of symptoms for the minority of adults (5 % or less) who develop symptoms. HBsAg-positive blood units may not be used for transfusion purposes.

If the initial HBsAg test is positive, it must be repeated in duplicate and a confirmatory (i.e., neutralization) test must be performed. If the confirmatory test is positive, the donor is considered infected (acute or chronic) with HBV and must be permanently deferred. If the initial HBsAg test is positive but the confirmatory testing is not (i.e., an unconfirmed positive), the donor does not need to be permanently deferred if the anti-HBc test is also negative; however, the collected blood product(s) will be discarded. The donor is temporarily deferred for 8 weeks and may be reinstated if the next HBsAg test is negative.

In addition, some blood banks are instituting NAT for HBV DNA to detect early and current infection, but it is not required by the FDA. The ARC implemented HBV MP-NAT (triplex TMA) in 2009, in addition to the existing tests for HBsAg and anti-HBc; results from over 6.5 million donors indicated that a small number of donors (2) were detected who had early infection that was missed by serologic testing [27]. There were no NAT-negative samples that were HBsAg positive.

HCV

The serologic testing algorithm for HCV is identical to that for HIV (see above) except for the use of the recombinant immunoblot assay (RIBA) instead of WB. Serologically, antibody tests, including screening by enzyme immunoassay (EIA) and confirmation by recombinant immunoblot assay (RIBA), are generally effective, but seroconversion may not occur for up to 6 months [39], resulting in potentially long periods of acute infection that cannot be detected by serologic assays. In addition, RNA detection is variable, with the occurrence of "blips" of RNA in plasma (inconsistent presence) and periods where RNA is not detected (Constantine, personal observation). Currently, blood units are screened by serology (EIA) and screened by NAT, sometimes in a multiplex format (see below).

HTLV

Several EIA screening tests are available for donor screening. Included is the Avioq HTLVI/II Microelisa System that has been recently approved by the FDA for use to screen individual human donors, volunteer donors of whole blood and blood components, and other living donors for the presence of anti-HTLV-I/II in serum or plasma. As with HIV, repeatedly reactive donors are further tested by an HTLV-I or HTLV-1/2 WB confirmation test. Currently, NAT assays for HTLV are not commercially available and are not being used for donor screening.

The most common assays used to screen donor blood to detect antibodies to HTLV-I and HTLV-II in serum or plasma are serologic, but these do not discriminate the viruses. HTLV-I/II antibody detection methods are divided into two classes: screening tests such as EIA or ChLIA and confirmatory tests such as the WB, RIPA, and IFA. Generally, these screening assays are excellent for the detection of HTLV-I and HTLV-II infections. The WB is the most specific confirmatory serological assay due to the incorporation of both whole virus lysate and recombinant and synthetic peptide antigens. Molecular assays such as polymerase chain reaction (PCR) can detect HTLV nucleic acid and are particularly useful for resolving individuals with indeterminate WB results, but they are not approved for screening blood donors. The incorporation of antigens spiked with a recombinant transmembrane protein (r21e) and some that contain an HTLV-II viral lysate has increased sensitivity of confirmatory WB assays.

T. pallidum

Testing for *T. pallidum* is performed in blood banks and is required for whole blood donor testing. Screening tests include the rapid plasma reagin (RPR) test and the Venereal Disease Research Laboratory (VDRL) tests. Both tests are based on the detection of reagin, an antibody directed toward cardiolipin particles. A positive result is indicated by visible flocculation (or agglutination) of cardiolipin-coated carbon particles. The confirmatory test for syphilis is the FTA-ABS (fluorescent treponemal antibody absorption) test. If the RPR or VDRL screen is reactive or indeterminate, that donation must be discarded and the donor deferred unless a confirmatory FTA-ABS test is nonreactive.

If the FTA-ABS test is nonreactive, the donor may be reentered.

A serological test for syphilis (STS) on donated whole blood has been required since the 1950s and continues to be done because syphilis is a sexually transmitted disease, meaning that the prospective donor is at higher risk for other sexually transmitted diseases, such as HBV, HCV, and HIV. Currently, all blood donations are screened for *T. pallidum* using an STS.

WNV

WNV infection in blood donors is detected using NAT (description below); no serologic tests are approved for donor screening. A positive result precludes donation.

T. cruzi

Screening for *T. cruzi* is performed in blood banks by EIA or the recently approved Abbott PRISM ChLIA assay. RIPA, as a supplemental test, and PCR produce variable results and have low sensitivity, and the lack of international standards precludes PCR application into practice. All blood donors are screened for a past history of *T. cruzi* infection through medical history questioning before donation. Those who have a history are deferred from donating [20]. Those without a history are tested for antibodies to *T. cruzi* using an FDA-licensed EIA test. Those who are EIA reactive are retested in duplicate and repeatedly reactive donations are further tested by a supplemental RIPA that confirms the EIA result. The requirement for screening is that when a donor has been tested once and found to be negative or nonreactive, they need not be tested again. That is, donors need only be tested once for evidence of infection with *T. cruzi,* but it is up to each blood bank if it wishes to test donors every time they donate. PCR research methods are available for identifying *T. cruzi* infection [20], but they are not licensed for blood donor screening and thus are not used. The authors claim that the sensitivity is 0.5 parasites/20 mL and the target is kinetoplastic DNA. The only implicated products reported to transmit *T. cruzi* have been platelets, with no evidence of plasma or RBC [20].

Molecular Testing

HIV

NAT for detecting HIV viral RNA or DNA is now in wide use, particularly for monitoring viral load before and after treatment, and most are approved only for this application. They are often used as an initial test to detect HIV infection and to resolve inconclusive HIV antibody results. There are several NAT methods currently being used in non-blood bank clinical practice for monitoring (or confirming) HIV infection, including reverse transcriptase RT-PCR, nucleic acid sequence-based amplification (NASBA), transcription-mediated amplification (TMA), and branched-chain DNA. Details of some molecular methods and their formats are described below and in other chapters. For blood donor screening, NATs have been used to identify infected persons who are in the window period before HIV antibody becomes detectable. These tests have now replaced p24 antigen testing and are performed on pools of samples to decrease cost. The Aptima HIV-1 NAT (Gen-Probe), if positive, confirms infection. Amplification is by TMA and detection is by using probes in a hybridization protection assay (HPA). The test has inter- and intra-assay coefficients of variation (CVs) of about 5 % and 12 %, respectively, and the sensitivity is 100 copies/mL (98 % at 30 copies/mL). The cobas® Taq/Screen MPX test has been FDA licensed for the purpose of screening individual human donors, including donors of whole blood and blood components, and other living donors. It is also intended for use in testing plasma specimens to screen individual organ donors when specimens are obtained while the donor's heart is still beating. For donations of whole blood, blood components, and other living donors, plasma specimens may be tested individually or in pools, and results interpreted in conjunction with serology tests. The test detects HIV-1 RNA, HIV-1 group M RNA, group O RNA and HIV-2 RNA, as well as HCV RNA and HBV DNA.

Although the NAT strategy shortens the window period by several days and eliminates some infected blood units, it does not eliminate all infected units because of the 12-day eclipse period where even viral nucleic acids cannot be detected (see Fig. 8.1).

HBV

HBsAg and HBV DNA are the first viral markers to circulate in an individual infected with HBV. PCR and TMA-based NAT systems for HBV have been licensed by FDA for use in donor screening since 2005. While there are FDA-approved NAT systems available for testing blood donors, their use is currently considered optional. FDA regards HBV NAT as voluntary because the estimated individual and public health benefits of adding this test to available screening tests are thought to be very limited. This consensus decision was reached by FDA's Blood Products Advisory Committee, the Department of Health and Human Services' (DHHS) Advisory Committee on Blood Safety and Availability, and the DHHS Blood Safety Committee [40]. According to the FDA, this decision may be reconsidered (changed to mandatory NAT donor screening for HBV) based on experience with, and results of voluntary use of the test, further technology developments, and any other factors that might affect the health benefits expected from such testing. Until then, blood donations must still be tested for HBsAg and anti-HBc by non-NAT methods. On November 15, 2012, FDA released a draft guidance document in which it recommends that blood establishments consider adding an FDA-licensed HBV NAT to the screening tests now performed on whole blood and source plasma donations. While draft guidance is not a regulation, it represents FDA's current thinking on a matter and as such, it is likely that this recommendation will be implemented. A copy of the draft guidance is available in the November 15, 2012 Federal Register.

Anti-HBc confirmation is done by testing each individual reactive donation sample for DNA detection using NAT. HBV DNA detection by NAT for routine blood donor screening is done using TMA technology. Screening for DNA is performed in small MP of 16 donor samples using a combined test that detects HBV DNA as well as HIV and HCV RNA. NAT using TMA in MP of 16 reduces the window as compared to HBsAg detection by 4–7 days. The risk of HBV infection through blood transfusion is between 1 in 200,000 and 1 in 500,000 [26–28].

HCV

All donor units must be screened for the presence of antibodies to HCV (anti-HCV) and if the screening test is positive, it must be followed by appropriate confirmatory testing. Alternatively, donor specimens may be tested by NAT either individually or in MP. For conventional testing, if the initial screening test is negative, the unit is suitable for transfusion, but first, FDA recommends that it be retested using NAT. If the screening test is reactive, the test must be repeated in duplicate. If any one of the duplicate tests is reactive, the unit must be discarded as well as any existing components from prior donations. The details of HCV NAT are described below.

HTLV-I/II

There are no commercially available or FDA-licensed NAT for HTLV, and thus, it is not performed in blood banks.

T. pallidum

At present, there is no NAT for donor blood syphilis testing.

T. cruzi

There are currently no FDA-licensed NATs for use to detect *T. cruzi*.

WNV

NAT screening for WNV started in 2003 after 23 WNV blood transfusion-transmitted cases were confirmed in the previous year. The assays incorporate 6–24 minipools (MP-NAT) [41]. A retrospective individual testing of units in high-prevalence regions showed 14 viremic units that were missed in MP testing in the 2003 season in addition to 183 previously identified by MP-NAT [42]. The WNV was detected in 2003–2004 by routine testing; there were 540 positive donations of which 147 (27 %) were detected by individual testing [41]. AABB had guidelines for triggering NAT screening for WNV to close the gap of risk of transfusion from

MP-NAT screened units but each blood center could define and implement it differently based on their capacity or width of area it could cover; thus, the guidelines needed to be tighter [43]. In New York City, for example, the trigger was one positive MP-NAT, followed by a confirmed NAT which led to 20 excluded units. NAT of all units collected during July 1st through October 30th of 2010 showed that 2 donations could have been missed by the triggering system in place, which indicated that more revision of the guidelines is still required [44].

Multiplex NAT Approaches

While individual NAT assays are available for testing blood donors for HIV-1/2, HBV, and HCV, a more efficient approach results from the development of "multiplex" assays. These multiplex assays are FDA approved and available for use in blood banks to detect some of these viruses.

The PROCLEIX® HIV-1/HCV Assay and the PROCLEIX® ULTRIO® Assay (HIV-1/HCV/HBV) use the principle of TMA, while the cobas® TaqScreen MPX Test (HIV-1 Group M/HIV-1 Group O/HIV-2/HCV/HBV) uses PCR. For donor testing purposes, all tests have acceptable performance characteristics, including analytical sensitivity. In addition, all assays can be performed on fully automated platforms. If positive, all assays require further testing with individual discriminatory assays to demonstrate which viral nucleic acid has been detected.

Each molecular assay is described briefly below, but the reader is encouraged to review package inserts on the FDA's and company web pages for more detail, including specific procedures, instrumentation, limitations, and performance characteristics during clinical trials.

Readers should note that while NAT is available for HIV-1, HIV-2, HCV, and HBV, the FDA has not permitted blood banks to cease testing blood donations with traditional methods (EIA for screening, WB/IFA/RIBA for confirmation) with the exception that blood banks need no longer test donations for HIV p24 antigen.

Standard Reagents: Examples

West Nile Virus [45, 46]

Two NAT assays are FDA approved and available for use in blood banks to detect WNV. The Gen-Probe PROCLEIX WNV Assay uses the principle of TMA, while the cobas® TaqScreen WNV Test uses real-time PCR. Both tests are essentially equivalent in their performance characteristics, including their analytical sensitivity. In addition, both assays can be performed on fully automated platforms, and their costs are similar.

PROCLEIX® WNV Assay: Principle

Gen-Probe's PROCLEIX® WNV Assay is used with the PROCLEIX® System and the PROCLEIX® TIGRIS System and is a qualitative in vitro assay system for the direct detection of WNV RNA in human plasma. It is approved for donor screening to detect WNV RNA in plasma specimens from human donors, as individual specimens or in MP of up to 16 equal single specimen aliquots.

The assay involves three main steps in a single tube: sample preparation, WNV RNA target amplification by TMA, and detection of the amplification products (amplicon) by HPA. During sample preparation, RNA is isolated from specimens via target capture. The specimen is treated with detergent to solubilize the viral envelope, denature proteins, and release viral genomic RNA. "Capture oligonucleotides" that are homologous to highly conserved regions of the WNV are hybridized to the WNV RNA target if present, in the test specimen. The hybridized target is captured onto magnetic microparticles that are separated from the specimen in a magnetic field; wash steps remove extraneous components from the reaction tube. Target amplification occurs via TMA, using two enzymes, MMLV reverse transcriptase (RT) and T7 RNA polymerase. The RT generates a DNA copy of the target RNA sequence, while the T7 RNA polymerase produces multiple copies of the RNA amplicon from the DNA copy. Detection is carried out by HPA using single-stranded nucleic acid probes with chemiluminescent labels that are complementary to the amplicon. Labeled nucleic acid probes hybridize specifically to the amplicon, and a chemiluminescent signal is produced by the hybridized probe; it is measured in a luminometer and reported in Relative Light Units (RLU).

An internal control (IC) is added to each test specimen, positive and negative controls (as required), and calibrators. The IC in the assay controls for specimen processing, amplification, and detection steps. The IC signal is discriminated from the WNV signal by the differential kinetics of light emission from probes with different labels. IC-specific amplicon is detected using a probe with rapid emission of light (flasher signal), while the amplicon specific to WNV is detected using probes with relatively slower kinetics of light emission (glower signal). The Dual Kinetic Assay (DKA) differentiates between the signals from flasher and glower labels. Positive and negative calibrators are run in triplicate at the beginning of each run. Each run can have up to 100 tests, including calibrators.

PROCLEIX® WNV Assay: Interpretation of Results

In this assay, a run is valid if four of the six calibrator replicates are valid (2/3 negative and 2/3 positive replicates), and the calibrators meet acceptance criteria specified in the package insert. All specimens in an invalid run must be retested. Cutoff values for the assay are automatically calculated for IC (flasher) and test (glower) specimens in a valid run. A specimen is reactive or nonreactive depending on the analyte signal to cutoff ratio, the relationship between the IC signal and cutoff, and the IC RLU value. A nonreactive specimen, whether from a single donor or a donor pool, requires no further testing. A reactive specimen from a single donor requires no further testing. If a reactive specimen were from a pool, then each individual specimen in the pool must be tested and interpreted individually. Any reactive result should be resolved according to the resolution algorithm for reactive specimens in the package insert.

There are assay- and instrument-specific differences in the performance of the WNV assay using the automated TIGRIS® system (e.g., using controls in addition to calibrators, different software, different RLU values for interpretation), but the essential principles are the same. There also are differences in assay interpretation, owing to the differences in performance and use of controls. Each TIGRIS® run must have a set of Assay Calibrators (positive and negative, in triplicate) at the beginning and a set of TIGRIS® Controls (positive and negative, in singlet) at the end. Each run can have up to 500 tests. These differences are fully described in the package insert.

PROCLEIX® WNV Assay: Analytical Sensitivity

The limit of detection (LOD) was evaluated using three reference standards (Table 8.2).

PROCLEIX® WNV Assay: Clinical Performance

The clinical specificity of the PROCLEIX® WNV Assay was determined in prospectively collected voluntary blood donor specimens, tested as 16-sample pools and as individual plasma samples. Specificity was calculated from 16,885 16-sample pools and 43,503 individual specimens. All 16 samples from a reactive pool were tested individually. Reactive samples, whether from pooled or individual testing, were retested with the PROCLEIX WNV Assay, and results compared with a validated alternate NAT and a commercial

Table 8.2 LOD using reference standards

	PROCLEIX® system	PROCLEIX® TIGRIS®
Health Canada WNV Reference Standard (Canadian Blood Services)	100 % @ 100 copies/mL	100 % @ 100 copies/mL
	100 % @ 30 copies/mL	100 % @ 30 copies/mL
	97 % @ 10 copies/mL	91 % @ 10 copies/mL
	53 % @ 3 copies/mL	58 % @ 3 copies/mL
West Nile Virus RNA Qualification Panel QWN701 (BBI Diagnostics)	98 % @ 100 copies/mL	100 % @ 100 copies/mL
	99 % @ 30 copies/mL	97 % @ 30 copies/mL
	89 % @ 10 copies/mL	82 % @ 10 copies/mL
Center for Biologics Evaluation and Research (CBER)/FDA West Nile Virus Panel (produced for CBER by BBI Diagnostics)	100 % @ ≥100 copies/mL	100 % @ ≥100 copies/mL

serologic IgM assay. Of the 16,885 pools, 16,855 were nonreactive (true negative). Thirty pools were reactive in the PROCLEIX WNV Assay, and of these, 21 pools contained at least 1 reactive sample when the pool members were tested individually. The 21 reactive pools were considered true positive pools; the results were confirmed as reactive by alternate NAT and/or positive for IgM antibody. Nine reactive pools were considered false positive because all individual specimens were nonreactive in the PROCLEIX WNV Assay. The overall specificity was 99.95 %.

Of the 43,503 individual donor specimens tested at four sites, 43,427 were nonreactive (true negative); there were 76 reactive specimens. Of these, 30 were confirmed by alternate NAT and/or IgM results (true positive) and the remaining 46 were considered false positive. The overall specificity was 99.89 %. Combining the results from 16-sample pools and individual donor testing, the overall specificity of the PROCLEIX WNV Assay in these studies was 99.91 %.

To test for cross-reactivity, specimens with various donor conditions were tested. No cross-reactivity or interference was observed in a large number of specimens from patients with a variety of conditions, including autoimmune diseases, infectious agents, other blood-borne pathogens, cancers, and liver diseases (see package insert). The assay did detect Kunjin virus, a WNV variant. Mostly comparable results (lack of cross-reactivity or interference) were observed in testing the assay on the PROCLEIX® TIGRIS® System.

For sensitivity, WNV known-positive samples obtained from a repository were tested with the PROCLEIX® WNV Assay. Specimens were tested neat and in a 1:16 dilution. Neat samples had known WNV RNA concentrations ≥100 copies/mL, and known-positive samples with WNV RNA copy levels less than 100 copies/mL after 1:16 dilution were included. The sensitivity of the assay was 100 % in neat known-positive samples and 91.6 % in diluted known-positive samples. All diluted samples with false-negative results were derived from samples that had low WNV viral loads. Assay sensitivity in diluted samples with copy levels ≥100 copies/mL was 100 %.

Assay clinical sensitivity in pooled samples was determined by testing 98 16-sample pools comprised 1–3 WNV known-positive samples and 13–15 negative samples. Pools contained individual specimens with viral concentrations ranging from 200 to 430,000 copies/mL. After pooling, 6 of the 98 pools had less than 100 copies/mL. The sensitivity of the assay in these 98 known-positive pools was 100 %.

cobas® TaqScreen WNV Test: Principle

The Roche Molecular Systems cobas® TaqScreen WNV Test is used with the cobas s 201 system and is a qualitative in vitro test for direct detection of WNV RNA in human plasma. It is approved as a donor screening test to detect WNV RNA in plasma from individual human donors. Donor plasma may be screened as individual specimens or pools of up to six equal aliquots of single specimens.

This test uses a generic nucleic acid preparation technique on the COBAS® AmpliPrep Instrument. WNV RNA is detected by automated, real-time PCR amplification on the cobas s 201 system. Reagents perform five sequential steps in the AmpliPrep. Protease solution digests proteins to promote viral lysis, inactivate nucleases, and facilitate RNA/DNA release from viral particles. Lysis Reagent induces viral lysis and nuclease inactivation by protein denaturation. RNA and DNA are released and bind to Magnetic Glass Particles, due to the net positive charge on the glass particle surface and lysis reagent-induced net negative charge of nucleic acids. Wash Reagent removes unbound substances, impurities, and PCR inhibitors. Purified nucleic acids are released from the Magnetic Glass Particles at elevated temperature with Elution Buffer.

After isolating the purified nucleic acids, the WNV Master Mix (MMX) is used to amplify and detect WNV RNA and an internal control (IC) RNA. With activation, the WNV MMX permits reverse transcription, followed by PCR amplification of a highly conserved region of WNV RNA and IC RNA using specific primers. Detection of the amplified DNA is performed by fluorescent signals from 5′-nucleolytic degradation of WNV and IC-specific probes, also present in the WNV MMX. Two fluorescent dyes are used: one labels the IC probe and a second labels the target-specific probe, permitting independent identification of WNV and IC.

Reverse transcription and PCR amplification are carried out in the same reaction mixture using a thermostable enzyme, Z05 DNA Polymerase. The enzyme produces a double-stranded DNA (amplicon) over multiple cycles, with each cycle doubling the amount of amplicon. This system allows simultaneous detection of the amplified WNV target at one wavelength and of the amplified IC nucleic acid at another wavelength. The system detects PCR products by measuring the fluorescence of the released reporter dyes representing WNV target and IC independently. A negative control and a positive control must be processed with each batch. A detailed description of the process and reagents is found in the product's package insert.

For the negative control to be valid, the test result must be nonreactive and the IC must be valid. For the positive control to be valid, the test result must be reactive, and the IC must be valid. If the IC is invalid, the result for the control is invalid. If the result for either the negative or the positive control is invalid, the entire batch is invalid and must be repeated. For a donor specimen to have a valid nonreactive test result, the specimen's IC must be valid; otherwise, the nonreactive result is invalid and the donor specimen must be retested. For a donor specimen to have a valid reactive test result, the specimen's IC may be either valid or invalid. Specimen results are valid only if the batch containing the specimen is valid. Donor results will be reported out by the system software as "Complete, Nonreactive," "Complete, Reactive," or "Complete, Unresolved" (viability time limit expired; see the cobas s 201 system Operator's Manual for a description of the viability time limit).

Donors that require additional testing include donor tubes whose pool or individual donation status is invalid (status of "Repeat Needed") and donor tubes included in a reactive pool (status of "Resolution Needed"). Invalid donor tubes require repeat testing as part of a repeat pool or a repeat single determination. Reactive pools require repeat testing of all specimens in that pool, individually. Any reactive individual specimen from that pool is reported as "Complete Reactive" and the remaining negative specimens in that pool are reported as "Complete, Nonreactive." If all individual donor specimens in a reactive pool subsequently test nonreactive, the specimens in that pool are all reported as "Complete, Nonreactive."

cobas® TaqScreen WNV Test: Analytical Sensitivity

The LOD was evaluated using four reference standards: the three standards named above and the Roche WNV Secondary Standard. Using the Health Canada Standard, the estimated 95 % detection rate was at 40.3 copies/mL, while the Roche Standard estimated a 95 % detection rate at 36.9 copies/mL. The QWN701 Standard estimated a 95 % detection rate of 3.8 copies/mL, while the CBER/FDA Panel indicated a detection of 100 % at 50 copies/mL.

cobas® TaqScreen WNV Test: Clinical Sensitivity

The clinical sensitivity of the test was evaluated by testing 315 WNV-positive clinical specimens (known WNV RNA positive by one of three nucleic acid methods). Three testing laboratories tested approximately 100 specimens, neat and diluted 1:6. The sensitivity with neat specimens in this study was 100 % and with 1:6 diluted specimens was 97.5 %. The 8 nonreactive, 1:6 diluted specimens, had viral loads less than 100 copies/mL.

cobas® TaqScreen WNV Test: Clinical Specificity

The clinical specificity of the test was evaluated by testing randomly selected whole blood donations at five sites (individual specimens and 6-donor pools). There were 86,935 evaluable donors from pooled testing and 10,375 evaluable donors from individual testing. The clinical specificity was 100 % for the pooled strategy and for individual testing.

cobas® TaqScreen WNV Test: Interference Studies

The specificity of the test was evaluated against 52 microorganisms, including 47 viral isolates, 4 bacterial strains, and 1 yeast isolate, added to normal, virus-negative human plasma and tested with and without WNV. Except for 4 isolates of the Japanese Encephalitis Virus (JEV) family, nonreactive results were obtained with all microorganism samples without added WNV and reactive results were obtained for all microorganism samples with added WNV. The four JEV family isolates were reactive in all eight testing replicates. These results were expected because these viruses share nucleotide sequence homology with WNV. Specimens from patients infected with a number of viruses were tested; results indicated nonreactive results on all specimens without added WNV and reactive results on all specimens with added WNV. Therefore, there was no interference with the assay using specimens positive for the viruses.

Viral Multiplex Assays

PROCLEIX® Multiplex Assays for HIV, HBV, and HCV: Principle [47, 48]

The PROCLEIX® HIV-1/HCV Assay and the PROCLEIX® ULTRIO® Assay are both qualitative in vitro nucleic acid assay systems for the detection of HIV-1/HCV or HIV-1/HIV-2/HBV/HCV, respectively, in plasma specimens from individual human donors; these can be used as either screening individual donor samples or pools of not more than 16 individual donors. The former is designed to be performed on the PROCLEIX® System (semi-automated) and the latter may be performed on both the PROCLEIX® System and the PROCLEIX®TIGRIS System (fully automated). These assays involve the same three main steps as the PROCLEIX® WNV assay described above in a single tube: sample preparation. RNA target amplification by TMA, and amplicon detection by HPA.

PROCLEIX® Multiplex Assays: Interpretation

Valid nonreactive specimens are considered nonreactive for viral nucleic acid. If the nonreactive specimen is a pool, each individual specimen in the pool is considered nonreactive and no further testing is required. Valid reactive specimens are considered reactive. If the reactive specimen is a pool, then each of the individual specimens in the pool must be tested individually with the multiplex assay. The nonreactive individual specimens are considered nonreactive. An individual specimen reactive with the multiplex assay must be tested further with the corresponding discriminatory assays. Specimens that are nonreactive in the PROCLEIX Assays or are reactive in the PROCLEIX assays but are not discriminated (nonreactive discriminatory result) and are also repeatedly reactive in a licensed donor screening test for antibodies should be further tested using an FDA-approved serologic assay (such as WB or IFA for HIV-1 or RIBA for HCV).

Table 8.3 Clinical performance of the PROCLEIX HIV-1/HCV NAT

		Specificity	Sensitivity
PROCLEIX®	Pool of 16	99.67 %	99.3 %
HIV-1/HCV	Individual	99.87 %	99.8 %
HIV-1 discriminatory	Individual	99.76 %	100 %
HCV discriminatory	Individual	99.71 %	99.6 %

PROCLEIX® Multiplex Assays: Analytical Sensitivity

Using the PROCLEIX® HIV-1/HCV assay, detection at 300 and 100 copies/mL of virus was 100 %. At 30 copies/mL, HIV-1 detection was 98.2 % and HCV detection was 93.2 %. With the PROCLEIX® ULTRIO® assay, detection of HIV-1 was 100 % at 300 copies/mL, 99 % at 100 copies/mL, and 92 % at 30 copies/mL. Detection of HCV was 100 % at 300 copies/mL, 100 % at 100 copies/mL, and 99 % at 10 copies/mL. Detection of HBV was 100 % at 45 copies/mL and 99 % at 15 copies/mL. TIGRIS® results were comparable. All these reported results were obtained with WHO Standards.

PROCLEIX® Multiplex Assays: Clinical Performance

Overall clinical sensitivity and specificity for the PROCLEIX® HIV-1/HCV Assay and the corresponding discriminatory assays are shown in Table 8.3.

Table 8.4 Clinical specificity for the PROCLEIX ULTRIO® Assay

	PROCLEIX	TIGRIS
Pool of 16	99.5 %	99.9 %
Individual	99.1 %	99.8 %
All combined	99.95 %	Not reported in package insert
HIV-1 discriminatory	99.8 %	
HCV discriminatory	98.1 %	
HBV discriminatory	99.8 %	

Clinical specificity for the PROCLEIX ULTRIO® Assay is shown in Table 8.4 for both the PROCLEIX® and the TIGRIS® systems.

In a head-to-head comparison between the PROCLEIX ULTRIO® Assay and the PROCLEIX® HIV-1/HCV Assay, both assays detected 100 % of HIV-1 RNA-positive specimens and 98.4 % of HCV RNA-positive specimens.

For the majority of diseases and conditions tested, no cross-reactivity or interference was observed. However, a small portion of these specimens had random, unexpected results in greater than 5 % of the samples tested. These occurrences are described in detail in assay package inserts. Also, in the PROCLEIX® HBV Discriminatory Assay, antinuclear antibody cross-reactivity may be observed on the PROCLEIX® System and interference may be observed in the PROCLEIX® TIGRIS® System.

cobas® TaqScreen MPX Test [49]: Principle and Interpretation

The cobas® TaqScreen MPX Test, used with the cobas s 201 system, is a qualitative multiplex test for the direct, simultaneous detection of HIV-1 Group M and Group O RNA, HIV-2 RNA, HCV RNA, and HBV DNA in human plasma. This test is used to screen plasma samples from individual human donors and donors of source plasma. Plasma may be screened as individual specimens or in pools of not more than six equal aliquots. This test is intended to be used in conjunction with licensed serology tests for HIV, HCV, and HBV.

To improve the efficiency of testing for multiple targets, a multiplex (MPX) PCR for simultaneous detection of multiple viruses was developed. In MPX PCR, more than one target sequence is amplified and detected by using multiple pairs of primers and probes in one reaction tube.

The cobas® TaqScreen MPX Test uses a generic nucleic acid preparation technique on the COBAS® AmpliPrep Instrument. HIV-1 Groups M and O RNA, HIV-2 RNA, HCV RNA, and HBV DNA are amplified and detected using automated, real-time PCR on the cobas s 201 system. The test incorporates an Internal Control (IC) for monitoring test performance in each individual test as well as the AmpErase enzyme to reduce potential contamination by previously amplified material (amplicon).

The cobas® TaqScreen MPX Test does not discriminate which virus was detected in a specimen. Any individual specimens found to be reactive should be further tested using the COBAS® AmpliScreen HIV-1, HCV, and HBV Tests for viral target identification (Discriminatory Testing). Individual viral identification procedures for HIV-1 Group O and HIV-2 are not available from Roche.

The cobas® TaqScreen MPX Test has four processes (all automated): specimen pooling and control pipeting; specimen preparation; amplification of nucleic acid and real-time detection of PCR products; and data management using proprietary software. The instrumentation is essentially the same as for the WNV assay (see above). Target and internal control nucleic acids are processed simultaneously. Two fluorescent dyes are used; one to label the IC and one to label all target-specific probes, allowing a distinction between target and IC signals. Individual targets cannot be distinguished, however. A detailed description of the process and reagents is found in the product's package insert. Interpretation of results also is essentially the same as for the WNV assay (see above).

cobas® TaqScreen MPX: Analytical Sensitivity

Testing showed average 95 % LOD as follows:

- HIV-1 Group O (49 IU/mL; converts to 29.4 copies/mL)
- HIV-1 Group M (89 copies/mL)
- HIV-2 (59 copies/mL)
- HCV (11 IU/mL; converts to 29.7 copies/mL)
- HBV (3.8 IU/mL; converts to 19 copies/mL)

The LOD testing for the cobas® TaqScreen MPX Test included WHO Standards for HBV and HCV and Roche Standards for HIV-1 Group M and Group O, and HIV-2 (from Boston Biomedica). Genotype/subtype sensitivity and inclusivity testing was performed with an array of clinical specimens and cultured isolates; results are presented in the package insert. Commercial seroconversion panels were tested for HIV-1 Group M, HCV, and HBV. Specimens were tested neat and diluted 1:6. The MPX assay was compared against the performance of various commercial or research antibody detection assays. HIV RNA was detected in neat and diluted specimens between 5 and 89 days before the antibody detection tests. HCV RNA was detected in neat and diluted specimens between 0 and 97 days before the antibody detection tests. In a few cases (1 of 20 panels or 5 %), the MPX test result detected HCV RNA on the same day as the antibody assays. HBV DNA was detected in neat specimens and diluted specimens before HBsAg detection (by EIA) in a majority of specimens tested, but in a substantial number of tests, HBV DNA was detected on the same day or after HBsAg detection.

cobas® TaqScreen MPX: Clinical Performance

Clinical specificity of the cobas® TaqScreen MPX Test was evaluated by testing plasma samples from randomly selected whole blood donations on both individual blood donations and pooled specimens. Clinical specificity was 99.98 %. Specimens from high-risk individuals were tested neat with the MPX Test. The MPX Test showed greater detection rate than three licensed discriminatory tests.

Specificity also was evaluated by testing 17 microorganisms, including viruses, bacteria, and yeast. The microorganisms did not cross-react with the MPX Test. When target virus was added to the microorganism samples, all tested reactive. The MPX Test was nonreactive for an array of disease states, including viral infections and autoimmune diseases. These disease states did not interfere with the sensitivity or specificity of the cobas® TaqScreen MPX Test.

Economics of Keeping the Blood Supply Safe

One important aspect of NAT specifically, and increased donor blood testing for transmissible agents in general, is the effect of these added tests on the cost of a unit of blood. This cost may be divided into the cost for procuring (collecting) that unit and the cost to the patient for being transfused with it.

Procurement cost includes recruiting and screening donors, collecting the blood, processing and testing the blood, and storing it until distribution. Procurement cost includes the cost of follow-up when a prospective donor's specimen is found to be positive for one or more infectious agents. Follow-up includes repeating the positive test(s), performing confirmatory tests on repeatedly reactive tests (if available), sequestering the blood, adding the donor to the donor deferral registry, notifying the donor of the positive testing, and tracing back and pulling units from prior donations that may still be in the inventory, a process called "lookback."

News reports in 2007 [50, 51] indicated the average procurement cost of blood rose between 1979 and 2000 from $32 to $96. By 2004, it reached over $200 (recall the first NAT approvals for HIV-1 and HCV donor screening assays were granted in 2002). Recent studies by Toner et al. [52]. and Shander et al. [53]. indicated average acquisition (procurement) cost for a unit of red blood cells in the USA ranged from $203 to $248. It appears that the rate of increase has stabilized since 2004. Each new donor test adds between $5 and $12 to the cost of that unit.

This procurement cost will be passed through to the patient being transfused and it represents one-fifth to one-quarter of the total cost charged to the patient. That total cost will then be passed through (in whole or in part) to insurers (private, government) as a hospitalization cost. There are geographical differences, of course, and according to Toner et al. [52], volume discounts for large teaching hospitals.

The public demands a safe blood supply. Absolute safety may not be possible unless and until methods are developed to treat a unit of blood in a manner that destroys all infectious agents without affecting the safety and effectiveness of the transfused unit. However, as FDA issues new donor testing mandates, in the face of newly recognized infectious agents and/or newer (presumably better) technologies, costs will rise again to meet those new mandates. Meantime, hospitals may each spend several millions of dollars annually on procuring and transfusing blood products. Stakeholders concerned about the rising cost of health care need to consider this in their deliberations about how society can best achieve seemingly contradictory goals—high-quality and affordable health care [54].

Regulatory Issues

Clinical trials for a NAT system useful for screening blood donors were carried out in the late 1990s. Trials incorporated several molecular diagnostic principles, including PCR and TMA. The earliest FDA license approvals were for testing source plasma. They included a 2001 approval to National Genetics Institute for its UltraQual HCV and HIV-1 RT-PCR assays. NAT screening of individual donor units was first FDA approved on 2/27/2002, granted to Gen-Probe, Inc. for its PROCLEIX HCV/HIV-1 multiplex assay, based on TMA. Individual sample test approvals soon followed to Roche Molecular Systems for its PCR-based tests for HCV (COBAS® AmpliScreen HCV, 2002) and HIV-1 (COBAS® AmpliScreen HIV-1, 2002). Since then, NAT assays for HBV and WNV have been developed and FDA approved. In particular, multiplex or combination tests are now available and used (examples above). Other molecular amplification modes (e.g., signal amplification) have been FDA approved for other uses, e.g., patient monitoring, but not donor screening.

More than 3,000 blood banks in the USA collect and process nearly 16 million units of blood, donated by volunteers every year. It is the responsibility of FDA's Center for Biologics Evaluation and Research to ensure the safety of the USA blood supply. FDA is charged with establishing standards for blood products and for regulating the collection, preparation, processing, and testing of whole blood and the components that can be made from it (RBC, PC, and FFP). FDA also is the responsible agency for plasma that is used for manufacturing fractionated biological products such as albumin and general or specific immune serum globulins. Finally, FDA regulates blood collection-related devices such as cell separation devices, blood collection containers, and screening tests used in the testing of blood products.

FDA uses a system of overlapping safeguards to protect the blood supply [55]. These include the following:

- Donor screening
  Donors are asked many questions about factors that may reflect the safety status of their blood. For example, donors with a history of IVDU are routinely deferred (donor deferral definitions are provided below). Since November 1999, questions have been asked about travel to and residence in Europe and the UK countries, including USA military personnel and their families stationed there, owing to the high risk of exposure to variant Creutzfeldt–Jakob Disease (vCJD). There are travel questions to elicit possible exposure to malaria and leishmaniasis, parasitic infections for which there are no current tests to detect infection. These questions are part of standardized Medical History Questionnaires used by all facilities in the USA that collect blood and blood products.
- Blood testing
  After donation, each unit of donated blood undergoes tests for infectious agents or the diseases they cause, including syphilis, HBV, HCV, HIV 1/2, HTLV I/II, WNV, and Chagas disease.
- Donor lists
  Blood banks must keep current a list of deferred donors and use it to ensure that they do not collect blood from anyone on the list.
- Quarantine
  Donated blood must be quarantined until tested and shown free of infectious agents.

- Problems and deficiencies
  Blood centers must investigate manufacturing problems, correct all deficiencies, and notify FDA when product deviations occur in distributed products.

If any one of these safeguards is breached, the blood product is considered unsuitable for transfusion and is subject to recall. In addition to employing these safeguards, FDA has substantial oversight of the blood industry. It inspects all blood facilities at least every 2 years, and "problem" facilities are inspected more often.

FDA mandates that all blood donors and blood units collected for allogeneic transfusion (donating blood for use by another person) whether by whole blood or apheresis collection must be screened/tested for infectious diseases that are known to be transmissible by blood transfusion. These include HBV, HCV, HIV 1/2, HTLV I/II, WNV, syphilis, and Chagas Disease.

Most source plasma is collected by a process called "serial plasmapheresis." If the source plasma is to be further manufactured into injectable products such as immune serum globulin or clotting factors (derivatives), the infectious disease donor screening and testing requirements are the same as for whole blood donations. As an added protection against infectious disease transmission, most plasma derivatives made from source plasma go through a pathogen inactivation process that may include any of the following: heat inactivation, solvent/detergent treatment, nanofiltration, chromatography, or cold ethanol fractionation.

If the plasma is collected for further manufacture into non-injectable/non-transfusable products such as diagnostic reagents, controls, or research material, the donors are exempt from strict adherence to the deferral regulations for infectious diseases.

Donors who are donating for transfusion for themselves (autologous donations) do not have to be deferred for a history of or a positive test for infectious diseases such as HCV, HBV, HIV, HTLV, or syphilis. However, their units of blood must be labeled with biohazard labels and must identify what disease or test was identified. In addition, the hospital or facility that will be transfusing these units must be willing to accept them into their facility and to store them in a manner that segregates the unit(s) from the general transfusion inventory. These units are not permitted to be released into the general transfusion inventory, and if not used by the donor/patient who donated the unit, the unit is discarded.

Donor Deferrals

A zero risk blood supply may not be possible. As biological products, blood and blood products always carry an inherent risk of transmitting infectious agents. FDA's role is to drive that risk to the lowest level reasonably achievable without unduly decreasing the availability of this lifesaving resource. A critical element of that risk reduction strategy is donor deferral. When a donor fails any element of the donor screening process (including infectious agent testing), the donor's blood is quarantined and one of the following three FDA donor deferral categories is applied:

Indefinite Deferral: The prospective donor is unable to donate blood for someone else for an unspecified period of time due to current regulatory requirements. For example, a prospective donor who states he lived in England in 1989 or a donor who gives a history of viral hepatitis after the age of 11 or a donor who gives a history of babesiosis or Chagas Disease would be deferred indefinitely. This donor would not be able to donate blood until the current requirement changes. This donor may be eligible for autologous blood donation, e.g., for elective surgery.

Permanent Deferral: The prospective donor will never be eligible to donate blood for someone else. For example, a prospective donor who states that he has HCV or the test for HBsAg is confirmed to be positive will be permanently deferred. In addition, some permanent deferrals may result from the testing performed on a previous donation. These donors also may be eligible to donate autologous blood.

Temporary Deferral: The prospective donor is unable to donate blood for a limited period of time. For example, a prospective donor who has received a transfusion within the last 12 months would be deferred for 12 months from the date of the transfusion or a donor who tests positive for WNV would be deferred for at least 120 days.

American Association of Blood Banks

AABB [56, 57] is an international professional association of blood centers, transfusion and transplantation services, and individuals involved in transfusion medicine. It provides a voluntary inspection/assessment and accreditation (I&A) program for its member institutions that meets the requirements of the federal CMS (Centers for Medicare and Medicaid Services) and CLIA '88 (Clinical Laboratory Improvement Amendments of 1988) regulations. The basis for the AABB I&A program is the AABB Standards for Blood Banks and Transfusion Services. Since 1957, these standards and guidelines have been periodically revised to reflect new scientific data, changing FDA regulations and good manufacturing practice. The guidelines set forth in the Standards reflect current FDA regulations. Although the AABB I&A program is voluntary, and adherence to the established standards does not carry regulatory impact, it is viewed as an industry standard both in the USA and internationally and is considered the standard of practice in the blood banking/transfusion medicine community.

College of American Pathologists

College of American Pathologists (CAP) is another professional organization that provides guidelines of practice for blood banks and transfusion services and their guidelines for donor screening and donor testing follow the FDA regulations for compliance. Like AABB, CAP provides a voluntary inspection and accreditation program for its members on a 2-year inspection cycle that is also approved by CMS for compliance with the CLIA 88 regulations. Since the CAP accreditation program encompasses the entire clinical laboratory, not just the blood bank, CAP accreditation is used by many hospital-based donor centers and transfusion services instead of or in addition to AABB accreditation.

How Nucleic Acid Testing Has Changed Medical Practice

There is unequivocal evidence that the incorporation of molecular methods (NAT) has significantly improved blood screening for infectious agents and has resulted in a decrease in transfusion-transmitted infections. Not only has this substantially addressed the detection of HIV early infection (shortened the window period), but has now been applied to decrease the number of infectious units for HBV, HCV, and WNV. Noteworthy is that only NAT is available to detect infectious units for WNV. Collectively, the detection of infections from these viruses has saved numerous lives as compared with the use of serologic assays alone, especially when considering the millions of blood units transfused annually in the USA. It shouldn't be overlooked that NAT is also used throughout the world (even in some resource-limited countries) to screen blood and detect early infection. However, NAT has not replaced the use of serologic assays because they are efficient and effective for detecting the majority of infections, and because the chance of false-negative NAT, although small, is not zero. It is evident that as new NAT assays are developed for additional infectious agents, they also will be implemented to decrease transfusion-related infections. Importantly, the availability of automated instrumentation has allowed these tests to be used in blood banks, even if pooling strategies must be used to lower costs.

NAT has also been invaluable in the diagnostic arena and for monitoring infected persons (viral load monitoring). Although not the purpose of this chapter, NAT has contributed substantially and vastly in medical practice. In addition, point of care NAT assays are being refined and will assist for protecting the blood supply in geographic locations that cannot support current instrumentation or ones that do not have adequate infrastructure.

Molecular methods will continue to improve to push the limits of sensitivity, and it is certain that additional multiplexing formats with enhanced detection will be implemented for efficiency and cost-savings. Although there are limitations to NAT, including the detection of infection during the eclipse period, false-negative results, higher costs, and increased requirements for regulations, there is no question that NAT has contributed substantially to the safety of the blood supply, and that these methods will continue to be used.

Future Directions

Methods for the detection of infectious diseases in human blood perpetually change to offer improvement in test indices (sensitivity, specificity, predictive values). In addition, quality assurance measures continue to be refined and expanded, leading to a lesser number of errors (both technical and transcriptional). Testing technologies for HIV, for example, set the stage for newer and better methods for all blood-borne infectious agents. These technologies have evolved from 1985 when the first screening test was introduced for HIV, have been supplemented with exquisite technologies to detect viral proteins and viral RNA, and are still becoming better to challenge even better sensitivity. After 28 years of evolution of blood screening tools for infectious agents, it is certain that the current methods will continue to improve.

In addition, new methods are being pursued, such as immune-PCR, a method that has the potential to decrease the eclipse period for early HIV detection [5, 6, 58]. This technique exploits the large number of p24 antigen molecules/virion in plasma (~3,000) as a target in comparison with just two copies of viral RNA; that is, there are a larger number of targets to detect. Accordingly, a sensitive technique such as immune-PCR that detects protein rather than RNA has been shown to detect less than one virion (due to the many p24 protein molecules) [6]. This technique is a signal amplification method that couples PCR with serologic detection of viral protein. Other newer techniques, as described by Azzazy (Chap. 10) for HCV, have the potential to increase the analytical sensitivity of assays for all the threatening agents. Also, newer molecular tests are being considered to further increase the sensitivity of detecting infectious agents. In 2011, it was reported that, among nearly four million blood samples analyzed, DNA-based assays were more effective than conventional tests at detecting HIV, HCV, and HBV in newly infected donors [26]. In addition, new DNA molecular tests have shown utility over conventional microscopy-based testing for the detection of malarial and Babesia infections [59].

Of major concern are the large number of potentially infectious agents that may be transmitted through blood but that are not currently being monitored. New threats include Chikungunya virus (from Africa) that would include specific IgM assays to detect infection in plasma or cerebrospinal fluid (CSF); Babesia, a protozoan parasitic infection linked to at least ten deaths through blood transfusions starting in 2006 [60]; and dengue virus, a mosquito-borne disease that kills 25,000 people a year worldwide (and is being increasingly found in returning travelers). The latter has resulted in the ARC currently using an investigational test to screen blood for dengue in Puerto Rico (although it is not yet approved), and showed that a new genetic test was ten times more sensitive in detecting dengue than conventional blood assays [61]. Recently, concern has been raised about the transmissibility of xenotropic murine leukemia virus (XMRV), a retrovirus that may be linked to chronic fatigue syndrome [62]. A few years ago, researchers identified 68 emerging infectious agents with the potential to threaten the blood supply [60]. Current techniques and perhaps newer ones will need to be developed in order to identify an increasingly high number of blood-borne pathogens. Future efforts will need to address the number of specific tests that must be performed to address an ultimately safe blood supply. Undoubtedly, multiplex testing will have a significant role in blood bank testing efficiency and for cost considerations, but maintaining the sensitivity for each agent will continue to be a challenge.

References

1. Facts about the blood supply. http://www.redcrossblood.org/learn-about-blood/blood-facts-and-statistics. Retrieved 27 July 2012.
2. Weusten JJ, van Drimmelen HA, Lelie PN. Mathematic modeling of the risk of HBV, HCV, and HIV transmission by window-phase donations not detected by NAT. Transfusion. 2002;42(5):537–48.
3. Constantine NT, Saville RD, Dax EM. Retroviral testing and quality assurance: essentials for laboratory diagnosis. Ann Arbor, MI: Malloy Printers; 2005.
4. Branson BM, McDougal JS. Establishing the diagnosis of HIV infection. In: Dolin R, Masur H, Saag M, editors. AIDS therapy. 3rd ed. Philadelphia, PA: Churchill-Livingstone and Elsevier Inc.; 2008. p. 1–22.
5. Barletta JM, Edelman DC, Constantine NT. Lowering the detection limits of HIV-1 viral load using real-time immuno-PCR for HIV-1 p24 antigen. Am J Clin Pathol. 2004;122:20–7.
6. Barletta J, Bartolome A, Constantine NT. Immunomagnetic quantitative immuno-PCR for detection of less than one HIV-1 virion. J Virol Methods. 2009;157:122–32.
7. Wainberg MA, Brenner BG. The impact of HIV genetic polymorphisms and subtype differences on the occurrence of resistance to antiretroviral drugs. Mol Biol Int. 2012;2012:256982.
8. Alter HJ, Klein HG. The hazards of blood Transfusion in historical perspective. Blood. 2008;112(7):2617–26.
9. Rao MR, Abdollah B, Naficy AB, Darwish MA, Darwis NM, Schisterman E, Clemens JD, Edelman R. Further evidence for association of hepatitis C infection with parenteral schistosomiasis treatment in Egypt. BMC Infect Dis. 2002;2:29–34.
10. Chou R, Clark E, Helfand M. Screening for hepatitis C virus infection [Internet]. Rockville, MD: Agency for Healthcare Research and Quality (US); 2004. Systematic Evidence Reviews, No. 24. http://www.ncbi.nlm.nih.gov/books/NBK43248/.
11. Ribeiro MA, Martins ML, Teixeira C, Ladeira R, de Fátima OM, Januário JN, Proietti FA, Carneiro-Proietti AB. Blocking vertical transmission of human T-cell lymphotropic virus type 1 and 2 through breast-feeding interruption. Pediatr Infect Dis J. 2012;31(11):1139–43.
12. Blood safety: reducing the risk of transfusion-transmitted infections. http://www.unboundmedicine.com/redbook/ub/view/RedBook/187182/3/blood_safety:_reducing_the_risk_of_transfusion_transmitted_infections. Accessed 4 Aug 2012.
13. Roback JD, Combs MR, Grossman BJ, Hillyer CD, editors. Technical manual. 16th ed. Bethesda, MD: American Association of Blood Banks; 2008.
14. Rassi Jr A, Rassi A, Marin-Neto JA. Chagas disease. Lancet. 2010 April 17;375(9723):1388–402. Review.
15. Young C, Losikoff P, Chawla A, Glasser L, Forman E. Transfusion-acquired Trypanosoma cruzi infection. Transfusion. 2007 Mar;47(3):540–4.
16. Mascola L, Kubak B, Radhakrishna S, Mone T, Huntere R, Leiby DA, Kuehnert M, Moore A, Steurer F, Lawrence G, Kun H. Chagas disease after organ transplantation – Los Angeles, CA, 2006. MMWR Morb Mortal Wkly Rep. 2006;55:798–800.
17. Kun H, Moore A, Mascola L, Steurer F, Lawrence G, Kubak B, Radhakrishna S, Leiby D, Herron R, Mone T, Hunter R, Kuehnert M. Chagas disease in transplant recipients investigation team. Clin Infect Dis. 2009 Jun 1;48(11):1534–40.
18. Teizeira AR, Hecht MM, Guimaro MC, Sousa AO, Nitz N. Pathogenesis of chagas' disease: parasite persistence and autoimmunity. Clin Microbiol Rev. 2011 Jul;24(3):592–630. Review.
19. Bern C, Montgomery SP. An estimate of the burden of Chagas disease in the United States. Clin Infect Dis. 2009 Sep 1;49(5):52–4.
20. Galavíz-Silva L, Molina-Garza DP, González-Santos MA, Mercado-Hernández R, González-Galavíz JR, Rosales-Encina JL, Molina-Garza ZJ. Update on seroprevalence of anti-Trypanosoma cruzi antibodies among blood donors in northeast Mexico. Am J Trop Med Hyg. 2009 Sep;81(3):404–6.
21. Blumberg BS, Alter HJ, Visnich S. A "new" antigen in leukemia sera. JAMA. 1965;191:541.
22. MMWR. Public health service inter-agency guidelines for screening donors of blood, plasma, organs, tissues, and semen for evidence. MMWR Recomm Rep. 1991;40(RR-4):1–17.
23. Zou S, Notari EP, Musavi F, Dodd RY, ARCNET Study Group. Current impact of the confidential unit exclusion option. Transfusion. 2004 May;44(5):651–7.
24. Stramer S. Current risks of transfusion-transmitted agents – a review. Arch Pathol Lab Med. 2007;131:702–7.
25. Zou S, Dorsey K, Notari EP, Foster GA, Krysztof DE, Musavi F, Dodd RY, Stramer S. Prevalence, incidence, and residual risk of human immunodeficiency virus and hepatitis C virus infections among United States blood donors since the introduction of nucleic acid testing. Transfusion. 2010;50:1495–504.
26. Stramer SL, Wend U, Candotti D, Foster GA, Hollinger FB, Dodd RY, Allain JP, Gerlich W. Nucleic acid testing to detect HBV infection in blood donors. N Engl J Med. 2011;364:236–47.
27. Stramer SL, Zou S, Notari EP, Foster GA, Krysztof DE, Musavi F, Dodd RY. Blood donation screening for hepatitis B virus markers in the era of nucleic acid testing: are all tests of value? Transfusion. 2012;52:440–6.
28. Infectious disease testing. http://www.redcrossblood.org/hospitals/infectious-disease-testing Accessed 26 July 2012.
29. Proietti FA, Carneiro-Proietti ABF, Catalan-Soares BC, Murphy EL. Global epidemiology of HTLV-I

infection and associated diseases. Oncogene. 2005; 24:6058–68.
30. Kaidarova Z, Murphy EL. HTLV-I and –II seroprevalence among United States blood donors, 2000–2009. Retrovirology. 2011;8 suppl 1:A74.
31. Montgomery S, Brown J, Kushneri M, Smith TL, Crall N, Lanciotti S, Macedo de Oliveira A, Boo T, Marfin AA, 2003 West Nile Virus Transfusion-associated Transmission Investigation Team. Transfusion-associated transmission of West Nile Virus, United States 2003 through 2005. Transfusion. 2006;46(12):2038–46.
32. Custer B, Agapova M, Bruhn R, Cusick R, Kamel H, Tomasulo P, Biswas H, Tobler L, Lee TH, Caglioti S, Busch M. Epidemiologic and laboratory findings from 3 years of testing United States blood donors for Trypanosoma cruzi. Transfusion. 2012;52(9):1901–11.
33. Bern C, Montgomery SP, Katz L, Caglioti S, Stramer SL. Chagas disease and the US blood supply. Curr Opin Infect Dis. 2008 Oct;21(5):476–82.
34. Rosenberg E, Brennan C, Claessens C, Constantine N, Murphy G, Owen S, Werner B, Yao J, Yen-Lieberman B, Branson B, Garrett P, Howell R. Criteria for laboratory testing and diagnosis of HIV infection. CLSI, M53-P, 30(21), ISBN: 1-56238-735-9, 2011.
35. Hare, CB, Pappalardo, BL, Busch MP, Phelps B, Alexander SS, Ramstead C, Levy JA, Hecht, FM. Negative antibody test results among individuals treated with antiretroviral therapy (ART) during acute/early infection. International AIDS Society Meeting, Bangkok, Thailand, 11–16 July, 2004. Poster MoPeB3107.
36. Fiebig EW, Wright DJ, Rawal BD, et al. Dynamics of HIV viremia and antibody seroconversion in plasma donors: implications for diagnosis and staging of primary HIV infection. AIDS. 2003;17:1871.
37. Lindback S, Thorstensson R, Karlsson AC, et al. Diagnosis of primary HIV-1 infection and duration of follow-up after HIV exposure. AIDS. 2000;14:2333.
38. Petersen LR, Satten GA, Dodd R, Busch M, Kleinman S, Grindon A, Lenes B. Duration of time from onset of human immunodeficiency virus type 1 infectiousness to development of detectable antibody. The HIV Seroconversion Study Group. Transfusion. 1994 Apr; 34(4):283–9.
39. Lu SN, Tung HD, Chen TM, Lee CM, Wang JH, Hung CH, Chen CH, Changchien CS. Is it possible to diagnose acute hepatitis C virus (HCV) infection by a rising anti-HCV titre rather than by seroconversion? J Viral Hepat. 2004 Nov;11(6):563–70.
40. FDA website. http://www.fda.gov/BiologicsBloodVaccines/BloodBloodProducts/ pprovedProducts/LicensedProductsBLAs/BloodDonorScreening/InfectiousDisease/ucm077899.htm.
41. Stramer SL, Fang CT, Foster GA, Wagner AG, Brodsky JP, Dodd RY. West Nile Virus among blood donors in the United States, 2003 and 2004. N Engl J Med. 2005;353:451–9.
42. Busch MP, Caglioti S, Robertson EF, McAuley JD, Tobler LH, Kamel H, Linnen JM, Shyamala V, Tomasulo P, Kleinman SH. Screening the blood supply for West Nile virus RNA by nucleic acid amplification testing. N Engl J Med. 2005;353:460–7.
43. Kleinman SH, Williams JD, Robertson G, Caglioti S, Williams RC, Spizman R, Morgan L, Tomasulo P, Busch MP. West Nile virus testing experience in 2007: evaluation of different criteria for triggering individual-donation nucleic acid testing. Transfusion. 2009;49:1160–70.
44. Francis RO, Strauss D, Williams JD, Whaley S, Shaz BH. West Nile Virus infection in blood donors in the New York City area during the 2010 seasonal epidemic. Transfusion. 2012;52(12):2664–70. doi:10.1111/j.1537-2995.2012.03639.x.
45. PROCLEIX package insert from FDA approval site. http://www.fda.gov/downloads/BiologicsBloodVaccines/BloodBloodProducts/ApprovedProducts/LicensedProductsBLAs/BloodDonorScreening/InfectiousDisease/UCM090247.p.
46. cobas® TaqScreen WNV Test labeling package insert from FDA approval site. http://www.fda.gov/downloads/BiologicsBloodVaccines/BloodBloodProducts/ApprovedProducts/LicensedProductsBLAs/BloodDonorScreening/InfectiousDisease/UCM091938.p.
47. PROCLEIX HIV-1/HCV package insert from FDA approval site. http://www.fda.gov/BiologicsBloodVaccines/BloodBloodProducts/ApprovedProducts/LicensedProductsBLAs/Blood Donor Screening/InfectiousDisease/ucm092022.htm.
48. PROCLEIX ULTRIO PLUS Assay package insert from FDA approval site. http://www.fda.gov/BiologicsBloodVaccines/BloodBloodProducts/ApprovedProducts/LicensedProductsBLAs/BloodDonorScreening/InfectiousDisease/ucm080466.htm.
49. COBAS TaqScreen MPX Test package insert from FDA approval site. http://www.fda.gov/downloads/BiologicsBloodVaccines/BloodBloodProducts/ApprovedProducts/LicensedProductsBLAs/BloodDonorScreening/InfectiousDisease/UCM176443.
50. Engel M. Making the blood supply safe also makes it more expensive. Los Angeles Times. 2007. Retrieved 27 July 2012. http://articles.latimes.com/2007/sep/02/local/me-bloodside2.
51. Rauber C, Robertson K. Rising price of blood puts squeeze on hospitals. San Francisco Business Times. 2007. Retrieved 27 Mar 2012. http://www.bizjournals.com/sanfrancisco/stories/2007/01/29/story14.html.
52. Toner RW, Pizzi L, Leas B, Ballas SK, Quigley A, Goldfarb NI. Costs to hospitals of acquiring and processing blood in the US: a survey of hospital-based blood banks and transfusion services. Appl Health Econ Health Policy. 2011;9(1):29–37.
53. Shander A, Hofmann A, Ozawa S, Theusinger OM, Gombotz H, Spahn DR. Activity-based costs of blood transfusions in surgical patients at four hospitals. Transfusion. April 2010;50:753–65.

54. Custer B. The cost of blood: did you pay too much or did you get a good deal? Transfusion. April 2010;50:742–4.
55. Testimony on FDA's regulation of blood, blood products, and plasma by Michael A. Friedman, M.D., FDA Lead Deputy Commissioner, before the House Committee on Government Reform and Oversight, Subcommittee on Human Resources and Intergovernmental Relations, June 5, 1997. http://www.hhs.gov/asl/testify/t970605a.html.
56. American Association of Blood Banks. Standards for blood banks and transfusion services. 27th ed. Bethesda, MD: AABB; 2011.
57. Roback JD, editor. Technical manual. 17th ed. Bethesda, MD: AABB; 2011.
58. Constantine NT, Zhao RY. Molecular-based laboratory testing and monitoring for human immunodeficiency virus infections. Clin Lab Sci. 2005;18(4):263–70.
59. Sanjai Kumar, Academy of Science meeting, ref: Nature Med., 19, 2011.
60. Landro L. New threats to U.S. blood supply. http://online.wsj.com/article/SB10001424052748704792104575264600619273586.html. Accessed 31 July 2012.
61. Stramer S. Reported at meeting of Academy of Science, ref-Nature Med, 17, 2011.
62. Keeping the U.S. blood supply safe. p. 14–16. http://www.mlo-online.com/features/2010_july/0710_10.pdf.

Part III

Genetics

Chromosome Microarrays

9

Umut Aypar, Swaroop Aradhya, Hutton Kearney, Christa Martin, Sarah South, and Eric C. Thorland

Background

Since the late 1960s, conventional G-banded karyotype analysis has been the gold standard for the detection of genetic etiologies in patients with unexplained developmental delay/intellectual disability (DD/ID), autism spectrum disorders (ASD), and multiple congenital anomalies (MCA) due to its ability to interrogate the entire genome in a single assay. While chromosome studies have significant diagnostic utility, chromosomal variation smaller than 5–10 megabases (Mb) is often not visible. Whole genome chromosomal microarray (CMA) analysis has revolutionized the field of clinical cytogenetics due to the significantly increased whole genome resolution it provides. This increased resolution has allowed the definition of many new clinical syndromes and has provided vast improvements in the diagnostic yield (12–15 % versus ~4 %). As a result, CMA testing has now replaced chromosome analysis as the first-tier test in this patient population.

History of Chromosomal Microarray Testing

The transition from genome-wide cytogenetic analysis carried out by G-banded chromosome studies to DNA-based molecular cytogenetic methods first occurred with the advent of comparative genomic hybridization (CGH). This technique, originally developed for use in cancer cytogenetics, was the first DNA-based test to enable copy number detection of losses and gains across the entire genome in a manner similar to a G-banded karyotype [1]. However, whereas G-banding analysis is a highly subjective method reliant on an individual's chromosome analysis skills, CGH has the advantage of being an objective test with results based on computationally generated signal intensity ratios between two DNA samples. CGH is based on a comparative hybridization between a test and a control sample. The two DNA samples are differentially labeled with two different fluorescent dyes and

U. Aypar, Ph.D.
Department of Laboratory Medicine and Pathology, Mayo Clinic, Rochester, MN, USA

S. Aradhya, Ph.D.
Neurogenetics, Array Services, Genedx, Gaithersburg, MD, USA

H. Kearney, Ph.D., F.A.C.M.G.
Cytogenetics, Mission Health Hospital, Asheville, NC, USA

C. Martin, Ph.D.
Emory Genetics Laboratory, Emory University, Atlanta, GA, USA

S. South, Ph.D.
ARUP Laboratories, Department of Pediatrics, University of Utah, Salt Lake City, UT, USA

E.C. Thorland, Ph.D. (✉)
Clinical Cytogenetics Laboratory, Department of Laboratory Medicine and Pathology, Mayo Clinic, Rochester, MN, USA
e-mail: thorland.erik@mayo.edu

W.E. Highsmith Jr. (ed.), *Molecular Diagnostics: 12 Tests That Changed Everything*, Molecular and Translational Medicine, DOI 10.1007/978-1-4614-8127-0_9,

then hybridized to target DNA in the form of normal metaphase chromosome preparations on a glass slide. Losses or gains are detected by comparing the ratio of the intensities of the two fluorescent dyes along the length of each chromosome. Where the ratio is equal between the test and control sample, the test sample is considered to have normal copy number for that region of the genome. If the ratio of the test DNA is decreased compared to the normal DNA, then this result is indicative of a deleted region. Conversely, if the ratio of the test DNA is increased compared to the normal DNA, a duplication is present.

While this transformative method proved to be extremely useful in defining deleted and duplicated regions in highly complex cancer genomes, its utility was deemed limited for the detection of constitutional copy number changes due to its relatively low resolution. Since the target DNA for traditional CGH is metaphase chromosomes, the resolution is only 5–10 Mb, similar to that attained with a G-banded karyotype. However, the immense potential for CGH in constitutional studies was recognized as an objective method for assessing copy number across the genome if the resolution could be improved beyond that of G-banding. Such a goal was attained when the target for CGH assays was changed from metaphase chromosomes to mapped DNA sequences printed on glass slides. The creation of these DNA "microarrays" provided the opportunity for significant increases in resolution for the detection of copy number changes far beyond that of G-banded chromosomes and traditional CGH.

The initial phase of the human genome project focused on building a physical map of the genome using large fragments of human sequence cloned into vectors such as bacterial artificial clones (BAC) and P1 clones. These large insert clones were used to generate a tiling path of overlapping clones for each chromosome of the human genome and were used as the input for the sequencing process. The earliest array comparative genomic hybridization (array CGH) technologies took advantage of this physical map and used these genomic clones as the target DNA. The first reported use of array CGH employed an array with BAC and P1 clones from chromosome 20 to assess gains and losses in breast tumors [2]. As the technology to produce microarrays improved, the number of BAC clones that could be spotted on a slide increased, eventually reaching tens of thousands of clones. For example, an array with approximately 2,400 BAC clones spaced at regular intervals across the genome had an estimated 1.4 Mb genome-wide resolution for the detection of deletions and duplications, while a subsequent array developed with 32,433 BAC clones tiling across the human genome achieved the first microarray with submegabase resolution [3, 4]. While genome-wide array CGH with genomic clones produced exciting results and was quickly integrated into research studies for copy number analyses, its incorporation into clinical cytogenetic testing was much more gradual for multiple reasons. First, arrays containing a large number of genomic clones were challenging to manufacture in a standardized manner at quality suitable for clinical testing. Second, since understanding the complexity of copy number variation (CNV) across the human genome was in its infancy, clinical laboratories were reluctant to carry out testing which could generate results that were difficult to interpret from a clinical perspective. A solution to these issues was the creation of "targeted" arrays, which contained a limited number of genomic clones corresponding to regions of the genome that were already known to be associated with disease. This single array test can be equated to examining hundreds of disease loci using individual fluorescence in situ hybridization (FISH) probes. The use of such targeted arrays in clinical cytogenetic laboratories quickly began to replace individual FISH tests for subtelomere and centromere imbalances and syndromes associated with recurrent microdeletions and microduplications [5–7].

Beginning in 2006, a handful of commercial vendors began manufacturing microarrays for array CGH using synthetic oligonucleotides ranging in size from 20 to 60 base pairs synthesized in situ. The use of oligonucleotide probes specific to particular regions of the human genome overcame some of the issues with genomic clone arrays since they were much

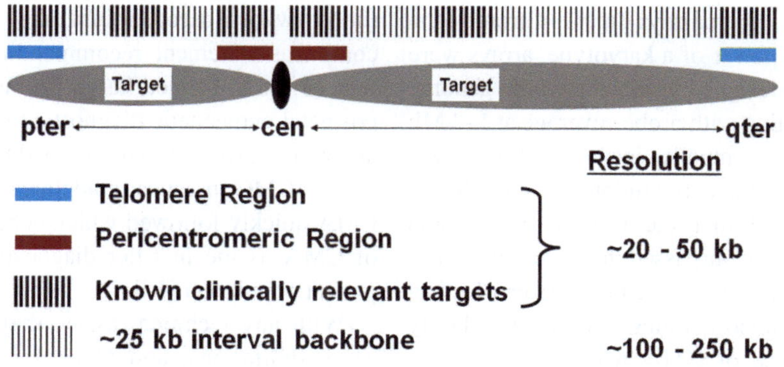

Fig. 9.1 Customized oligonucleotide probe coverage allowing for higher density probe coverage in regions of known clinical significance

easier to manufacture in a quality-controlled manner and could be printed at much higher density compared to BAC-based arrays. In addition, the oligonucleotides could be designed to avoid repetitive elements in the human genome adding specificity to the hybridization process. The first oligonucleotide arrays contained 40,000–60,000 probes, but this number soon increased from hundreds of thousands to greater than one million probes today. Oligonucleotide arrays soon became widespread and are now the standard due to the excellent data quality and resolution afforded by these arrays. In addition, some manufacturers of oligonucleotide arrays allowed customization of the individual probes printed on the arrays. The ability to pick probes precisely at the genomic regions of interest provided a powerful means to develop arrays suited for clinical genetic testing. In this manner, arrays with whole genome backbone probe coverage but higher density coverage targeted to regions or genes of known clinical significance could be carefully developed (Fig. 9.1). Lastly, manufacturers also provided complete kits for the DNA labeling and hybridization steps that streamlined the process and generated consistent high quality data. These advantages provided clinical laboratories with the tools needed to assess genome-wide copy number changes by DNA microarray technology in a quality controlled and highly reproducible manner [8, 9].

Clinical Applications

The use of CMA technology has revolutionized the diagnostic yield of clinical cytogenetic testing. Although CMA parallels G-banded chromosome analysis in providing genome-wide assessment of copy number aberrations, it far surpasses it in the resolution that can be obtained for detecting deletions and duplications: a standard G-banded karyotype (550 band resolution) has been estimated to have a resolution of 5–10 Mb, while routine CMA can detect imbalances down to 50 kb and smaller, depending on probe coverage—resulting in more than a 100-fold improvement [9]!

CMA was first incorporated into clinical testing using arrays with targeted coverage of known clinically relevant regions, such as syndromes associated with recurrent microdeletions/duplications and subtelomeric and pericentromeric regions. Early reports demonstrated that the use of such an array could detect clinically relevant genomic alterations in ~5–9 % of patients referred for clinical testing [5, 6]. Although these targeted arrays could circumvent the need for multiple FISH tests and identify cryptic imbalances of targeted regions, they were not a replacement for a G-banded karyotype, since there were still large gaps in probe coverage across the genome.

To create microarrays that mirrored the genome-wide power of a karyotype, arrays were subsequently designed to include whole genome coverage, starting with probe coverage at 1–3 Mb intervals and eventually including tiling path coverage across the entire unique genome. It was quickly realized that the use of such whole genome arrays far surpassed the power of a traditional karyotype; a significant number of clinically relevant abnormalities were identified only through the use of CMA when the G-banded karyotype was normal. Furthermore, Miller et al. [10]. reviewed 33 CMA studies encompassing 21,698 subjects and determined that CMA detected clinically relevant imbalances in ~12.2 % of individuals with idiopathic DD/ID, ASD, and/or MCA. This diagnostic yield far surpassed that of previous testing strategies, such as targeted analysis of subtelomeric regions, which was shown to have an ~2.5 % yield in the same patient population [11, 12].

Multiple types of array platforms are currently being used as part of clinical testing, including those that include single nucleotide polymorphism (SNP) probes in addition to copy number probes. Arrays with SNPs have the added benefit of being able to detect certain classes of uniparental disomy (UPD) and regions that are identical by descent. For example, in a study by Bruno et al. [13], it was demonstrated that clinically significant abnormalities were identified in 0.5 % of cases that would not have been detected by the use of copy number probes alone. Given the various array platforms that have emerged, the American College of Medical Genetics (ACMG) published recommendations for the design and performance of arrays used for postnatal clinical CMA [14]. These guidelines suggested that gains and losses of 400 kb or larger should be able to be detected genome wide, and that probe enrichment be added for dosage-sensitive genes and known clinically relevant regions.

With the broad genetics community recognition of the added value of CMA over the current standard of care G-banded karyotype, as well as multiple published studies documenting a higher diagnostic yield from CMA, the International Standard Cytogenomic Array (ISCA) Consortium (https://www.iscaconsortium.org/) released a consensus statement recommending that CMA replace the G-banded karyotype as the first-tier postnatal cytogenetic diagnostic test in individuals with unexplained DD/ID, ASD, and/or MCA [10]. ACMG practice guidelines for postnatal CMA quickly followed which echoed the utility of CMA as the first-tier diagnostic test in this patient population [15].

With any technical assay, there are always some limitations, and CMA is no exception. Unlike chromosome and FISH analyses, which can detect both unbalanced and balanced rearrangements, CMA can only detect cytogenetic rearrangements that result in an *unbalanced* genomic complement. Therefore, CMA will not detect truly balanced rearrangements such as translocations or inversions. Given this limitation, CMA is not an appropriate test for certain clinical indications such as couples presenting with recurrent miscarriages where one of the individuals may be expected to carry a balanced rearrangement. In addition, since CMA results are generated from normalized ratios across the entire genome, this test cannot detect most cases of polyploidy (triploidy and tetraploidy) unless SNP probes are incorporated into the array design. Furthermore, since CMA utilizes extracted genomic DNA, it cannot provide any information about the mechanism of an imbalance. For example, a CMA result may show a loss of the terminal region of one chromosome and a gain of the terminal region of another chromosome, suggestive of an unbalanced translocation. However, only a chromosome study or metaphase FISH analysis can demonstrate the actual mechanism leading to the two imbalances, which has significant implications for genetic counseling and recurrence risks for the family.

Methodology and Standard Reagents

There are two main classes of chromosomal microarrays available from manufacturers today: (1) traditional arrays based on comparative

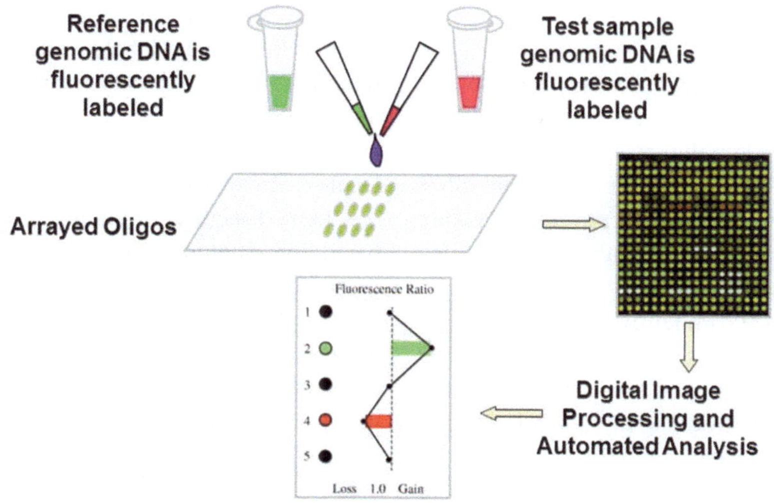

Fig. 9.2 Array CGH Methodology. Reference and test DNA samples are fluorescently labeled with two different dyes, combined and co-hybridized to arrayed oligonucleotides on the slide. Following hybridization, high-resolution scanning of each spot on the array allows for calculation of relative fluorescence ratios which are plotted to visualize copy number differences between the experimental and reference DNA samples

genomic hybridizations with DNA derived from both a reference genome and a patient genome on the same chip and (2) microarrays that require only patient DNA to generate intensity data that are subsequently compared to an in silico reference. Both of these technologies are discussed below.

Array CGH

In array CGH, the test and control DNA samples are labeled with two different fluorescent dyes. Cy5 and Cy3 dyes are the most widely used fluorescent labels. The fluorescent labeling is performed by random primer labeling using one of a variety of commercially available kits. The differentially labeled DNA samples are purified to remove excess unincorporated label. The labeled products are combined and co-hybridized to the microarray slide. The microarray is incubated for 24–40 h and then washed to remove unhybridized DNA. The washed slides are subsequently scanned on a high-resolution scanner to measure the fluorescence intensity for both dyes at each probe. The intensity data are imported into software that calculates the relative fluorescence ratios between the experimental and reference DNA samples at each probe spot. These data can then be plotted, typically on a log2 ratio plot, to visualize the relative intensity of fluorescence, or copy number, between the experimental and reference DNA samples (Fig. 9.2).

The quality of the array data depends on the specificity of the hybridization of the genomic DNA to the probe DNA. This specificity is influenced by the sequence content of the probe such that unique sequence will produce more reliable data than sequence containing repeats. To improve data quality, Cot-1 DNA is used to block nonunique DNA sequences and improve hybridization specificity to the probe sequences. The derivative of the log2 ratio (DLR score) is a metric often used to evaluate the quality of the array data. When the score is low, the array generally shows good hybridization and strong fluorescence values to produce readily interpretable data. High scores may reflect a poor DNA sample, increased background noise, poor specificity in probe hybridization, or other suboptimal hybridization conditions. In general, an array CGH protocol, once established, is generally very reproducible in a clinical or research setting.

SNP-Based Microarrays

SNP-based microarrays provide detection of copy number changes as well as genotype information at multiple polymorphic loci throughout the genome. There are several different SNP-based microarray platforms currently available, each with different methodologies for SNP allele discrimination.

SNP allele discrimination for single-channel microarrays (one-color microarrays), such as those manufactured by Affymetrix, is provided by differential hybridization to allele-specific probe targets. In brief, genomic DNA from the experimental sample is restricted by endonuclease digestion, ligated with PCR adapters, and amplified. Subsequently, fragmented PCR products are then TdT (terminal deoxynucleotidyl transferase)-end labeled with biotin and hybridized to the array. Arrays are washed and stained with a streptavidin conjugate and scanned. The individual probe intensity values indicate relative abundance when compared to other samples processed previously as a reference set. This data provides both relative copy number assessment as well as SNP-allele discrimination for those probe sets targeting biallelic SNPs.

In contrast to oligonucleotide arrays constructed by DNA synthesis directly on the array surface, bead-based arrays, such as those manufactured by Illumina, are made by attaching oligonucleotides to beads. A subset of these oligonucleotides are designed with the 3′ end terminating just before a biallelic SNP, the genotype of which can be interrogated as described below. Because the beads are randomly assembled onto the array for each experiment, the position of each bead must first be determined before use through a process of repeated hybridizations termed *decoding*. Once the decoding hybridization cycles are complete, whole-genome amplified genomic DNA from the experimental sample is hybridized directly to the array. Following sample hybridization, the arrays are washed and labeled. Genomic DNA from the experimental sample (now hybridized to the corresponding oligo-bound bead) is then used as a template for a single base extension reaction using differentially labeled nucleotides. If the sample is homozygous at the targeted locus, then only one of the two labeled nucleotides is introduced. If the sample is heterozygous, then both labels are incorporated. After this step, the arrays are washed, signals amplified, and further prepared for scanning. Normalized data are then compared to the expected normalized fluorescence intensity values from control experiments to determine chromosome copy number for an experimental specimen. Similarly, a SNP allele genotype for each targeted locus in the array is assigned by comparing the expected fluorescence ranges in each channel for homozygous and heterozygous calls.

While SNP-based arrays are used in some settings for specific resequencing applications, when used for genomic copy number assessment, SNP markers are usually generalized as present in a homozygous or heterozygous state. For most platforms, biallelic SNPs are arbitrarily denoted as “A” or “B,” and relative allele distribution is provided by either allele difference (A – B) plots or B-allele frequency plots (B/A + B), with the heterozygous population occupying the central position between the two homozygous allele states (Fig. 9.3). In addition to detection of regions with absence of heterozygosity (AOH), allele distribution plots have utility for supportive assessment of copy number state and detection/interpretation of mosaic states.

Chromosomal Microarray Resolution

The resolution of a CMA is one parameter used to define the utility of the microarray. In general, resolution refers to the minimum size of a genomic deletion or duplication that can be reliably detected. However, the measurement and expression of resolution is often a confusing topic. Resolution can be measured spatially by determining the number of probes over a given genomic distance (e.g., one probe every 1,000 base pairs or one million probes per genome). However, CMA technology generally requires data from several consecutive probes to accurately

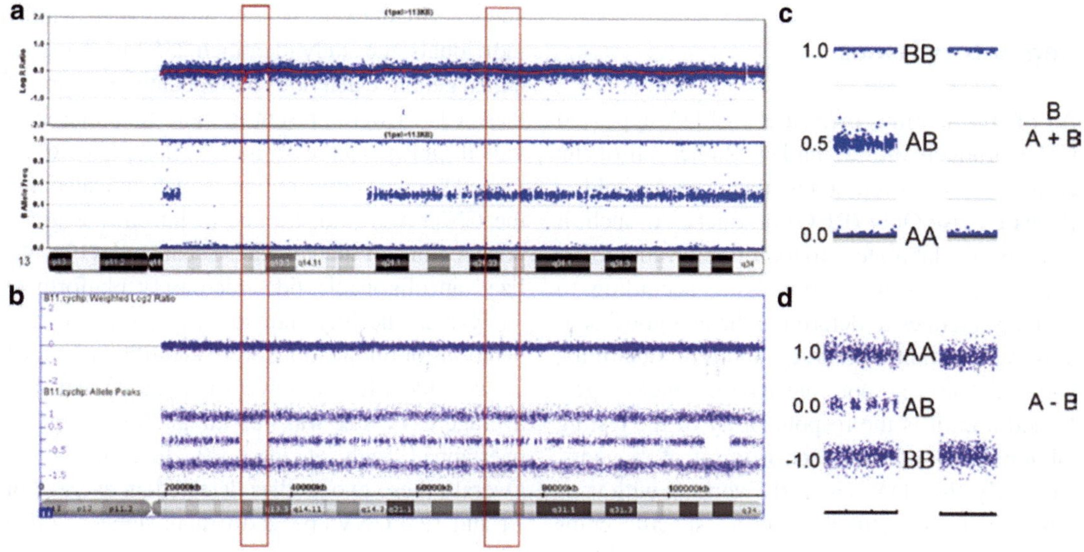

Fig. 9.3 Allele plots. (**a**) Screenshot of a chromosome 13 from a patient DNA sample run on the Illumina Quad610 array, and visualized in BeadStudio software. Top: Log R ratio plot shows a normal copy number state for the chromosome. Bottom: B-allele frequency plot shows a large region of homozygosity from bands 13q12.11 to 13q14.3. (**b**) Screenshot of a chromosome 13 from a patient DNA sample run on the Affymetrix CytoScan™ HD array and visualized in Affymetrix Chromosome Analysis Suite (ChAS) software. *Top*: Weighted log2 ratio plot shows a normal copy number state for the chromosome. *Bottom*: Allele difference plot shows 2 regions of homozygosity from bands 13q13.1 to q13.3 and 13q33.2 to q33.3. Panels C and D represent magnified views of the allele plots for each software, from the boxed regions in panels A and B. (**c**) B-allele frequency, as plotted in Illumina BeadStudio software. The Y-axis value is determined by the formula given on the right. Alleles are plotted as a frequency, determined by the number of B alleles compared with the total number of alleles (A + B). B-allele frequency of 1 indicates homozygosity for the B allele (2/2), a frequency of 0 indicates homozygosity for the A allele (0/2), and a frequency of 0.5 indicates a heterozygous genotype (1/2). (**d**) Allele difference, as plotted in Affymetrix Chromosome Analysis Suite (ChAS) software. The Y-axis value is determined by the formula given on the right. Alleles are plotted as the difference between the estimated number of A alleles and the estimated number of B alleles (A-B). Each allele corresponds to a value of 0.5. Values near 1 indicate homozygosity for the A allele (AA: [0.5 + 0.5] – [0] = 1), values near –1 indicate homozygosity for the B allele (BB: [0] – [0.5 + 0.5] = –1), and values near 0 indicate a heterozygous genotype (AB: [0.5] – [0.5] = 0)

determine copy number state. Chromosomal microarrays from different manufacturers may differ substantially in the number of consecutive probes required to make a high confidence copy number call due to differences in probe length, oligonucleotide synthesis technology, and assay protocols. Therefore, spatial resolution is only one factor in determining the true functional resolution of an array platform. Functional resolution can be defined as the minimum number of probes necessary to detect a copy number change with high confidence times the spatial resolution of the microarray. Only the functional resolution calculation should be utilized to compare the true resolution of microarray platforms between manufacturers and to determine the utility of any particular microarray.

Chromosomal microarrays can be designed with different levels of resolution at different genomic locations to suit particular applications. For example, particular genomic regions may be targeted with a higher number of probes to increase resolution in regions of known clinical significance to ensure reliable detection of copy number changes within these regions. In addition, very high density coverage of individual exons within selected genes allows for the detection of copy number changes affecting as little as a single exon. For further discussion on this topic, see section "*Single-Gene array CGH*."

Regulatory Issues

As of this writing, there are no FDA approved CMA products on the market. Rather, all of the chips from the different manufacturers are sold as Research Use Only (RUO) products. As such, it is up to each laboratory to thoroughly validate the performance of the entire assay according to CLIA guidelines to determine the analytical sensitivity, specificity, accuracy, and reproducibility, and establish the reportable and reference ranges. In addition, it is the responsibility of the testing laboratory to validate each new lot of reagents. Currently, the FDA is actively working with various chip manufacturers to bring specific chips through the FDA approval process. It is likely that additional regulatory guidance will be available in the near future.

Interpretation

Copy Number Variation in Humans

Analysis of sequence data from the Human Genome Project revealed extensive sequence variation in the human genome, including polymorphic sequences such as SNPs, variable number tandem repeats (VNTRs), short tandem repeats (STRs), and transposable elements (i.e., LINE and SINE elements). While SNPs were thought to be the predominant form of human variation, the advent of CMA technology revealed extensive structural variation, an entirely new level of genomic complexity which had largely been unrecognized.

Structural variation includes both balanced variation (chromosomal translocations and inversions) and unbalanced variation in the form of CNVs. CNVs include deletions, duplications, and insertions relative to the reference human genome and are typically defined as greater than 1 kb in size. In 2004, two independent studies reported the widespread presence of CNVs in phenotypically normal individuals [16, 17]. Iafrate et al. [16]. used BAC-based array CGH with BAC clones tiling the human genome at about 1 Mb intervals. Among 39 unrelated healthy individuals, the study identified 255 loci that contained genomic deletions or duplications. Many of these CNVs were present in more than one individual and greater than half of the CNVs overlapped known coding regions which indicated that the CNVs were not limited to intronic or gene-poor regions of the genome. Sebat et al. [17]. utilized an oligonucleotide microarray platform to analyze 20 healthy individuals. A total of 221 deletions or duplications were identified of which 76 were identified in only a single individual. The average CNV size was 465 kb, and these regions overlapped with at least 70 different genes. Overall, these two studies detected an average of 11 and 12.4 CNVs per individual, suggested that while these CNVs may not lead directly to genetic disease, structural variation may play a significant role in human phenotypic variation.

These initial studies were quickly replicated in larger populations using higher resolution CMAs which revealed even more extensive structural variation [18–22]. Subsequently, the Database of Genomic Variants (DGV; http://projects.tcag.ca/variation) was created to catalog the structural variation published in peer-reviewed studies. By 2006, 1,237 CNVs covering an estimated 143 Mb of genomic sequence were cataloged in DGV [23]. An aggregation of this data revealed that genomic variation (as measured by the total number of base pairs affected) due to CNVs in the human genome was greater than the variation contributed by SNPs. The CNVs in the database averaged 118 kb with a median size of about 18 kb. This discrepancy between the mean and the median was largely due to the differences in the methods of discovery with each having particular biases toward specific types and sizes of CNVs [23]. As the resolution of the technologies improved, the number of CNVs identified per person increased from tens [16, 17] to hundreds [18, 24, 25]. Most recently, even higher resolution arrays based on SNP-CNV genotyping [26] and paired-end sequencing [27] have shown that approximately 5 % of the human genome is involved in CNVs and at the time of this writing, DGV contains 66,741 reported CNVs distributed over nearly 16,000 individual loci.

Our understanding of the contributions of CNVs to normal human variation and to disease phenotypes is still evolving. Many disorders associated with recurrent CNVs have been described in abnormal patient populations, such as Prader–Willi and Williams syndromes. It remains challenging to distinguish between normal and disease-causing CNV when performing CMA studies on patients with abnormal phenotypes. Therefore, significant efforts are ongoing to classify CNVs with regard to their frequency and clinical significance (See section "Interpretation of Chromosomal Microarrays" for additional discussion).

Interpretation of Chromosomal Microarray Data

As alluded to in earlier sections of this chapter, the interpretation of CNVs encountered during clinical cytogenetic testing can be very challenging due to the significant amount of CNV that is present in the general population. The results of high resolution CMA testing in a clinical setting typically include 10–30 independent CNV calls per individual, each of which must be evaluated independently for their potential clinical significance. In many ways, the interpretation of novel CNVs parallels that of variants of undetermined significance that are often encountered in whole gene sequencing assays [28]. Various CNV classification schemes have been devised to facilitate consistency for assessment of the pathogenicity of a CNV and reporting its clinical consequences between laboratories performing clinical CMA testing. The ACMG has recently published guidelines for this classification [14]. The three main categories for classification include pathogenic, uncertain clinical significance, and benign. Depending upon the specific information available in the medical literature, the classification of uncertain clinical significance may be further specified as either likely pathogenic or likely benign, indicating the degree of uncertainty.

The primary considerations for the classification of a CNV are its size and genomic content. In general, the larger the size of a CNV, the more likely it is to have pathogenic consequences. However, it is clear that very small CNVs with a critical gene can be pathogenic, and very large CNVs in gene-poor regions may be benign. Therefore, analysis of the genomic content is ultimately the most critical factor. This requires continual familiarization with established microdeletion/microduplication syndromes and monitoring of the rapidly expanding medical literature for the description of new syndromes. Since an identified CNV may involve one or more genes, evaluation of the individual genes as well as the region as a whole must be considered. In addition, the identification of multiple CNVs may result in a combinatorial effect on the clinical outcome [29]. The location of the multiple CNVs may also suggest the mechanism of rearrangement [30]. For example, the identification of a terminal deletion on one chromosome and a terminal duplication on another may suggest the presence of an unbalanced translocation. In this situation, additional chromosome or FISH studies are necessary to identify and characterize the translocation since this mechanistic information has significant implications for recurrence risk in the family.

The evaluation of genomic content is greatly aided by numerous online resources. Useful databases include, but are not limited to, those that focus on specific syndrome annotation, specific gene annotation, CNV annotation in the general population, and CNV annotation in various patient populations. It is also recommended that individual laboratories maintain an internal database of detected CNVs. Comparison of prospective findings with an internal database in addition to the public databases is often informative since CNVs may be both platform- and population specific.

Two major databases for syndrome annotation are GeneReviews (http://www.ncbi.nlm.nih.gov/sites/GeneTests/review?db=GeneTests) and the Online Mendelian Inheritance in Man (OMIM) database (https://www.omim.org). A number of databases annotate genes and transcripts including the National Center for Bioinformatics (NCBI) Reference Sequences (RefSeq) (http://www.ncbi.nlm.nih.gov/refseq), Entrez gene entry (http://www.ncbi.nlm.nih.gov/gene), and GeneCards (http://www.genecards.org/). A PubMed search should also be considered to capture additional information, particularly more recent literature that may not yet have been updated in the relevant databases.

Two current patient databases for whole-genome microarray analysis are DECIPHER, an acronym for Database of Chromosomal Imbalance and Phenotype in Humans Using Ensembl Resources [31] (http://decipher.sanger.ac.uk/), and the ISCA clinical CNV database (http://www.ncbi.nlm.nih.gov/dbvar/studies/nstd37/; https://www.iscaconsortium.org). Both databases have been created from consortiums of clinical diagnostic laboratories with the patients presenting with primarily neuro-developmental conditions or congenital anomalies. The DGV referred to earlier in this chapter (http://projects.tcag.ca/variation/) houses a database of structural variation, including CNVs, identified primarily in the general population collected as control cohorts for various studies and published in peer-reviewed literature [16, 32].

A number of considerations should be taken into account when using databases of CNVs in the general population and affected individuals. In patient databases, the particular CNV in question may not be the only CNV observed in the patient, and a review of all the CNVs for a given patient is important. The term general population rather than normal population is appropriate, as "normal" is relative to the phenotype in question and review of the primary literature may be required to determine what phenotypic data, if any, was chosen for inclusion in the particular study. Factors such as incomplete penetrance, variable expressivity, age of onset, and parent of origin imprinting effects also need to be considered. When comparing a CNV in a patient to an outside database, careful comparison of the size and gene content of the CNV is critical, particularly since probe placement, type, and density on various array platforms can generate differences in the reported size of identical CNVs. In addition, many of the CNVs reported from bacterial artificial chromosome or low-resolution platforms may both underestimate or overestimate the size of a detected CNV. Finally, for X-linked CNVs, the sex of the individual in the database must be taken into account.

Large research studies surveying CNVs in the general population may have used CNV calling algorithms that are less stringent than those used in clinical laboratories, and the majority of CNVs in these studies have not been experimentally validated with another method. Therefore, a CNV detected in only a single study should be considered with increased caution. Numerous studies may also involve the same study cohort (i.e., the HapMap collection), so the identification of the same CNV in multiple studies, while useful for validation of the CNV, should not be misinterpreted as multiple independent individuals carrying the CNV.

The University of California Santa Cruz (UCSC) genome browser (http://www.genome.ucsc.edu/) is a particularly useful tool for both the visualization of the genomic interval of a CNV as well as a direct portal to many of these other online resources [33]. This tool allows many different tracks of data to be visualized together in a user-defined configuration in the context of the relevant genomic interval. Tracks for databases, such as ISCA, DECIPHER, the DGV, OMIM, and GeneReviews, and different gene sets, such as RefSeq genes, are all available. In addition, genomic architecture information may be visualized such as segmental duplications that may mediate copy number changes and are often themselves variable in copy number. In addition, links to a large selection of resources such as PubMed, mouse model data, expression data, and more are available. Although these tracks within the UCSC browser enable a quick visual graphic of the various resources and overview of the relevant information, linking out to the home database for any relevant information may also be appropriate to ensure the most complete and up-to-date information is utilized.

The ISCA Consortium has also created an evidence-based review process and a database (http://www.ncbi.nlm.nih.gov/projects/dbvar/ISCA) specifically to document and characterize any evidence for or against dosage sensitivity of individual genes and genomic regions [34].

The primary source for this evidence is peer-reviewed literature. The evidence is compiled and evaluated before haploinsufficiency, and triplosensitivity scores are assigned to indicate varying amounts of evidence that an individual CNV is associated with a particular clinical phenotype. This database is available as an additional resource to aid in the interpretative assessment of CNVs containing particular genes and genomic regions and their association with specific phenotypes. Through the public Web site, users are also encouraged to comment on particular genomic regions, provide additional evidence supporting or refuting dosage sensitivity, and to suggest genomic regions for immediate evaluation.

After careful evaluation of all of the available data, the clinical significance of a small number of CNVs in any given case may remain uncertain. In these situations, evaluation of samples from the biological parents may provide additional data for the interpretation of clinical significance. If the same CNV is inherited from a phenotypically normal parent, it is generally taken as evidence that the CNV is more likely to be benign. However, incomplete penetrance or variable expressivity of the phenotype must also be considered in this situation. In contrast, if the CNV occurred de novo, the CNV is more likely to be pathogenic. However, the background mutation rate for CNV formation in humans is unknown. Thus, de novo events are not always pathogenic. In addition, non-paternity should also be considered.

Interpretation of Homozygosity Detected by SNP-Based Arrays

The use of SNP-based microarrays allows for both copy number assessment (as outlined previously) and detection of genomic regions with absence of heterozygosity (AOH). The following discussion focuses on AOH observed as long contiguous stretches of homozygosity (LCSH) with diagnostic utility in the constitutional setting. While detection of LCSH rarely results in an immediate and definitive diagnosis, it can prompt additional testing, potentially leading to a diagnosis of a disorder of imprinting or recessive disease [35].

Uniparental Disomy

Uniparental disomy (UPD) is defined as the inheritance of both homologues of a chromosome from a single parent [36, 37]. Before the routine use of SNP-based microarrays, UPD was only detected when found with: (1) a hallmark cytogenetic finding (mosaic trisomy, marker chromosome, or other structural rearrangement such as a Robertsonian translocation), (2) clinical manifestation of an imprinting disorder [38], or (3) homozygosity for a recessive allele with only a single carrier parent [37]. With SNP-based microarrays, many more UPD events are detected by recognition of the hallmark patterns of homozygosity [35, 39]. One or more regions of LCSH found isolated to a single chromosome, particularly when longer than 10–15 Mb [39], can be a hallmark of uniparental disomy (UPD).

There are two well-accepted mechanisms explaining UPD involving a whole chromosome: (1) trisomy rescue, the most frequently observed mechanism and (2) monosomy rescue [40]. Additionally, somatic events can produce segmental UPD (involving only part of a chromosome) [41]. Non-mosaic trisomies and monosomies involving most chromosomes are incompatible with survival, and surviving zygotes have typically experienced a "rescue" event [42]. This involves secondary mitotic segregation errors to restore disomy or structural reduction of a trisomic chromosome (usually by conversion to a marker or ring chromosome). When the remaining disomic chromosomes are derived from the same parent, the result of this rescue event is uniparental disomy. For trisomy rescue, depending on the origin of the trisomy (e.g., meiosis I or II error) and the number and position of meiotic exchanges, the UPD chromosomes may be completely heterodisomic, completely isodisomic, or mixed hetero/isodisomic [35]. It is important to recognize that not all UPD events have regions of isodisomy (homozygosity) detectable by SNP-based microarrays. Therefore, these arrays cannot detect all UPD events. For example, trisomy rescue following a meiosis I error in the absence of recombination can generate uniparental heterodisomy for the entire chromosome. These events are only detectable through trio analysis to demonstrate that there is no contribution of that chromosome from one of the parents. Monosomy rescue mechanisms will generate only whole-chromosome uniparental isodisomy. Therefore, the detection of whole chromosome isodisomy indicates that a UPD event has occurred.

Segmental isodisomy occurs in mitotic division and results in only a portion of a chromosome (usually terminal) with uniparental inheritance. Because segmental UPD mechanisms generate only regions of uniparental isodisomy, the location of the LCSH (isodisomy) relative to any imprinted loci should be considered [43]. In contrast to whole-chromosome UPD, only the loci involved in the isodisomic segment are at risk for imprinted disorders if segmental UPD is confirmed as the mechanism underlying the LCSH.

When LCSH patterns detected by SNP-based microarray suggest UPD, further molecular analysis is necessary for UPD confirmation and/or determination of parent of origin. LCSH involving a chromosome associated with disorders of imprinting should be strongly considered for UPD confirmatory testing, especially when the patient presents with clinical features consistent with the syndrome in question. For reviews on UPD mechanisms and syndromes, see [40–42, 44–48].

Parental Consanguinity

When multiple LCSH regions are found throughout the genome, the findings are generally assumed to represent genomic regions identical by descent (IBD), with associated concerns for recessive disorders mapping to the homozygous intervals. The closer the biological relationship of the proband's parents, the greater the proportion of their shared alleles, and therefore, the greater the proband's risk of inheritance of two deleterious recessive mutations [49–51]. In addition to suspicion for recessive disease, genomic homozygosity found in excess of 12–25 % may trigger a suspicion for parental consanguinity or incest [52].

Autozygosity Mapping

Excessive homozygosity is not, by itself, an abnormal finding, but may suggest a recessive disease etiology. Whether found to be a result of parental consanguinity or UPD, all LCSH segments have the potential to harbor homozygous recessive mutations, and as such, are candidate regions for homozygosity/autozygosity mapping. The term autozygosity refers to homozygosity of alleles that are identical by descent (inherited from a common ancestor), as contrasted with homozygosity identical by state (random inheritance). The genetic basis of numerous recessive disorders has been elucidated through autozygosity mapping in consanguineous families [53–56]. While it is generally not feasible in the setting of a routine diagnostic investigation to pursue gene discovery efforts, autozygosity mapping restricted to known disease genes has proven diagnostic utility [57, 58]. When provided a specific and unique clinical indication, or a differential diagnosis which suggests one of several recessive disorders, it is relatively straightforward to map candidate genes to determine whether they are found in a region of LCSH [55, 57]. Finding a gene of interest in an LCSH may help to prioritize additional single gene testing.

Mitochondrial Disorders

Array CGH can also be applied to the analysis of the mitochondrial genome. Mitochondrial deletions are associated with a variety of disorders, including Kearns–Sayre syndrome (KSS), Pearson syndrome, and progressive external ophthalmoplegia (PEO) [59]. The mitochondrial genome is a 16.6-kb circular fragment that exists in multiple copies within each mitochondrion. Each cell has several mitochondria, and this population varies by tissue type and by the age of an individual. For instance, muscle may have several thousand mitochondria per cell whereas blood cells may have a few hundred. Due to the varying number of mitochondria among tissues, DNA from the reference genome may not contain the same amount of mitochondrial DNA as the patient sample. However, relative copy number of the mitochondrial DNA between the patient and control can still be represented on the log2 plot and partial deletions of the mitochondrial genome in the patient sample can be clearly visualized.

An additional complicating factor affecting mitochondrial copy number analysis is heteroplasmy. This term refers to the occurrence of a deletion or mutation in only a proportion of the mitochondria in an individual cell. This proportion can vary between cells in the same tissue and between different tissues. While analysis of copy number of the mitochondrial genome by array CGH is interrogating the aggregate copy number in a pool of cells, relative heteroplasmy levels can still be determined in that pool of cells. Given these complexities, determining the copy number of mitochondrial genome sequence is challenging. However, one group has shown that array CGH is a robust method for evaluating deletions in the mitochondrial genome [60] and such testing is now performed routinely in several laboratories. In these laboratories, array CGH analysis of mitochondrial disorders typically includes interrogation of the mitochondrial genome as well as the nuclear genes that control mitochondrial function.

Single-Gene Array CGH

Copy number analysis at the exon level for single genes has traditionally been done by multiplex ligation-dependent amplification analysis (MLPA), Southern blot, or quantitative polymerase chain reaction (qPCR). However, the recent availability of custom designed CGH arrays has enabled the design of arrays with dense probe coverage at very specific regions of the genome. Such array designs can be used quite effectively for the detection of small deletions or duplications that disrupt one or more exons within the coding regions of individual genes or panels of genes and have proven very useful for identifying exonic copy number mutations in a variety of disorders [61–65].

These targeted copy number arrays are particularly useful in conjunction with gene sequencing assays for disorders in which loss-of-function mutations are expected to result in a particular phenotype. The relative frequency of deletions and duplications and the inheritance pattern for a particular gene may dictate how and when array testing is most effectively utilized. Autosomal dominant disorders are prime candidates for this type of technology, and many exonic copy number mutations have been identified in disorders such as aniridia, Rubenstein–Taybi syndrome, or Alagille syndrome [61]. Testing algorithms for autosomal recessive disorders may also benefit from copy number arrays, particularly when only a single pathogenic mutation is identified by sequencing or when deletion mutations are frequent (e.g., in the *DHCR7* or *NPHP1 genes*). Exonic deletions and duplications have been reported in a variety of X-linked disorders as well, including adrenal hypoplasia, Rett syndrome, and Duchenne muscular dystrophy [61, 65, 66].

Single-gene copy number analysis by exon array CGH requires a different approach to array design compared to that necessary for whole genome cytogenetic analysis. When determining probe coverage across a gene, important considerations include the variety of transcripts or splice variants, variability in exon size and the number of probes required to reliably detect a copy number change of each exon, and probe coverage in the promoter, untranslated, and intronic regions (Fig. 9.4).

The concept of resolution, as described earlier in this chapter, requires some modification in the context of exon-level array CGH. The resolution of an array intended for single-copy number analysis must take into account the number of probes placed at each exon and the number of exons covered. Single gene CGH analysis requires high density probe coverage at each exon to maximize sensitivity. At the resolution of a single exon, at least three or four probes are required to reliably detect deletions or duplications, and most published array designs describe placing at least seven or more probes per exon [61].

Intronic sequences may also be targeted on an array used for single gene analysis. The addition of intronic probes offers better delineation of the breakpoints of a deletion or duplication and may add additional confidence to a copy number change impacting only a single exon, particularly when that exon is very small. In addition,

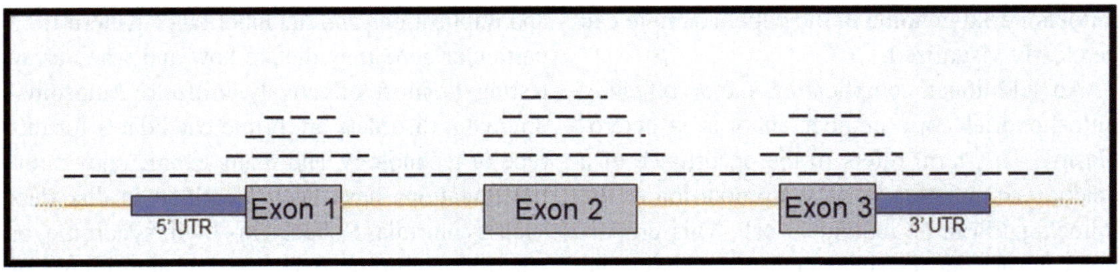

Fig. 9.4 Illustration of theoretical gene showing array CGH probe coverage. Backbone probe coverage spans the entire gene, including the promoter, untranslated regions, and introns, with individual exons specifically covered at higher density

probe placement within intronic sequences immediately flanking exons is useful when deletion or duplication breakpoints are found very close to an exon and may disrupt splicing.

While array CGH is quickly replacing MLPA and qPCR for single-gene copy number analysis in the clinical setting, there are certain limitations that must be brought to attention. Many genes have GC-rich regions, particularly in promoter sequences and the first exon. Probe design and performance in these regions can be difficult and may lead to suboptimal array performance. However, the probe performance in these regions is reproducible across hybridization experiments, and this reproducibility must be taken into account during analysis of any gene. In rare cases, nearly all probes within a gene can show poor performance, likely due to high GC content (examples include *STK11*, *MEN1*, and *SHH*). For such genes, MLPA may be a better method for copy number analysis because it can interrogate a single base and is not subject to the problems associated with high GC content.

How Chromosome Microarrays Have Changed Medical Practice

A "Genotype-First" Approach to the Diagnosis of Patients with Developmental Disorders

Prior to the advent of chromosome studies as a clinical diagnostic tool, syndromes were defined by the clinical assessment of patients with similar constellations of phenotypic features. The era of clinical cytogenetics began with a "phenotype-first" approach when it was recognized that Down syndrome, a syndrome that had been recognized on a clinical basis since the 1800s, was caused by an additional copy of chromosome 21 by Lejeune in 1959 [67]. Shortly after this discovery, the chromosomal causes of several additional clinically described syndromes were described (such as Klinefelter and Turner syndromes). A "genotype-first" approach was first applied when the ability to identify multiple patients with the same cytogenetic abnormality permitted the definition of new clinical syndromes such as Patau and Edwards syndromes in association with trisomy 13 and trisomy 18. With the advent of G-banded chromosome studies in the 1970s and high resolution chromosome studies in the 1980s, the detection of aneuploidy and large, recurrent structural rearrangements in association with groups of patients with shared clinical features allowed for the cytogenetic definition of many novel syndromes.

FISH technology that came into routine use in the 1990s also allowed for the discovery of the underlying cytogenetic abnormalities associated with syndromes, such as Williams syndrome, that were too small to be seen by routine chromosome studies. Overall, the syndromes that could be detected by chromosome and FISH studies were limited in number and were often defined by distinctive phenotypic features that allowed clinical diagnoses to be made readily. In these situations, the clinical recognition of a syndrome was critical, and chromosome or FISH testing was often utilized as a tool to confirm the clinical diagnosis—a phenotype-first approach.

As FISH testing became more routine, screening the end of chromosomes, the subtelomeric regions, became a tool for detecting chromosomal rearrangements involving the ends of all chromosomes. This screening technique also allowed for a genotype-first approach for defining syndromes and making clinical diagnoses—individuals were grouped by common structural rearrangements and when common clinical features could be assigned, a novel clinical syndrome could be described [68].

Since the advent of CMA technology and its application as a routine research and clinical tool, many new syndromes have been discovered. However, the smaller size and fewer genes contained within many of the recently described microdeletion syndromes are often associated with less severe or distinctive phenotypes and are associated with significantly more clinical variability—both in terms of variable expressivity and incomplete penetrance. In fact, many of these syndromes such as the 1q21.1 microdeletion/duplication syndromes are associated with a surprisingly wide range of clinical phenotypes [69, 70] that can confound clinical diagnosis and make a genotype-first approach an extremely useful tool. In addition, many of these new genomic disorders have very similar or overlapping phenotypes, making a specific clinical diagnosis and ordering a specific test to confirm that diagnosis much more difficult. Therefore, the use of CMA testing allows a clinician to interrogate the entire genome with a single test and to have a very high diagnostic yield (12–15 %) based on a single screening technique.

Additional advantages to a genotype-first approach to clinical diagnosis include the definition of the entire spectrum of phenotypic variability associated with a particular genotype and earlier diagnosis of a syndrome. Using a phenotype-first approach, patients are diagnosed based on a set of distinct clinical features. However, patients without one or more features may not be tested for a particular syndrome defined by those features. Without this testing, the true phenotypic variability associated with a particular genotype would go unrecognized. Therefore, the genotype-first approach offered by CMA testing is an objective means of collecting patient cohorts with the same genotype which subsequently allows the complete phenotypic spectrum of a syndrome to be defined. In addition, the application of a genomic screen such as CMA testing in patients with nonspecific findings may prevent a stepwise "diagnostic odyssey" that can be expensive, time consuming, and frustrating for the patient and family. Finally, early diagnosis, possibly before all features of a syndrome have developed, may allow early clinical or therapeutic intervention and the opportunity for genetic counseling regarding the developmental expectations and milestones for the patient and recurrence risk counseling for family.

Future Directions

CMA testing has replaced G-banded chromosome analysis in individuals with unexplained DD/ID, ASD, or MCA and provided significant increases in diagnostic yield for this patient population due to its higher resolution. While this transition took over 30 years to complete, recent technological advances in sequencing technologies may soon displace CMA as the first-tier test in this patient population. These advances will likely allow for the detection of all types of structural variation (both balanced and unbalanced) at base pair resolution revealing a complete picture of an individual's chromosomal structure. This information will lead to additional, exciting discoveries regarding the contribution of structural variation to human disease and yield further improvements in patient care.

References

1. Kallioniemi A, Kallioniemi OP, Sudar D, et al. Comparative genomic hybridization for molecular cytogenetic analysis of solid tumors. Science. 1992; 258:818–21.
2. Pinkel D, Segraves R, Sudar D, et al. High resolution analysis of DNA copy number variation using comparative genomic hybridization to microarrays. Nat Genet. 1998;20:207–11.
3. Snijders AM, Nowak N, Segraves R, et al. Assembly of microarrays for genome-wide measurement of DNA copy number. Nat Genet. 2001;29:263–4.

4. Ishkanian AS, Malloff CA, Watson SK, et al. A tiling resolution DNA microarray with complete coverage of the human genome. Nat Genet. 2004;36:299–303.
5. Lu X, Shaw CA, Patel A, et al. Clinical implementation of chromosomal microarray analysis: summary of 2513 postnatal cases. PLoS One. 2007;2:e327.
6. Shaffer LG, Kashork CD, Saleki R, et al. Targeted genomic microarray analysis for identification of chromosome abnormalities in 1500 consecutive clinical cases. J Pediatr. 2006;149:98–102.
7. Wong A, Vallender EJ, Heretis K, et al. Diverse fates of paralogs following segmental duplication of telomeric genes. Genomics. 2004;84:239–47.
8. Aradhya S, Cherry AM. Array-based comparative genomic hybridization: clinical contexts for targeted and whole-genome designs. Genet Med. 2007;9:553–9.
9. Baldwin EL, Lee JY, Blake DM, et al. Enhanced detection of clinically relevant genomic imbalances using a targeted plus whole genome oligonucleotide microarray. Genet Med. 2008;10:415–29.
10. Miller DT, Adam MP, Aradhya S, et al. Consensus statement: chromosomal microarray is a first-tier clinical diagnostic test for individuals with developmental disabilities or congenital anomalies. Am J Hum Genet. 2010;86:749–64.
11. Ravnan JB, Tepperberg JH, Papenhausen P, et al. Subtelomere FISH analysis of 11 688 cases: an evaluation of the frequency and pattern of subtelomere rearrangements in individuals with developmental disabilities. J Med Genet. 2006;43:478–89.
12. Ballif BC, Sulpizio SG, Lloyd RM, et al. The clinical utility of enhanced subtelomeric coverage in array CGH. Am J Med Genet A. 2007;143A:1850–7.
13. Bruno DL, Stark Z, Amor DJ, et al. Extending the scope of diagnostic chromosome analysis: detection of single gene defects using high-resolution SNP microarrays. Hum Mutat. 2011;32:1500–6.
14. Kearney HM, Thorland EC, Brown KK, Quintero-Rivera F, South ST. American College of Medical Genetics standards and guidelines for interpretation and reporting of postnatal constitutional copy number variants. Genet Med. 2011;13:680–5.
15. Manning M, Hudgins L. Array-based technology and recommendations for utilization in medical genetics practice for detection of chromosomal abnormalities. Genet Med. 2010;12:742–5.
16. Iafrate AJ, Feuk L, Rivera MN, et al. Detection of large-scale variation in the human genome. Nat Genet. 2004;36:949–51.
17. Sebat J, Lakshmi B, Troge J, et al. Large-scale copy number polymorphism in the human genome. Science. 2004;305:525–8.
18. Tuzun E, Sharp AJ, Bailey JA, et al. Fine-scale structural variation of the human genome. Nat Genet. 2005;37:727–32.
19. Sharp AJ, Locke DP, McGrath SD, et al. Segmental duplications and copy-number variation in the human genome. Am J Hum Genet. 2005;77:78–88.
20. Conrad DF, Andrews TD, Carter NP, Hurles ME, Pritchard JK. A high-resolution survey of deletion polymorphism in the human genome. Nat Genet. 2006;38:75–81.
21. Hinds DA, Kloek AP, Jen M, Chen X, Frazer KA. Common deletions and SNPs are in linkage disequilibrium in the human genome. Nat Genet. 2006;38:82–5.
22. McCarroll SA, Hadnott TN, Perry GH, et al. Common deletion polymorphisms in the human genome. Nat Genet. 2006;38:86–92.
23. Freeman JL, Perry GH, Feuk L, et al. Copy number variation: new insights in genome diversity. Genome Res. 2006;16:949–61.
24. Redon R, Ishikawa S, Fitch KR, et al. Global variation in copy number in the human genome. Nature. 2006;444:444–54.
25. Korbel JO, Urban AE, Affourtit JP, et al. Paired-end mapping reveals extensive structural variation in the human genome. Science. 2007;318:420–6.
26. McCarroll SA, Kuruvilla FG, Korn JM, et al. Integrated detection and population-genetic analysis of SNPs and copy number variation. Nat Genet. 2008;40:1166–74.
27. Kidd JM, Cooper GM, Donahue WF, et al. Mapping and sequencing of structural variation from eight human genomes. Nature. 2008;453:56–64.
28. Richards CS, Bale S, Bellissimo DB, et al. ACMG recommendations for standards for interpretation and reporting of sequence variations: revisions 2007. Genet Med. 2008;10:294–300.
29. Girirajan S, Eichler EE. Phenotypic variability and genetic susceptibility to genomic disorders. Hum Mol Genet. 2010;19:R176–87.
30. South ST. Chromosomal structural rearrangements: detection and elucidation of mechanisms using cytogenomic technologies. Clin Lab Med. 2011;31:513–24. vii.
31. Firth HV, Richards SM, Bevan AP, et al. DECIPHER: database of chromosomal imbalance and phenotype in humans using ensembl resources. Am J Hum Genet. 2009;84:524–33.
32. Zhang J, Feuk L, Duggan GE, Khaja R, Scherer SW. Development of bioinformatics resources for display and analysis of copy number and other structural variants in the human genome. Cytogenet Genome Res. 2006;115:205–14.
33. Fujita PA, Rhead B, Zweig AS, et al. The UCSC genome browser database: update 2011. Nucleic Acids Res. 2011;39:D876–82.
34. Riggs ER, Church DM, Hanson K, et al. Towards an evidence-based process for the clinical interpretation of copy number variation. Clin Genet. 2012;81:403–12.
35. Kearney HM, Kearney JB, Conlin LK. Diagnostic implications of excessive homozygosity detected by SNP-based microarrays: consanguinity, uniparental disomy, and recessive single-gene mutations. Clin Lab Med. 2011;31:595–613. ix.
36. Engel E. A new genetic concept: uniparental disomy and its potential effect, isodisomy. Am J Med Genet. 1980;6:137–43.

37. Spence JE, Perciaccante RG, Greig GM, et al. Uniparental disomy as a mechanism for human genetic disease. Am J Hum Genet. 1988;42:217–26.
38. Nicholls RD, Knoll JH, Butler MG, Karam S, Lalande M. Genetic imprinting suggested by maternal heterodisomy in nondeletion Prader-Willi syndrome. Nature. 1989;342:281–5.
39. Papenhausen P, Schwartz S, Risheg H, et al. UPD detection using homozygosity profiling with a SNP genotyping microarray. Am J Med Genet A. 2011; 155A:757–68.
40. Lapunzina P, Monk D. The consequences of uniparental disomy and copy number neutral loss-of-heterozygosity during human development and cancer. Biol Cell. 2011;103:303–17.
41. Kotzot D. Complex and segmental uniparental disomy (UPD): review and lessons from rare chromosomal complements. J Med Genet. 2001;38:497–507.
42. Robinson WP. Mechanisms leading to uniparental disomy and their clinical consequences. Bioessays. 2000;22:452–9.
43. Geneimprint. 2012. http://www.geneimprint.com/site/genes-by-species.Homo+sapiens. Accessed 10 Dec 2012.
44. Kotzot D. Complex and segmental uniparental disomy updated. J Med Genet. 2008;45:545–56.
45. Yamazawa K, Ogata T, Ferguson-Smith AC. Uniparental disomy and human disease: an overview. Am J Med Genet C Semin Med Genet. 2010;154C: 329–34.
46. Liehr T. Cytogenetic contribution to uniparental disomy (UPD). Mol Cytogenet. 2010;3:8.
47. Engel E. Uniparental disomy revisited: the first twelve years. Am J Med Genet. 1993;46:670–4.
48. Engel E. A fascination with chromosome rescue in uniparental disomy: Mendelian recessive outlaws and imprinting copyrights infringements. Eur J Hum Genet. 2006;14:1158–69.
49. Modell B, Darr A. Science and society: genetic counselling and customary consanguineous marriage. Nat Rev Genet. 2002;3:225–9.
50. Stoll C, Alembik Y, Dott B, Feingold J. Parental consanguinity as a cause of increased incidence of birth defects in a study of 131,760 consecutive births. Am J Med Genet. 1994;49:114–7.
51. Stoltenberg C, Magnus P, Skrondal A, Lie RT. Consanguinity and recurrence risk of birth defects: a population-based study. Am J Med Genet. 1999;82: 423–8.
52. Schaaf CP, Scott DA, Wiszniewska J, Beaudet AL. Identification of incestuous parental relationships by SNP-based DNA microarrays. Lancet. 2011;377: 555–6.
53. Sheffield VC, Nishimura DY, Stone EM. Novel approaches to linkage mapping. Curr Opin Genet Dev. 1995;5:335–41.
54. Lander ES, Botstein D. Homozygosity mapping: a way to map human recessive traits with the DNA of inbred children. Science. 1987;236:1567–70.
55. Alkuraya FS. Homozygosity mapping: one more tool in the clinical geneticist's toolbox. Genet Med. 2010; 12:236–9.
56. Highsmith Jr WE, Burch LH, Zhou Z, et al. Identification of a splice site mutation (2789 +5 G>A) associated with small amounts of normal CFTR mRNA and mild cystic fibrosis. Hum Mutat. 1997;9:332–8.
57. Alkuraya FS. Autozygome decoded. Genet Med. 2010;12:765–71.
58. Genomic Oligoarray and SNP array evaluation tool v1.0. http://www.ccs.miami.edu/cgi-bin/ROH/ROH_analysis_tool.cgi. Accessed 10 Dec 2012.
59. DiMauro S, Hirano M. Mitochondrial DNA Deletion Syndromes. In: Pagon RA, Bird TD, Dolan CR, Stephens K, Adam MP, editors. GeneReviews. Seattle, WA: University of Washington; 1993.
60. Chinault AC, Shaw CA, Brundage EK, Tang LY, Wong LJ. Application of dual-genome oligonucleotide array-based comparative genomic hybridization to the molecular diagnosis of mitochondrial DNA deletion and depletion syndromes. Genet Med. 2009;11:518–26.
61. Aradhya S, Lewis R, Bonaga T, et al. Exon-level array CGH in a large clinical cohort demonstrates increased sensitivity of diagnostic testing for Mendelian disorders. Genet Med. 2012;14:594–603.
62. Piluso G, Dionisi M, Del Vecchio BF, et al. Motor chip: a comparative genomic hybridization microarray for copy-number mutations in 245 neuromuscular disorders. Clin Chem. 2011;57:1584–96.
63. Boone PM, Bacino CA, Shaw CA, et al. Detection of clinically relevant exonic copy-number changes by array CGH. Hum Mutat. 2010;31:1326–42.
64. Wong LJ, Dimmock D, Geraghty MT, et al. Utility of oligonucleotide array-based comparative genomic hybridization for detection of target gene deletions. Clin Chem. 2008;54:1141–8.
65. Saillour Y, Cossee M, Leturcq F, et al. Detection of exonic copy-number changes using a highly efficient oligonucleotide-based comparative genomic hybridization-array method. Hum Mutat. 2008;29: 1083–90.
66. del Gaudio D, Yang Y, Boggs BA, et al. Molecular diagnosis of Duchenne/Becker muscular dystrophy: enhanced detection of dystrophin gene rearrangements by oligonucleotide array-comparative genomic hybridization. Hum Mutat. 2008;29:1100–7.
67. Lejeune J, Gauthier M, Turpin R. Human chromosomes in tissue cultures. C R Hebd Seances Acad Sci. 1959;248:602–3.
68. Phelan MC, Rogers RC, Saul RA, et al. 22q13 deletion syndrome. Am J Med Genet. 2001;101:91–9.
69. Mefford HC, Sharp AJ, Baker C, et al. Recurrent rearrangements of chromosome 1q21.1 and variable pediatric phenotypes. N Engl J Med. 2008;359:1685–99.
70. Brunetti-Pierri N, Berg JS, Scaglia F, et al. Recurrent reciprocal 1q21.1 deletions and duplications associated with microcephaly or macrocephaly and developmental and behavioral abnormalities. Nat Genet. 2008;40:1466–71.

BRCA1 and *BRCA2* Testing in Inherited Breast Cancer

10

Karla R. Bowles and Eric Rosenthal

Background

The Clinical Problem

Although breast cancer is most common in more-developed countries, it is a global problem, comprising 22.9 % of all cancers in women, excluding noninvasive skin cancers, and 13.7 % of all cancer deaths in women [1]. Excluding non-melanoma skin cancers, breast cancer is the most common cancer in women and the most common cause of cancer death in women worldwide. The USA has the world's highest annual incidence of breast cancer. Estimates for 2011 are for the diagnosis of 232,620 new cases and 39,900 deaths [2].

As is the case for most types of cancer, it has long been known that individuals with a close relative who has had breast cancer have an increased risk of developing breast cancer themselves. The magnitude of this increased risk is two- to threefold when the affected relative is "first degree," i.e., a parent, sibling, or child [3]. The basis for this familial risk is thought to be due to a combination of environmental, lifestyle, and genetic factors. In most cases, the genetic factors are believed to involve interactions between many different genes, each of which individually contributes a relatively small component of the risk. However, mutations in a set of genes that function as tumor suppressors can have a much greater impact on cancer risk. Families in which these mutations are being passed down from generation to generation often have especially striking breast cancer histories, including not only a high incidence of breast cancer but also features such as women diagnosed at unusually young ages, men with breast cancer, and individuals with diagnoses of more than one primary tumor.

A subset of women with breast cancer also has personal and/or family histories of ovarian cancer. Ovarian cancer is a much less common, but more deadly cancer. It is estimated that there will be 21,990 cases diagnosed in the USA in 2011, with 15,460 deaths [2]. Accumulated observations of numerous families with a multigenerational pattern of breast and ovarian cancer, including breast cancer diagnoses under age 50, individuals with multiple primary breast cancers or breast and ovarian cancer, and male breast cancer, eventually led to the recognition of the genetic condition Hereditary Breast and Ovarian Cancer syndrome (HBOC) and a competitive search for the responsible genes. The search was eventually successful, resulting in the isolation of the gene *BRCA1* in 1994 [4] and *BRCA2* in 1995 [5].

By one estimate, approximately 7 % of breast cancers and 10 % of ovarian cancers are due to inherited mutations in tumor suppressor genes [6], the vast majority of which occur in *BRCA1* and

K.R. Bowles, Ph.D. (✉) • E. Rosenthal, Ph.D., Sc.M
Myriad Genetic Laboratories, Inc., Salt Lake City, UT, USA
e-mail: kbowles@myriad.com

W.E. Highsmith Jr. (ed.), *Molecular Diagnostics: 12 Tests That Changed Everything*, Molecular and Translational Medicine, DOI 10.1007/978-1-4614-8127-0_10,

BRCA2. There are many other genes, some of which function in the same molecular pathways as *BRCA1* and *BRCA2*, also known to have a link to an increased risk for breast cancer and/or ovarian cancer. Depending on the specific gene involved, there may also be increased risk for other malignancies. Examples include *TP53*, *PTEN*, *CDH1*, *CHEK2*, *ATM*, *STK11*, *RAD51*, and *PALB2* [7, 8]. The four DNA mismatch repair genes, *MLH1*, *MSH2*, *MSH6*, and *PMS2*, which primarily increase risks for colon and endometrial cancer, are responsible for a small percentage of hereditary ovarian cancer as well [9]. However, due to the relatively high prevalence of *BRCA1* and *BRCA2* mutations in most populations, and their large impact on breast and ovarian cancer risk, *BRCA1* and *BRCA2* are widely considered to be the most significant and clinically relevant genes for both hereditary breast and hereditary ovarian cancer. Therefore, genetic testing for patients considered to be at risk for HBOC will almost always start with *BRCA1* and *BRCA2*. If no mutations are found, a minority of patients may go on to have testing for mutations in other genes.

It is estimated that 1:500 to 1:100 individuals carry mutations in *BRCA1* or *BRCA2* [10–12]. The prevalence of mutations is higher in some ethnic populations, most notably Ashkenazi Jews, where 1:40 individuals carry one of three discrete "founder" mutations (187delAG and 5385insC in *BRCA1* and 6174delT in *BRCA2*) that are very common in this population [13]. Based on these figures, we can estimate that there are approximately 300,000 female mutation carriers in the USA. The discovery of these genes has provided an opportunity to identify these individuals, who are at a high risk for both breast and ovarian cancer, and take steps to reduce their risk through both prevention and early detection. A greater understanding of the molecular function of *BRCA1* and *BRCA2* also holds promise in the development of more effective treatment options for those patients who do develop cancer.

Molecular Biology

BRCA1 and *BRCA2* are classic tumor suppressors—genes that protect cells from the changes that trigger transformation to a cancer. Many tumor suppressors function to maintain the integrity of the cell's DNA, and although the full scope of their function is not yet completely understood, it is clear that *BRCA1* and *BRCA2* play a major role in DNA repair, specifically repair of double-stranded DNA breaks by a mechanism known as homologous recombination. Cells that lack functional *BRCA1* or *BRCA2* protein accumulate DNA damage that disrupts other genes, including those that regulate normal cell growth. Both *BRCA1* and *BRCA2* interact with a host of other proteins to carry out their DNA repair activity, as well as other steps in cell proliferation (i.e., cell cycle progression, transcription, and mitotic spindle formation). Several reviews are available for more detailed discussion of the molecular biology of these genes [14–16]. It is not known why the tumor suppressor roles of *BRCA1* and *BRCA2* are focused primarily, but not exclusively, in preventing breast and ovarian cancer.

The basis for the increased risk of cancer in patients who inherit a single nonfunctional copy of *BRCA1* or *BRCA2* is thought to be via the "two-hit model" of tumor suppressor gene inactivation, first described for the retinoblastoma tumor suppressor gene [17]. As with other autosomal genes—all genes other than those found on the X and Y chromosomes—everyone is usually born with two copies of the *BRCA1* and *BRCA2* genes. Complete loss of *BRCA1* or *BRCA2* function would normally only occur as a result of sporadic loss of both copies of either gene from a cell (i.e., as a result of environmental insult or DNA replication error). Random loss of both copies of either gene in a single cell is a relatively rare event, but individuals born with one copy of either gene that is already nonfunctional are at much higher risk of losing all *BRCA1* or *BRCA2* function as a result of sporadic loss of their one remaining functional copy.

HBOC is a "dominant" genetic condition, meaning that someone has the condition if they inherit a single damaged copy of *BRCA1* or *BRCA2* from either parent. While rare, it is possible for an individual to inherit nonfunctional copies of either *BRCA1* or *BRCA2* from both of their parents (homozygosity/compound heterozygosity), with generally disastrous results.

In the case of *BRCA1*, homozygosity/compound heterozygosity for two mutations is widely assumed to be an embryonic lethal condition [18]. In the case of *BRCA2*, homozygosity/compound heterozygosity may either be embryonically lethal or lead to Fanconi Anemia, resulting in bone marrow failure and hematological malignancies during childhood, as well as a variety of congenital physical anomalies, although there may be rare exceptions [19, 20].

Breast cancers arising in *BRCA2* mutation carriers do not appear to have any distinctive pathological features. In contrast, a majority of breast tumors in *BRCA1* mutation carriers lack estrogen and progesterone receptors and do not over-express HER2/neu. This "triple-negative breast cancer" (TNBC) pathology is linked to a set of additional characteristics known as a basal phenotype. These characteristics are also present in breast tumors that arise as a result of sporadic loss of *BRCA1* function [21–23].

Clinical Applications

At this time, the clinical utility associated with the identification of *BRCA1* and *BRCA2* mutation carriers is focused primarily on identifying individuals at high risk for breast and ovarian cancer and targeting them with interventions aimed at prevention and early detection. There has been a steady accumulation of published evidence supporting risk-reducing strategies for *BRCA1/2* mutation carriers in the years since clinical testing for *BRCA1* and *BRCA2* first became available in the mid-1990s. While there is still progress to be made, the weight of this evidence has been a key driver behind the incorporation of *BRCA1/2* testing into clinical practice. For those interested in a more comprehensive discussion of the clinical applications of *BRCA1* and *BRCA2* testing, there are many excellent reviews available [7, 24, 25].

Figure 10.1 dramatically illustrates the increase in cancer risk for women with mutations in *BRCA1* and *BRCA2*. The increased breast cancer risk for women under age 50 is particularly striking. This figure shows the upper estimates of cancer risk in mutation carriers, but the aggregate

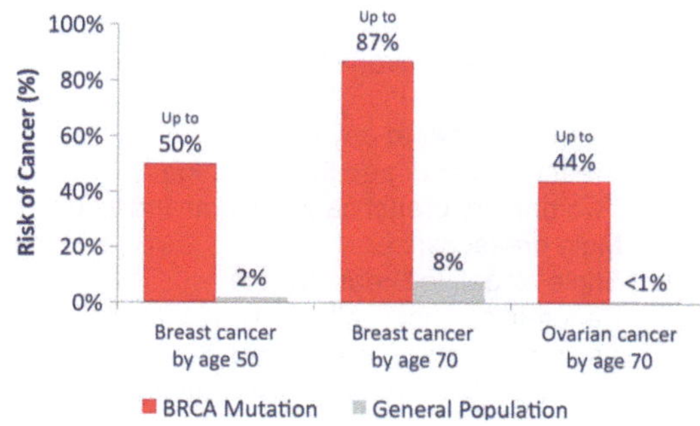

Fig. 10.1 Mutations in *BRCA1* and *BRCA2* lead to dramatic increases in risk for breast and ovarian cancer in women

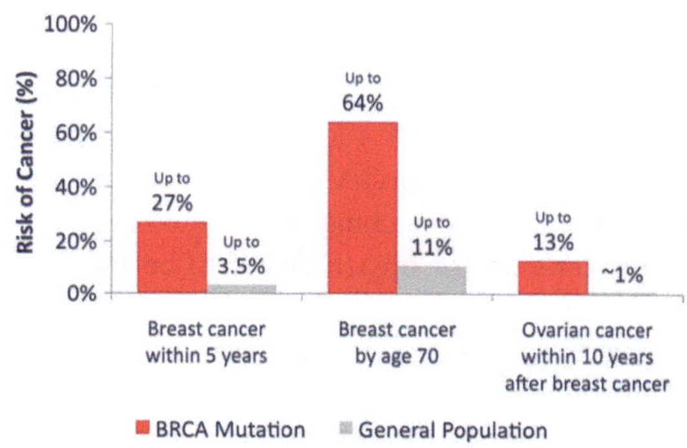

Fig. 10.2 Mutations in *BRCA1* and *BRCA2* dramatically increase the risk for a second cancer in women with a breast cancer diagnosis

outcome of various studies indicates that the breast cancer risk to age 70 may actually fall somewhere between 45 and 87 %. The breast cancer risk associated with *BRCA2* mutations is lower than that associated with *BRCA1*, and *BRCA2* mutation carriers are diagnosed at somewhat older ages than carriers of mutations in *BRCA1* [13, 26–31]. Ovarian cancer risk estimates also differ between the genes, with ranges to age 70 of 28 to 44 % for *BRCA1* mutation carriers and 11 to 27 % for *BRCA2* mutation carriers [26, 28, 29, 31–33]. It is important to note that two other cancers related to ovarian cancer, fallopian tube and papillary serous peritoneal carcinoma, are also much more common in *BRCA1* and *BRCA2* mutation carriers [34–36].

Female mutation carriers have greatly increased risks for additional primary breast and ovarian cancers after an initial breast cancer, as illustrated in Fig. 10.2 [29, 37, 38]. There are data for *BRCA1* mutation carriers showing that

For the purposes of these clinical indications, breast cancer includes both invasive cancer and ductal carcinoma *in situ*, and ovarian cancer includes cancer of the fallopian tubes and primary peritoneal cancer.

- Ovarian cancer at any age
- Breast cancer at age 50 or younger
- Two primary breast cancers in an individual or family
- Male breast cancer
- Triple Negative Breast Cancer
- Pancreatic cancer with an additional HBOC-associated cancer (breast, ovarian or pancreatic cancer)
- Ashkenazi Jewish with an HBOC-associated cancer (breast, ovarian or pancreatic cancer)
- A previously identified BRCA mutation in the family

Fig. 10.3 Clinical indications for identifying patients for evaluation for genetic testing for mutations in *BRCA1* and *BRCA2* (as of 2011)

younger ages of diagnosis for the first breast cancer may be associated with higher risks for second primaries [39, 40]. Presumably, there is also an increased risk for breast cancer after a diagnosis of ovarian cancer in a mutation carrier, but data are lacking because it is much more common for breast cancer to be the first diagnosis.

There are conflicting data on the risks for malignancies other than breast and ovarian cancer in individuals with mutations in *BRCA1* and *BRCA2*. At this time, it seems clear that there is an increased risk for pancreatic cancer, which is estimated to be up to 7 % by age 80 for *BRCA2* mutation carriers [37, 41], but this risk may be considerably higher in *BRCA2* mutation carriers where a family history of pancreatic cancer is present [42]. There are less data for *BRCA1* [43], but the National Comprehensive Cancer Network (NCCN) has recently added a personal or family history of pancreatic cancer to the list of factors for consideration when targeting patients for both *BRCA1* and *BRCA2* testing [24]. Male carriers of mutations in *BRCA1* and *BRCA2* are thought to have an elevated risk for prostate cancer, with estimates ranging from 1.8- to 4.6-fold over the general population [37, 43, 44].

Guidance for the selection of patients who are appropriate candidates for *BRCA1* and *BRCA2* testing is available in the form of guidelines from numerous professional societies [7, 45]. Typical clinical indications are presented in Fig. 10.3. When a patient has one or more of the characteristics listed, or has a close blood relative who has any of these characteristics, further clinical evaluation by a qualified healthcare professional to determine the appropriateness of genetic testing for mutations in *BRCA1* and *BRCA2* is warranted.

The first individual in a family to be tested can be either affected with a *BRCA1*/2-associated cancer, or unaffected, but it is advantageous to begin with an affected family member. This is because affected family members, especially those with the most striking clinical features, are the individuals most likely to be positive for a clinically significant mutation, and once a mutation has been identified in a family member, testing for relatives is much less expensive and more easily interpretable. This is often a confusing concept for healthcare providers and patients, and a much more detailed discussion is presented below in the section Interpretation. Although there are significant benefits to first performing testing in affected patients, obstacles often make this impossible. The family members who are the best candidates for testing may be deceased or unavailable for other reasons, unwilling to participate, or lacking insurance coverage. There are cases where family members are not in communication for either logistical or psychosocial reasons. There is no question that failures in family communication reduce the potential clinical benefit from all types of genetic testing, including that done for *BRCA1* and *BRCA2*, and developing strategies to overcome these challenges would have a major impact on public health.

Medical management options for women with mutations in *BRCA1* and *BRCA2* include both

	Procedure	Age to Begin	Frequency
Breast cancer surveillance	Breast self-exam	18 yrs	Monthly
	Clinical breast exam	25 yrs	Twice a year
	Mammography	25 yrs	Yearly
	MRI	25 yrs	Yearly
Ovarian cancer surveillance	Pelvic exam	35 yrs in patients not electing RRBSO	Twice a year
	TVUS and CA-125*	35 yrs in patients not electing RRBSO	Twice a year

*Very limited data to support efficacy

Fig. 10.4 Current surveillance recommendations for women with mutations in *BRCA1* and *BRCA2*. *Very limited data to support efficacy

cancer prevention strategies and surveillance for early detection. The most effective, albeit crude, prevention strategy is the removal of the at risk tissues before cancer develops, through risk reducing mastectomy (RRM) and removal of the ovaries and fallopian tubes, known as risk reducing bilateral salpingo-oophorectomy (RRBSO). Both of these procedures have been shown to reduce the risk of the associated cancers by 90 % or more in *BRCA1* and *BRCA2* mutation carriers [35, 46–53]. Neither intervention is 100 % effective because it is not possible to remove all breast tissue from the chest wall during RRM, and a risk for primary peritoneal cancer remains after RRBSO. Premenopausal RRBSO carries an additional benefit for women who do not opt for RRM, as it is associated with an up to 68 % decline in the risk for breast cancer, presumably due to the reduction in lifetime estrogen exposure, which is a well-established risk factor for breast cancer in women with and without *BRCA1* and *BRCA2* mutations [49, 51].

An alternative prevention strategy is chemoprevention. Tamoxifen, which is used widely to treat estrogen receptor-positive breast cancers, is a drug that interferes with the ability of estrogen to stimulate breast cell growth. Tamoxifen has also been shown to reduce the risk of developing breast cancer in the general population, and there is some evidence that it may be effective in *BRCA1* and *BRCA2* mutation carriers as well [54, 55]. A similar situation is seen with oral contraceptives, which have been shown to reduce ovarian cancer risk in the general population, and this also seems to be the case in *BRCA1* and *BRCA2* mutation carriers [56, 57]. One consideration in regards to chemoprevention options is whether or not even a significant impact on cancer risk (i.e., a 50 % reduction) is truly adequate in mutation carriers, given the very high level of baseline risk.

The goal of more aggressive surveillance is the earliest possible detection of breast and ovarian cancers, since early stage cancers generally have a better prognosis than advanced tumors. Surveillance guidelines for women with *BRCA1* and *BRCA2* mutations are shown in Fig. 10.4. Note that these recommendations are not only for more intensive screening but also for the initiation of screening at younger ages, since breast cancers are diagnosed at substantially younger ages in mutation carriers. There is mounting evidence that breast screening using magnetic resonance imaging (MRI) is more effective than mammography and ultrasound, and annual breast MRI is now recommended for all mutation carriers [58, 59]. On the other hand, there is currently no evidence that ovarian cancer screening using existing protocols combining transvaginal ultrasound and serum CA-125 measurements is an effective strategy for early stage ovarian cancer detection and there are no proven alternatives. For this reason, NCCN and other professional groups generally recommend RRSO for all *BRCA1* and *BRCA2* mutation carriers, ideally between age 35 and 40, or whenever childbearing is complete [24]. Choosing between RRM and surveillance, with or without chemoprevention, is a more complex decision. Most patients will find breast surgery much more demanding than an RRBSO, both psychosocially and physically. Since there is mounting evidence supporting the efficacy of a well-executed breast surveillance program in the early detection of breast cancer it is not surprising that studies have found a much higher uptake for RRSO than for RRM [60–62].

Women with mutations in *BRCA1* and *BRCA2* are typically very interested in lifestyle modifications that could lower their risk for breast and ovarian cancer. However, unlike certain other common cancers that are strongly linked to specific lifestyle factors over which patients have a great deal of control, such as smoking and lung cancer, or sun exposure and skin cancer, only small effects on risk in the general population have been documented from factors such as smoking, alcohol use, exercise, childbearing, breast feeding, and diet [63]. The potential impact of these factors in modifying risk in *BRCA1* and *BRCA2* mutation carriers has been investigated, and there are indications of a similar impact on mutation carriers. However, as with chemoprevention, the question is whether or not even a twofold reduction in cancer risk is enough when the baseline risk is so high [64–66].

Many women undergo genetic testing for *BRCA1* and *BRCA2* mutations only after a diagnosis of breast or ovarian cancer. Increasingly, testing is being offered at the time of diagnosis, particularly for new breast cancer patients, who may benefit from knowing their mutation status before proceeding with surgery, radiation, and reconstruction. This provides mutation carriers the opportunity to opt for bilateral mastectomies, even if a unilateral lumpectomy or mastectomy would have been adequate for treatment of the existing cancer. Studies have shown that 50 % or more patients newly diagnosed with unilateral breast cancer opt for bilateral mastectomies if it is possible to determine that they carry a deleterious mutation before surgery [67, 68]. Providing them with this opportunity requires that patients who are appropriate candidates for testing are identified quickly and counseled about their options early in their treatment. Samples from patients who opt for testing under these circumstances must be sent to the laboratory and processed quickly.

So far, only breast cancer risk management strategies in women have been discussed, although 50 % of all *BRCA1* and *BRCA2* mutation carriers are men. Male mutation carriers have a risk for breast cancer that is greatly elevated over men in the general population. This has best been characterized for *BRCA2*, where the breast cancer risk is estimated to be 7–8 % to age 80 [18, 43, 44, 69]. There is less data for *BRCA1*, with an estimate of a 1.8 % risk to age 80 [69]. Although these numbers are low compared with the breast cancer risks for women, they represent a very large increase over the 0.1 % risk for men in the general population. Therefore, male mutation carriers should have semiannual clinical breast exams, training in breast self-exams and consideration of mammography in the presence of characteristics such as gynecomastia [70]. As discussed earlier, *BRCA1* and *BRCA2* mutations also increase the risk for prostate cancer, but there are no specific screening recommendations [70]. Pancreatic cancer risk is also increased for both male and female mutation carriers, but there are no proven methods for screening or prevention, and the only protocols currently available are investigational. Participation in these protocols may be particularly appropriate for patients with a family history that includes pancreatic cancer [71].

There is growing evidence that the identification of *BRCA1* and *BRCA2* mutation carriers will have clinical utility in guiding chemotherapy decisions for patients with breast and ovarian cancer, and possibly pancreatic cancer as well. The role of *BRCA1* and *BRCA2* in repair of double-strand DNA breaks suggests that tumors that arise in cells lacking *BRCA1* or *BRCA2* function may be particularly susceptible to certain chemotherapy agents that kill tumor cells by causing lethal levels of DNA damage. There is evidence that this is the case with cisplatin treatment for breast and ovarian tumors in *BRCA1* mutation carriers [72, 73]. There is also a great deal of excitement surrounding ongoing clinical trials investigating the use of PARP inhibitors to treat breast and ovarian cancers in mutation carriers, as well as patients whose cancers developed due to sporadic inactivation of *BRCA1*. These drugs inhibit the activity of poly ADP-ribose polymerase (PARP), a protein that participates in an alternative pathway that can substitute for the *BRCA1* and *BRCA2* pathway in DNA repair. Tumors arising through loss of *BRCA1* or *BRCA2* function appear to be highly sensitive to PARP inhibition, presumably because this results in a lethal inability to repair certain types of DNA damage [74–76].

Methodology and Technical Interpretation

Comprehensive genetic analysis of *BRCA1* and *BRCA2* is currently capable of identifying both small DNA mutations, such as single nucleotide substitutions or small deletions/insertions, and larger genomic rearrangements spanning one or more exons. In a previous study, 90.1 % of mutations identified within a high-risk patient cohort were small nucleotide changes that were detectible by sequencing analysis, and the remaining 9.9 % were larger genomic deletions or insertions that were only detectible through large rearrangement analysis [77]. However, there may have been some selection bias for large rearrangements within this group as large rearrangements are more common within *BRCA1* than *BRCA2*, and *BRCA1* mutations are predicted to be more common within a high-risk group due to the higher penetrance of *BRCA1* mutations in comparison with *BRCA2*. The proportion of large rearrangements varied by ethnicity. Within the same high-risk group, large rearrangements represented 9.6 % of mutations identified in Western/Northern Europeans, 21.4 % of mutations identified in individuals of Latin American/Caribbean descent, and 8.3 % of mutations identified in individuals of African ancestry.

Detection of Point Mutations and Small Deletions/Insertions Using DNA Sequence Analysis

DNA sequence analysis is a powerful genetic analysis tool considered to be the gold standard for detecting single base substitutions and small deletions/insertions in genomic DNA. In brief, genomic DNA regions corresponding to the *BRCA1* and *BRCA2* genes are amplified using the Polymerase Chain Reaction (PCR) [78]. PCR primers are designed to anneal within the gene introns, allowing for amplification of all coding regions and small portions of each flanking intron. Partial intronic amplification is required in order to allow genetic analysis of intron/exon splice junctions, mutations of which can result in abnormal protein production and/or function. Each coding exon is PCR amplified using one or more primer pairs, depending on the size of the exon. If multiple primer pairs are required to amplify a larger exon, primer pairs are designed to overlap each other, allowing for full coverage of the exon. Full sequence analysis of the *BRCA1* and *BRCA2* genes currently analyzes approximately 15,600 coding base pairs and an additional 1,650 adjacent intronic base pairs.

PCR primers contain M13 sequence tails in order to facilitate subsequent sequencing analysis. Resulting PCR products are cycle sequenced in both the forward and reverse orientations using dye-primer chemistry [79]. PCR products are denatured and fluorescently labeled M13 primers annealed in the presence of all four deoxynucleotides (dATP, dGTP, dCTP, and dTTP) and only one of four dideoxynucleotides (ddATP, ddGTP, ddCTP, or ddTTP), which terminates extension once incorporated into the sequencing product. As only one dideoxynucleotide can be added to each reaction, four reactions (one for each dideoxynucleotide) are required in order to generate a complete unidirectional sequence. These four reactions are subsequently combined and analyzed on an automated capillary electrophoresis DNA sequencer (e.g., an ABI3730 from Applied Biosystems), which produces a sequencing chromatogram (Fig. 10.5). Computerized analysis of the resulting chromatograms is initially performed, followed by visual inspection and confirmation of

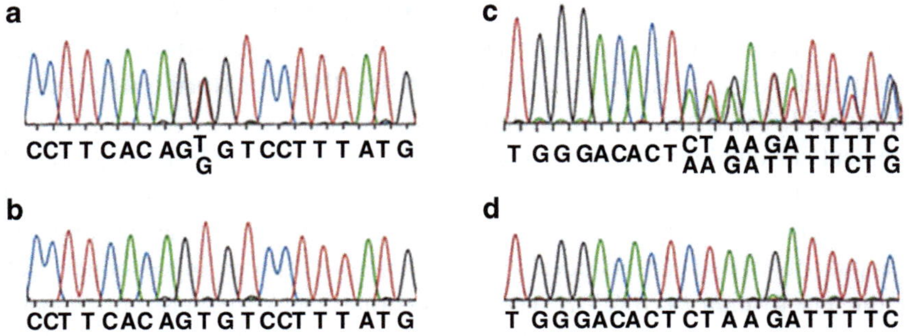

Fig. 10.5 *BRCA1* sequencing chromatograms. (**a**) A heterozygous single nucleotide substitution at nucleotide position 300 (300T>G; C61G). (**b**) No mutation detected at nucleotide position 300. (**c**) A heterozygous two nucleotide deletion at positions 187–188 (187delAG; reverse complement). (**d**) No deletion detected at nucleotide positions 187–188 (reverse complement)

computer-generated sequence results. All patient sequencing results are compared with a known normal control sequence in order to identify sequence variants. Reportable sequence variants are confirmed by repeated PCR amplification of the relevant gene region and subsequent sequencing analysis.

For autosomal genes, DNA variants can be present on either one copy of the gene (heterozygous) or both copies of the gene (homozygous). The heterozygous deleterious *BRCA1* mutation C61G (300T>G; GenBank # HSU14680) is an example of a single base substitution that is easily detectable by sequencing analysis (Fig. 10.5) [80]. This common mutation is caused by the substitution of the nucleotide deoxyguanosine (G) for deoxythymidine (T) at nucleotide position 300 (300T>G), resulting in the replacement of the amino acid cysteine by glycine in the BRCA1 protein product. Highly penetrant deleterious *BRCA1* and *BRCA2* mutations are always observed in the heterozygous state, which is easily detected as a double peak on sequencing chromatograms with one peak representing the wild-type allele and the other peak representing the variant allele.

The deleterious *BRCA1* Ashkenazi founder mutation 187delAG is an example of a small deletion that is also detectable by sequencing analysis (Fig. 10.5) [81]. This mutation is caused by the deletion of two nucleotides, deoxyadenosine (A) and deoxyguanosine (G) from nucleotide positions 187 and 188. As a single codon is composed of three nucleotides, deletions or insertions composed of nucleotide numbers that are not a multiple of three are predicted to result in a shift of the translation reading frame and most commonly, premature protein truncation. As with single nucleotide substitutions, highly penetrant small deletions and insertions are observed in the heterozygous state, which is easily detectable as two overlapping sequences on sequencing chromatograms.

Detection of Large Genomic Rearrangements

The identification of large genomic rearrangements, including deletions and insertions, is technically complex and multiple methodologies may be utilized. In cases where the DNA breakpoints of the rearrangement are previously known and well characterized, recombination-specific PCR analysis can be performed. In short, PCR primers are designed to specifically amplify both the wild-type allele and the allele carrying the large rearrangement, based on prior knowledge of the specific DNA breakpoints. One multiplex PCR reaction, including primer pairs for both the wild-type and deleterious alleles, is performed and the resulting PCR products analyzed and separated by size on a capillary electrophoresis instrument. Visual inspection of resulting chromatograms (Fig. 10.6) readily identifies both wild-type and deleterious alleles. Bins representing the expected

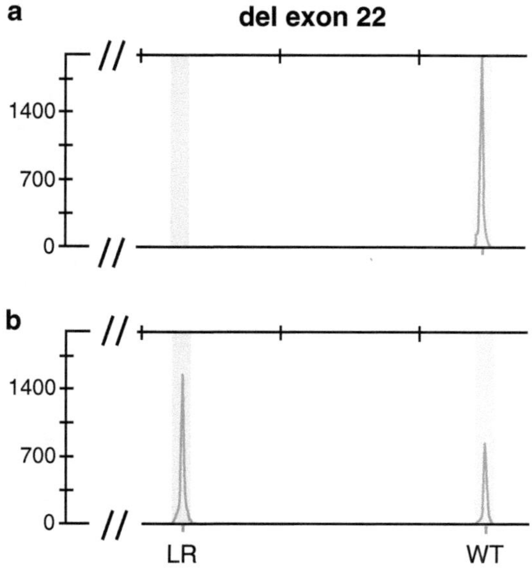

Fig. 10.6 Illustration of recombination-specific PCR analysis chromatograms. The *shaded bins* (LR) indicate the expected locations of peaks resulting from the presence of a large rearrangement. Wild-type peaks (WT) are expected to be observed in all individuals, as HBOC is an autosomal dominant disease. Signal intensity is indicated on the *y*-axis. (**a**) Testing results from an individual with no large rearrangement detected. (**b**) Testing results from an individual with a 510 bp deletion of exon 22

sizes of the wild-type and deleterious alleles for each large rearrangement are defined. Mutation-negative individuals are expected to have peaks only within the wild-type bins. Individuals heterozygous for a large rearrangement have peaks within both the wild-type bin and the bin corresponding to the specific large rearrangement.

In cases where the exact nature of the large rearrangement is unknown, analysis of the entire *BRCA1* and *BRCA2* coding regions is required. Multiple methodologies, including but not limited to Multiplex Ligation-dependent Probe Amplification (MLPA) [82] and quantitative PCR analysis, have been utilized. For example, during multiplexed quantitative PCR analysis, the *BRCA1* and *BRCA2* exon and promoter regions are PCR amplified using multiple fluorescently labeled primer pairs. Multiplex PCR products are analyzed on a capillary electrophoresis instrument and resulting signals for each amplicon are normalized and displayed on a scatter plot (Fig. 10.7) in order to detect copy number variation. Data points with values of approximately 1 indicate that a particular exon is present in the expected two copies (i.e., a normal result). Deletions are demonstrated on the scatter plot as one or more data points, corresponding to one or more exons, with values of approximately 0.5, indicating that only one copy is present. Duplications are shown as data points with values of approximately 1.5, demonstrating the presence of three exon copies.

While the interpretation of multi-exon deletions and duplications is relatively straightforward, caution must be used when analyzing large rearrangement data indicative of a single exon deletion. Large rearrangement analyses are often highly reliant upon the efficient annealing of PCR primers or other probes in order to yield an accurate result. Small sequence changes, such as a single nucleotide polymorphism (SNP) located at a PCR primer or probe annealing site, have the potential to result in decreased annealing, leading to a false-positive single exon deletion call even though both alleles are present within the genomic DNA sample. Due to this potential issue, sequencing analysis of all PCR primer and probe annealing sites is recommended in order to confirm that interfering SNPs are not present.

Regulatory Compliance

Clinical diagnostic testing is regulated by multiple agencies within the USA. On the national level, clinical laboratory testing, excluding research testing, is regulated by the Centers for Medicare & Medicaid Services (CMS) through the Clinical Laboratory Improvement Amendments (CLIA), and CLIA accreditation is required of clinical laboratories. This helps ensure that laboratory testing meets minimum standards for quality. Many clinical laboratories also participate in the College of American Pathologists (CAP) accreditation program, which is designed to improve laboratory standards of excellence above and beyond the minimal requirements established by CLIA. In addition to accreditation at the national level, licensure is

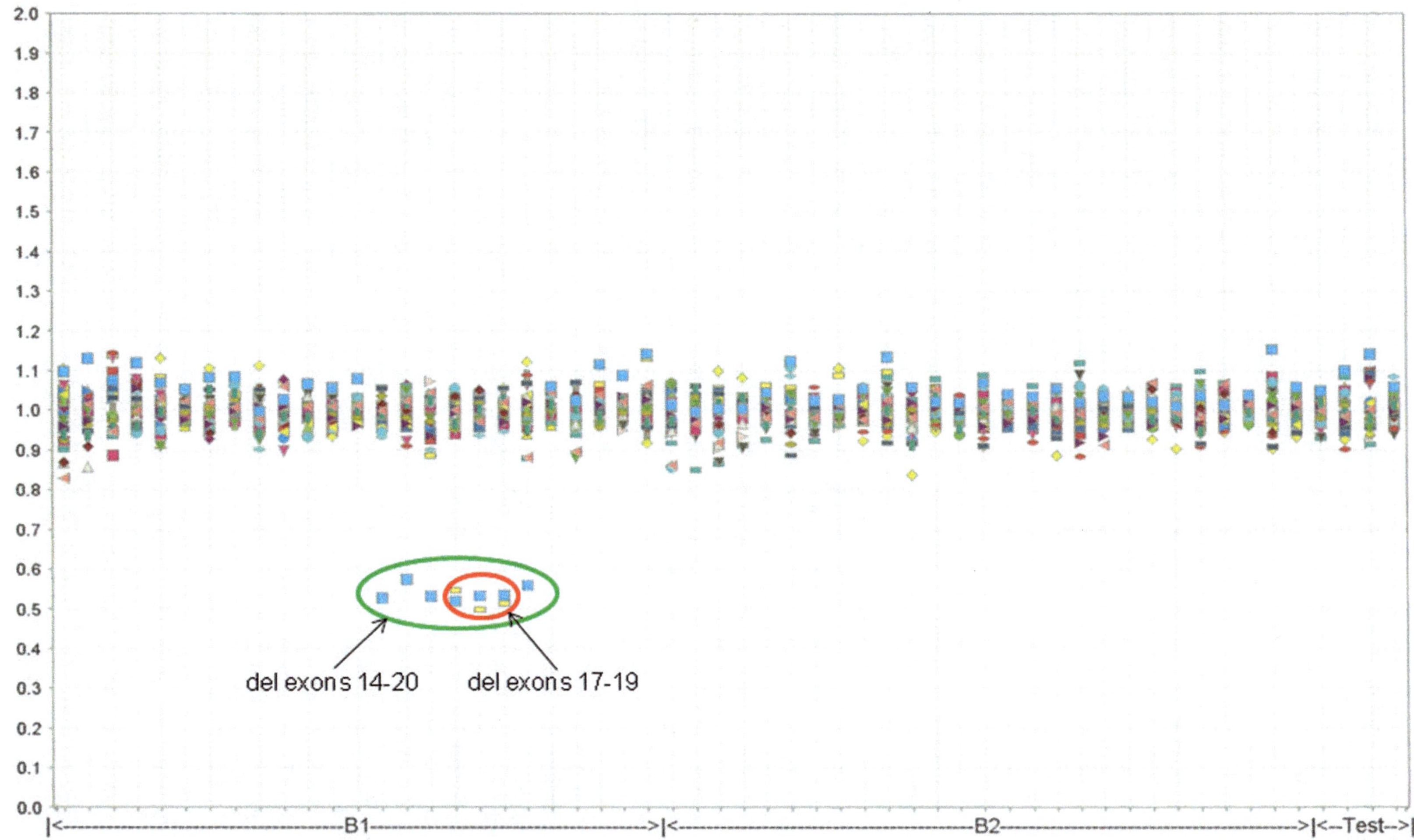

Fig. 10.7 A *BRCA1*/*BRCA2* multiplex quantitative PCR analysis data plot. The *BRCA1* (B1) and *BRCA2* (B2) genes are indicated on the *x*-axis, as well as three additional control genes shown in the "Test" region. Exons are ordered per gene 5′–3′. Normalized signal strength is shown on the *y*-axis. Signal intensities of ~1 indicate two copies of the exon are present, whereas values of ~0.5 or 1.5 indicate a deletion or duplication of one exon copy, respectively. A positive control sample (*light blue squares*) with a deletion of *BRCA1* exons 14–20 is *circled* in *green*. A patient sample (*yellow rectangles*) with a deletion of *BRCA1* exons 17–19 is *circled* in *red*

sometimes required by individual states in order to allow for laboratory operation within the state or to allow samples from within the state to be processed by a laboratory located outside of the state. The regulation of clinical diagnostic testing is constantly evolving to address changes in patient care expectations and available testing technologies.

CAP accreditation requires that laboratories meet high standards for laboratory quality to ensure that appropriate clinical management can be provided based on generated test results, and CAP regulations apply to all aspects of the clinical laboratory. Validation of all clinical laboratory tests is required, and test validation can be divided into three key components: (1) technical validation, (2) process validation, and (3) clinical validation. Through technical validation, the laboratory establishes that it can generate an accurate, reproducible result. A successful process validation shows that samples flow efficiently through all laboratory processes, as expected. Clinical validations are designed to demonstrate that the test offered has clinical utility, as specified by the laboratory.

Once a test is fully validated and made available to patients, continuous quality control is essential. Quality control requirements are extensive and encompass reagent and equipment qualification, instrument maintenance, and use of appropriate positive and negative assay controls. Documentation of all key quality control measures is essential to maintaining accreditation. Laboratory personnel are essential for maintaining quality, and all employees are required to meet minimal educational requirements specific to their duties. Employees must undergo initial training as well as yearly competency assessments, and they must participate in an established continuing education program.

CAP assesses quality through multiple mechanisms including laboratory inspections and proficiency testing. A biannual inspection performed by a team of practicing laboratory professionals chosen by CAP assesses adherence to CAP and CLIA regulations. Deficiencies identified during the inspection are documented and must be corrected within a specified time period in order to maintain accreditation. During years in which a CAP inspection does not occur, laboratories are required to perform and document self-inspection. Deficiencies identified during self-inspections must be corrected in a timely manner. Quality is also assessed through proficiency testing. At least twice per year, all accredited laboratories must perform proficiency testing for each laboratory test offered. Whenever possible, proficiency testing should be performed by obtaining samples through a proficiency testing program, such as that offered by CAP. Blinded samples with a known result are sent to the laboratory for testing. Samples are tested by the laboratory using its normal processes and results reported to the testing agency in order to determine accuracy. If samples are not available through an agency offering proficiency testing, samples can be obtained through either inter-laboratory exchange or by blinding of internal laboratory samples through a Quality Assurance department or third party, if necessary.

Interpretation

The clinical interpretation of *BRCA1* and *BRCA2* comprehensive genetic analysis test results can be highly complex and must take into account the personal and family history of the patient tested. Whenever possible, genetic testing should be targeted to a family member whose personal history is more suggestive of HBOC, i.e., a female family member affected with breast cancer before the age of 50 or ovarian cancer at any age, or a male family member with breast cancer at any age. However, in many cases, family members meeting these criteria are unavailable for testing, and testing must be performed for other family members

Interpretation of a Negative Comprehensive Test Result

Although families segregating a germline *BRCA1* or *BRCA2* mutation have a significantly increased incidence of breast and/or ovarian cancer in comparison with the general population, not all individuals with high-risk personal and family histories carry a deleterious mutation in one of these genes. Failure to identify a disease-causing *BRCA1/BRCA2* mutation in a high-risk affected individual may be due to either technical or genetic reasons. While comprehensive testing, including sequencing and large rearrangement analysis, identifies the vast majority of mutations in these genes, not all mutations are detectable. For example, only a small portion of each intron is sequenced; thus, mutations lying deep within an intron are not detectable. Promoter and enhancer mutations may also not be detectable by sequencing due to the limited region being analyzed, and while most large rearrangements can be identified through methods, such as multiplexed quantitative PCR analysis, it is possible that certain large rearrangements, such as gene inversions, are not captured. Therefore, there is a small chance that a disease-causing *BRCA1/BRCA2* mutation could go undetected. In addition, mutations in genes other than *BRCA1* and *BRCA2* are associated with increased risk of cancer; therefore, a negative comprehensive test result does not exclude the possibility of a familial mutation within another gene, and it must be viewed in light of an individual's personal and family history. Individuals with personal and family histories indicative of high cancer risk should be clinically managed as high-risk patients regardless of a negative test result. Studies indicate that high-risk probands testing negative for a *BRCA1/BRCA2* deleterious mutation still have a significantly increased risk of breast cancer [3, 83]. However, it is important to note that negatively testing probands do not appear to be at a significantly increased risk of ovarian cancer in comparison with the general population.

In cases where the patient tested is unaffected, the interpretation of a negative comprehensive test result is more complicated as the patient could test negative for either genetic or technical reasons (see above). Testing of an additional affected high-risk family member may help to clarify results in this case. Should a disease-associated mutation be identified in this family member, in most cases (excluding rare situations where more than one disease-associated mutation is present within the same family), the unaffected family member would be assumed to be a true negative for the familial mutation. If a disease-associated mutation is not identified in the affected family member, the test result is uninformative and all family members should be clinically managed based on personal and family history.

Interpretation of Site-Specific Test Results

Once a disease-associated mutation is identified in an individual, additional family members may be appropriate for testing. First- and second-degree relatives have a 50 % and 25 % chance of carrying the deleterious mutation, respectively. Individuals testing positive for a familial mutation are considered to have HBOC and its associated cancer risks. Thus, regardless of personal cancer history, these individuals should be clinically managed as high risk.

Unaffected individuals testing negative for the familial mutation are considered true negatives and are assumed to have cancer risks similar to the general population unless the individual's noncarrier parent has a strong personal and/or family history of cancer. In rare instances, an individual may have the potential to inherit both a deleterious *BRCA1* and *BRCA2* mutation. This is more common in individuals of Ashkenazi descent due to the high frequency of three founder mutations within this population. Individuals inheriting both a *BRCA1* and a *BRCA2* disease-associated mutation do not appear to have more severe cancers than those carrying one mutation alone. In most instances, individuals carrying two disease-associated mutations (one in *BRCA1* and one in *BRCA2*) inherit one mutation from each parent. However, it is possible to inherit both mutations from the same parent.

Affected family members testing negative for a familial mutation most likely represent phenocopies. Due to the high frequency of breast cancer within the female population, it is not uncommon for affected family members to test negative for a familial mutation. However, caution must be used, especially if the proband and family members are tested at different laboratories, that the testing methodology used is able to detect the familial mutation. Technical issues, such as the occurrence of a SNP lying within a PCR primer-binding site, may cause a false-negative result. Whenever possible, a DNA sample from a mutation-positive family member should be submitted along with the patient sample, if the familial mutation was identified by a different laboratory.

Clinical Interpretation of Genetic Variants

Genetic testing, including sequencing and large rearrangement analyses, identifies multiple types of variants which must be assigned a clinical interpretation. Based upon variant classification recommendations by the American College of Medical Genetics [84], a five-tier variant classification system is currently utilized within the USA for *BRCA1*/*BRCA2* analysis. While, these five tiers have been designated in different ways by various groups [77, 85], they are generally composed of the following five categories:

1. Deleterious Mutation (Pathogenic)
2. Suspected Deleterious Mutation (Likely Pathogenic)
3. Variant of Uncertain Clinical Significance (Uncertain)
4. Genetic Variant, Favor Polymorphism (Likely Not Pathogenic or of Little Clinical Significance)
5. Genetic Variant, Polymorphism (Not Pathogenic or of No Clinical Significance)

As always, any classification of any variant is dependent upon the scientific information available at the time of classification. Should new information become available, the classification of a variant can change.

"Deleterious" or "Suspected Deleterious" Mutations

Sequencing or large rearrangement mutations that have been demonstrated or are strongly predicted to result in HBOC are classified as either "Deleterious" or "Suspected Deleterious." Mutations classified as "Deleterious" typically are either of a variant type that is strongly predicted to result in abnormal protein production or function (i.e., large rearrangements, frameshifts, or protein-truncating mutations) or have multiple lines of evidence, such as segregation, functional, or statistical analyses, that demonstrate that they are associated with increased cancer risk. "Suspected Deleterious" mutations also have extremely strong evidence to indicate that they are associated with increased cancer risk. However, this evidence is weaker.

Deleterious mutations in *BRCA1* and *BRCA2* are associated with different cancer risks. In general, *BRCA1* mutations confer greater breast and ovarian cancer risks in comparison with *BRCA2* mutations, and mutations in both genes demonstrate age-related penetrance. Mutation risks conferred by a deleterious mutation are specific to the particular mutation; and at the present time, there are insufficient data to determine the exact penetrance/risk of most mutations. However, more generalized risk estimates have been determined for mutations in either gene (see above). Given these risks, the identification of a deleterious *BRCA1* or *BRCA2* mutation warrants increased clinical surveillance and/or preventative surgeries [70]. Clinical management of HBOC is patient specific and should be based upon personalized interaction between patient and healthcare provider.

As HBOC is an autosomal dominant syndrome, first-degree relatives (i.e., full-siblings, parents, and children) of individuals carrying a deleterious mutation have a 50 % chance of also carrying the mutation and its associated increased cancer risks. Therefore, genetic testing is recommended for these individuals. Once the familial mutation is identified, genetic testing for the specific familial mutation can be performed for additional family members at a significantly reduced cost. Given the high frequency of three founder mutations in the Ashkenazi population (i.e., 187delAG and 5385insC in *BRCA1* and 6174delT in *BRCA2*), it is recommended that individuals of Ashkenazi descent be tested for all three founder mutations in addition to a previously identified familial mutation. Due to psychological and privacy issues associated with genetic testing and given that *BRCA1/BRCA2* deleterious mutations very rarely result in pediatric cancers, testing of asymptomatic minors for a familial mutation is strongly discouraged. While preimplantation diagnosis for a deleterious mutation is available in some laboratories, most families do not actively pursue this testing.

Implications of Deleterious and Suspected Deleterious Mutations with Reduced Penetrance

Statistical analyses of deleterious and suspected deleterious mutations have identified a small percentage of mutations that confer a significantly increased risk of cancer in comparison with the general population but a lower risk in comparison with other *BRCA1* and *BRCA2* deleterious/suspected deleterious mutations [77]. These variants represent low penetrance alleles. It is believed that while these mutations disrupt normal protein production and/or function, some residual production/function remains. This residual protein production/function is predicted to be mutation-specific, and currently there is insufficient data to determine the exact cancer risks conferred by these mutations. Statistical variant classification techniques currently utilized may not be sufficiently sensitive to identify alleles that confer a very low level of risk due to lack of data required for analysis of each specific variant. As low penetrance alleles do not convey the same level of risk as other deleterious mutations, standard HBOC clinical management recommendations may not apply for these mutations; therefore, clinical management should be strongly based on the patient's personal and family history.

Variants Classified as "Polymorphisms" or "Favor Polymorphisms"

Person-to-person genetic variation is expected, and most genetic differences between individuals are not associated with disease. Sequencing analysis frequently identifies small DNA changes in the *BRCA1* and *BRCA2* genes that are not associated with increased cancer risk. Variants classified as "Polymorphisms" typically are either of a variant type that is strongly predicted not to affect protein production or function (i.e., silent variants that most likely do not affect splicing) or have multiple lines of evidence, such as segregation, functional, or statistical analyses, that demonstrate that they are benign. Interestingly, while variants predicted to result in premature protein truncation are usually assumed to be deleterious, some *BRCA2* variants resulting in premature protein truncation have been shown to represent benign polymorphisms. *BRCA2*-truncating variants located near the 3′ terminus of the gene have been shown not to be associated with a significantly increased risk of cancer [86], indicating that the C terminus of the protein is not necessary for normal protein function. There is currently insufficient data to determine if the *BRCA1* C terminus is necessary for proper function.

Variants classified as "Favor Polymorphisms" also have strong evidence to indicate they are benign. However, this evidence is weaker than that used to classify polymorphisms. As variants classified as Polymorphisms or Favor Polymorphisms are expected to be benign, clinical management of an individual identified with one or more of these variants should be based on personal and family clinical history and not on the presence of the variant itself. In most cases, testing of additional family members is not warranted or recommended. However, limited family testing is sometimes offered for "Favor Polymorphisms" that are still being investigated in hopes of obtaining an eventual reclassification. This type of testing is for reclassification purposes only, and it should not be used to guide clinical management.

Variants of Uncertain Clinical Significance

A "Variant of Uncertain Clinical Significance (VUS)" is currently identified in approximately 3 % of patients undergoing genetic analysis for HBOC [77]. This variant category is mainly comprised of missense variants, small in-frame deletions or insertions, and intronic variants with unknown splicing effects, although other variant types are included within this classification category. VUSs have insufficient data to determine if they affect protein production or function; therefore, it is not known if they have the potential to convey an increased risk of HBOC. In the absence of a deleterious or suspected deleterious mutation, clinical management of an individual identified with a VUS should be based upon personal and family history and not the presence of the VUS. Genetic testing of additional family members for the purpose of guiding clinical management is inappropriate and strongly discouraged. However, testing of select family members may aid in the eventual reclassification of a variant to a more definitive classification category (see below). Therefore, genetic testing is frequently offered to key family members who may be informative for reclassification purposes only.

Approaches to Variant Reclassification

The value of *BRCA1* and *BRCA2* genetic testing lies in the ability of the test to produce a clinically actionable test result. While the initial classification of a variant as a VUS may be unavoidable, great strides are taken with the ultimate goal of providing a definitive classification and clinical interpretation for each variant observed. To this end, multiple variant reclassification techniques can be utilized. While variations of some of these techniques have been utilized by geneticists for many years, others have only become feasible within recent years due to the large data set required for their development and use. It is expected that as technology continues to advance and more data becomes available, new reclassification techniques will be developed and improvements made to existing techniques.

Structural and Functional Analyses

One method of determining the clinical effect of a variant is to examine its effect on protein structure and function. However, this is complicated for *BRCA1* and *BRCA2* variants as the functional roles of BRCA1 and BRCA2 have not been fully elucidated. BRCA1 has been shown to perform multiple functions necessary for transcriptional regulation, DNA repair through DNA damage-induced nuclear signaling, and the maintenance of cell-cycle control and centrosome number [87–92]. Multiple assays have been designed to assess the effects of *BRCA1* missense variants on normal protein function. These assays include, but are not limited to, those designed to measure variant effects on centrosome number control [89], homologous recombination [93], transcription, protein folding, and phosphopeptide binding [94].

BRCA2 is necessary for homologous recombination-dependent DNA repair and centrosome number control. As with BRCA1, multiple assays have been developed to determine variant effects on normal BRCA2 protein function. These techniques include homologous recombination and centrosome amplification assays [95]. In addition, analysis of the BRCA2 crystal structure can sometimes be utilized to determine the effect that a variant may have on BRCA2 function.

While these BRCA1 and BRCA2 functional assays have proven useful in a research setting, they are currently not utilized for missense variant reclassification in the absence of other supportive data as they have been tested on a limited number of variants. Analysis of a large number of variants of known clinical classification would be required to assess and be confident in their clinical utility as their current error rate is unknown. In addition, due to the complexity and labor-intensive nature of these assays, they are currently not practical in a large-scale diagnostic setting, and there is much that is still not known about the functional roles of BRCA1 and BRCA2. Therefore, it is not certain that these assays provide accurate measures of all BRCA1 and BRCA2 protein functions in all cell types. Despite these limitations, functional analyses can often be used as supportive evidence for reclassification when additional data from other reclassification methodologies is available.

While current protein function assays are of limited value for variant reclassification, biochemical analyses of potential mRNA splicing variants can be invaluable, but they must be viewed conservatively. Analysis of patient mRNA or a minigene assay demonstrating a particular variant results in abnormal mRNA splicing provides strong evidence that the variant is deleterious. However, caution must be used in interpreting the data. It is important that the assay show that the variant allele produces only abnormal mRNA transcripts. If the variant allele produces some level of normally spliced transcript, one cannot exclude the possibility that the allele may represent a polymorphism of limited clinical significance or a low penetrance allele. At the present time, there is insufficient information to determine the level of normal *BRCA1* or *BRCA2* mRNA expression or BRCA1 and BRCA2 protein production required for normal cellular function. Splicing variants that result in the production of an abnormal transcript that maintains a normal translation reading frame must also be interpreted with caution as these transcripts have the potential to produce a functional protein, albeit of abnormal length.

Segregation Analysis

Segregation analysis, which measures whether or not a variant segregates with cancer in one or more families, represents the gold standard for determining whether or not a genetic variant is associated with disease. It has traditionally relied upon obtaining one or more large pedigrees with multiple affected family members available for analysis. However, as families for *BRCA1*/*BRCA2* genetic testing are ascertained due to high incidence of breast and/or ovarian cancers which can be fatal, often times there are insufficient numbers of affected family members available for testing. In addition, due to age related penetrance, young unaffected family members are not particularly informative. Due to these limitations, modifications that allow for analysis of multiple small families must be made to the traditional segregation analysis approach. Thus, active participation of multiple families carrying the same variant is required before a variant can be reclassified.

In rare instances, a single family may be ascertained that is of sufficient size to theoretically allow for reclassification of a variant in the absence of additional data from other families carrying the same variant. However, these data must be used with extreme caution. While statistical evidence from one family may indicate that a particular variant segregates with cancer and is therefore deleterious, one cannot definitively exclude the possibility that the variant is benign but lies *in cis* (i.e., on the same allele) with a deleterious mutation that is not detectable by the current assay.

Conservation Analysis

Evaluation of species conservation can provide data that are useful for variant reclassification. The premise behind this type of analysis is that if a particular amino acid is important for protein function, it will be conserved within numerous species. Functionally significant amino acids are predicted to be highly conserved and are either identified in multiple species, or if replaced, are substituted by an amino acid with similar biochemical properties. In contrast, functionally insignificant amino acids are often replaced with biochemically dissimilar amino acids in other species or may be absent altogether. Multiple computational algorithms have been designed to evaluate the evolutionary/functional significance of an amino acid change through analysis of multiple species protein alignments. Two of the most common programs currently utilized are SIFT and PolyPhen-2 [96–98]. While these programs are often used in a research setting, their estimated error rates are too high to be used for standalone variant classification in a clinical setting.

Identification of Homozygous or Compound Heterozygous Individuals

Absence of *Brca1* expression in mice has been demonstrated to be embryonically lethal [99–103], and it is believed that normal *BRCA1* expression is also required for human embryonic development. While *BRCA1* mutations are relatively rare within most ethnic groups, two Ashkenazi founder mutations, 187delAG and 5385insC, occur with a relatively high frequency (1:40) within this ethnic group. Given the high frequency of these mutations, one would expect to identify Ashkenazi individuals who are homozygous or compound heterozygous for these two founder mutations. However, to date, homozygous or compound heterozygous individuals have not been observed, suggesting that homozygosity or compound heterozygosity for highly penetrant *BRCA1* deleterious mutations is most likely embryonically lethal [18, 104]. Similarly, homozygosity or compound heterozygosity for deleterious *BRCA2* mutations is most likely either embryonically lethal or results in childhood Fanconi anemia (FANC D1), which is an autosomal recessive disease resulting in developmental abnormalities, bone marrow failure, and early-onset leukemia or solid tumors [19, 20].

Given the severe phenotypes associated with homozygosity for a *BRCA1* or *BRCA2* deleterious mutation, observation of a homozygous variant in a healthy individual or an individual with later onset cancer provides significant evidence that the variant itself does not represent a deleterious mutation. Caution must be used in determining that a variant is truly homozygous. It is necessary to rule-out other possibilities, such as allelic drop-out during PCR amplification and sequencing. In addition, a hemizygous variant may appear to be homozygous due to a large genomic deletion on the allele opposite the variant. This would represent an *in trans* observation of the variant with a deleterious mutation (i.e., compound heterozygosity), which also provides strong evidence that the variant is benign and not associated with increased cancer risk. The phase (i.e., *in cis* or *in trans*) of a variant and a deleterious mutation can be determined using multiple methodologies. However, the gold standard for determining phase is family analysis. For example, if an individual is found to carry two variants and family analysis identifies one parent with each variant, then the variants lie *in trans*. If one parent carries both variants, then they lie *in cis*. Due to limited availability of family members, family analysis for determining phase is not always possible and other more complex methodologies for determining phase must be utilized.

Caution must be used when reclassifying a variant based upon a homozygous or compound heterozygous observation. The use of this reclassification technique assumes that deleterious mutations are highly penetrant. While most *BRCA1* and *BRCA2* deleterious mutations associated with significantly increased cancer risk are assumed to result in a nonfunctional or severely impaired protein, one cannot exclude the possibility that a *BRCA1* or *BRCA2* low penetrance deleterious mutation may retain partial functionality. Should this occur, homozygosity or compound heterozygosity with a second deleterious mutation may not necessarily result in embryonic lethality or Fanconi anemia (*BRCA2* only).

Mutation Co-occurrence and Phenotype Analyses

BRCA1 and *BRCA2* deleterious mutations are uncommon within the general population, excluding individuals of Ashkenazi descent, and it is very rare to identify a non-Ashkenazi individual carrying two deleterious mutations either within the same gene or one in each gene. The identification of multiple individuals carrying a particular variant in addition to a deleterious mutation provides supporting statistical evidence that the variant itself is not deleterious [105, 106]. Mutation Co-occurrence analysis analyzes the frequency at which a variant co-occurs with a deleterious mutation within the same individual in order to determine whether or not the variant may be deleterious.

Phenotype analysis is based upon a very simple premise. If a variant is deleterious, it should be identified more often in probands with strong personal and family histories of cancer. If a variant is not associated with increased risk of cancer, it should be identified more often in probands with less severe personal and family histories of cancer relative to other individuals who pursue genetic testing. Using statistical analysis based upon empirical data, phenotype data gathered from multiple probands carrying the same variant can be used to determine whether a variant represents a deleterious mutation or a benign polymorphism [107, 108].

How Genetic Testing for *BRCA1* and *BRCA2* Has Changed Medical Practice

Prior to the introduction of clinical genetic testing for mutations in *BRCA1* and *BRCA2*, the medical management of patients at risk for HBOC was surrounded by uncertainty. A young woman with a strong family history of breast and ovarian cancer had no way of knowing for sure if she shared the high risk apparently present in the family. Women being treated for early-onset breast cancer in one breast had limited knowledge to guide them about their risk for a subsequent breast cancer in either breast or ovarian cancer. The lack of a clear explanation for a pattern of cancers in the family not only posed medical management dilemmas, but exacted an emotional toll as well.

The identification of a *BRCA1* or *BRCA2* mutation in a patient provides guidance not only for their own future care but also permits relatives to utilize testing to determine, with a very high degree of certainty, their own level of risk. Thus, high risk medical management can be effectively targeted only to those family members who will benefit. While some uncertainty remains for women from families in which there is no detectable mutation in *BRCA1* or *BRCA2*, a negative result from analysis of these genes rules out the most common cause of a greatly increased risk for both breast and ovarian cancer.

Attitudes towards the integration of genetic testing into mainstream medical care have changed dramatically in the past 15 years, and the widespread utilization of *BRCA1* and *BRCA2* testing has been a key driver of increased awareness and acceptance among both healthcare providers and the public. *BRCA1* and *BRCA2* were the first genes for a common adult-onset disorder for which clinical testing was made available, and at the time, there was considerable debate about the wisdom of offering such a test in the absence of any proven interventions to prevent the adverse outcomes associated with having a mutation. There were concerns that the identification of a mutation would create enormous anxiety in patients, disrupt family dynamics, and lead to insurance, employment, and even social discrimination. The model originally proposed for the provision of *BRCA1* and *BRCA2* testing was based on what had been put in place for Huntington's Disease (HD), a severe genetic neurodegenerative condition for which there was, and still is, no effective prevention or treatment. Genetic testing for HD first became available in 1993, using a protocol that required multiple patient visits with a multidisciplinary team of healthcare providers, including neurologists, genetic counselors/medical geneticists, and mental health professionals. The focus of this process was not to provide the patient with a recommendation about testing, but to guide the patient to their own carefully considered decision, and assist them with the medical/psychosocial outcomes of that decision.

Over time, the protocols for providing *BRCA1* and *BRCA2* testing have diverged considerably from this original model. This is due in large part to the accumulated evidence that, in contrast to HD, there are highly effective medical management options available to mutation carriers. This supports a more "directive" approach on the part of healthcare providers, which may result in a clear recommendation to proceed with testing. The potential utility of the testing for guiding immediate treatment decisions, as discussed above, creates a need for streamlining the testing process. Also, since the testing has significant clinical utility, it is questionable whether or not concerns about the potential for emotional distress and discrimination should factor heavily into the decision-making process. While these issues should certainly be part of the informed consent process, the same can probably be said for any medical procedure. This evolution in the testing protocol for *BRCA1* and *BRCA2* has set a significant precedent for future genetic testing in cases where the results will guide effective medical management interventions.

Outside of testing performed in the prenatal setting, *BRCA1* and *BRCA2* analysis is probably the most familiar and frequently utilized genetic test in the USA. Over 600,000 individuals have been tested with either comprehensive analyses, targeted analysis for the Ashkenazi Jewish founder mutations or single-site testing for known family mutations.

Future Directions

The paradigm for genetic testing across all areas of medicine, including testing for hereditary cancer risk, is likely to change dramatically in coming years. A key driver of this change will be the ongoing development and validation of new technologies that greatly reduce the cost of analyzing genetic variation, the most prominent current example being next generation sequencing platforms that have already made it feasible to sequence entire exomes and even genomes. However, while the costs associated with acquiring sequence data are anticipated to drop significantly, the challenges associated with efficient and accurate data interpretation remain, and they pose an obstacle to the application of whole exome or genome sequencing in the clinical setting.

In the past, genetic tests such as *BRCA1* and *BRCA2* analysis have been selectively triaged to patients based on an assessment of their personal and family history. Earlier, we pointed out that although *BRCA1* and *BRCA2* are unquestionably the most important genes for both hereditary breast and hereditary ovarian cancer, there are many other genes that are also capable of modulating risk for these cancers. Mutations in some of these genes result in distinctive patterns of malignancy, i.e., testing for mutations in the gene *CDH1* may be a better choice than *BRCA1* and *BRCA2* for a family with a combination of diffuse gastric cancer and breast cancer, or testing for mutations in the four Lynch syndrome genes may be the best first option for a patient with ovarian cancer if her personal or family history includes early-onset colon and endometrial cancers. Due to current cost constraints, providers currently choose genetic tests targeting the gene or a limited panel of genes that fits best with the pattern of disease in a patient and his/her family. This is an imperfect exercise, as it is difficult to obtain an accurate family history for most patients, there is considerable overlap between the patterns of malignancy associated with different genes and our understanding of exactly which cancers are associated with which genes comes from studies that are often subject to ascertainment bias and may be too small to be definitive.

Technologies that dramatically reduce the cost of genetic analysis make it possible to simply test patients for variation in all of the genes that could possibly be relevant to the clinical issue at hand, be it a patient with early-onset breast cancer or a family history of ovarian and pancreatic cancer. A limited number of such multigene panels targeted to specific conditions are already clinically available (i.e., for X-linked mental retardation and muscular dystrophy) [109, 110], and many others are in development. The feasibility of a 40-gene panel for hereditary breast and hereditary ovarian cancer, including *BRCA1* and *BRCA2*, has been already demonstrated in the research setting [111], and panels are now available in the diagnostic setting. Some have suggested that whole genome sequencing is a viable alternative to the development of targeted multigene panels, and pilot projects are already underway to investigate this option.

These developments pose both tremendous opportunities and challenges for patients, healthcare providers, and clinical laboratories. More data, for more genes, will provide an opportunity to investigate gene–gene interactions, which could explain much of the variation in the clinical presentation of patients and families with mutations in genes like *BRCA1* and *BRCA2*. A higher percentage of patients tested will have at least some sort of informative result and our understanding of the natural history associated with mutations in different genes will improve. However, none of this will come to fruition without the development of mechanisms to collect, store, analyze, and annotate massive amounts of genetic and clinical information. It seems inevitable that the overall interpretation of the data from this testing will require constant re-evaluation, as variants of uncertain significance will be abundant in all patients undergoing testing for large numbers of genes, or entire genomes, and even the overall interpretation of clearly deleterious mutations will be subject to modification as we learn more about modifier effects of variants in other genes.

Some additional areas of excitement for the future of clinical *BRCA1* and *BRCA2* genetic testing include: (1) hope that current clinical trials will demonstrate the effectiveness of targeted therapy (e.g., the platinum-based and PARP inhibitor chemotherapies) for the treatment of cancer in mutation carriers, as well as the possible future development of additional agents informed by an improved understanding of the molecular biology of these genes, (2) the development of more reliable strategies for the early detection of cancer, particularly ovarian cancer, (3) alternatives to surgical removal of the breasts and ovaries for cancer prevention, through chemoprevention and/or lifestyle modification, and (4) further education of providers and the public so that *BRCA1* and *BRCA2* testing is utilized appropriately and fully integrated into medical practice.

References

1. International Agency for Research on Cancer. World cancer report. 2008. http://www.iarc.fr/en/publications/pdfs-online/wcr/. Accessed 30 Aug 2011.
2. American Cancer Society. Cancer facts & figures 2011. 2011. http://www.cancer.org/Research/CancerFactsFigures/CancerFactsFigures/cancer-facts-figures-2011. Accessed 30 Aug 2011.
3. Metcalfe KA, Finch A, Poll A, et al. Breast cancer risks in women with a family history of breast or ovarian cancer who have tested negative for a BRCA1 or BRCA2 mutation. Br J Cancer. 2009; 100:421–5.
4. Miki Y, Swensen J, Shattuck-Eidens D, et al. A strong candidate for the breast and ovarian cancer susceptibility gene BRCA1. Science. 1994;266:66–71.
5. Wooster R, Bignell G, Lancaster J, et al. Identification of the breast cancer susceptibility gene BRCA2. Nature. 1995;378:789–92.
6. Claus EB, Schildkraut JM, Thompson WD, Risch NJ. The genetic attributable risk of breast and ovarian cancer. Cancer. 1996;77:2318–24.
7. Petrucelli N, Daly MB, Feldman GL. GeneReviews: BRCA1 and BRCA2 hereditary breast and ovarian cancer. 2011. http://www.ncbi.nlm.nih.gov/books/NBK1247/. Accessed 30 Aug 2011.
8. Wong MW, Nordfors C, Mossman D, et al. BRIP1, PALB2, and RAD51C mutation analysis reveals their relative importance as genetic susceptibility factors for breast cancer. Breast Cancer Res Treat. 2011;127:853–9.
9. Watson P, Vasen HF, Mecklin JP, et al. The risk of extra-colonic, extra-endometrial cancer in the Lynch syndrome. Int J Cancer. 2008;123:444–9.
10. Antoniou AC, Gayther SA, Stratton JF, Ponder BA, Easton DF. Risk models for familial ovarian and breast cancer. Genet Epidemiol. 2000;18:173–90.
11. Group ABCS. Prevalence and penetrance of BRCA1 and BRCA2 mutations in a population-based series of breast cancer cases. Br J Cancer. 2000;83:1301–8.
12. Kurian AW. BRCA1 and BRCA2 mutations across race and ethnicity: distribution and clinical implications. Curr Opin Obstet Gynecol. 2010;22:72–8.
13. Struewing JP, Hartge P, Wacholder S, et al. The risk of cancer associated with specific mutations of BRCA1 and BRCA2 among Ashkenazi Jews. N Engl J Med. 1997;336:1401–8.
14. Pellegrini L, Venkitaraman A. Emerging functions of BRCA2 in DNA recombination. Trends Biochem Sci. 2004;29:310–6.
15. Shuen AY, Foulkes WD. Inherited mutations in breast cancer genes–risk and response. J Mammary Gland Biol Neoplasia. 2011;16:3–15.
16. Wu J, Lu LY, Yu X. The role of BRCA1 in DNA damage response. Protein Cell. 2010;1:117–23.
17. Knudson Jr AG. Mutation and cancer: statistical study of retinoblastoma. Proc Natl Acad Sci USA. 1971;68:820–3.
18. Abkevich V, Zharkikh A, Deffenbaugh AM, et al. Analysis of missense variation in human BRCA1 in the context of interspecific sequence variation. J Med Genet. 2004;41:492–507.
19. Hirsch B, Shimamura A, Moreau L, et al. Association of biallelic BRCA2/FANCD1 mutations with spontaneous chromosomal instability and solid tumors of childhood. Blood. 2004;103:2554–9.
20. Wagner JE, Tolar J, Levran O, et al. Germline mutations in BRCA2: shared genetic susceptibility to breast cancer, early onset leukemia, and Fanconi anemia. Blood. 2004;103:3226–9.
21. Atchley DP, Albarracin CT, Lopez A, et al. Clinical and pathologic characteristics of patients with BRCA-positive and BRCA-negative breast cancer. J Clin Oncol. 2008;26:4282–8.
22. Rakha EA, Reis-Filho JS, Ellis IO. Basal-like breast cancer: a critical review. J Clin Oncol. 2008;26: 2568–81.
23. Turner NC, Reis-Filho JS. Basal-like breast cancer and the BRCA1 phenotype. Oncogene. 2006;25:5846–53.
24. National Comprehensive Cancer Network. Practice guidelines in oncology-V.1. 2011. http://www.nccn.org. Accessed 30 Aug 2011.
25. Nathanson KL, Domchek SM. Therapeutic approaches for women predisposed to breast cancer. Annu Rev Med. 2011;62:295–306.

26. Antoniou A, Pharoah PD, Narod S, et al. Average risks of breast and ovarian cancer associated with BRCA1 or BRCA2 mutations detected in case Series unselected for family history: a combined analysis of 22 studies. Am J Hum Genet. 2003;72:1117–30.
27. Begg CB, Haile RW, Borg A, et al. Variation of breast cancer risk among BRCA1/2 carriers. JAMA. 2008;299:194–201.
28. Chen S, Parmigiani G. Meta-analysis of BRCA1 and BRCA2 penetrance. J Clin Oncol. 2007;25:1329–33.
29. Ford D, Easton DF, Bishop DT, Narod SA, Goldgar DE. Risks of cancer in BRCA1-mutation carriers. Breast Cancer Linkage Consortium. Lancet. 1994; 343:692–5.
30. King MC, Marks JH, Mandell JB. Breast and ovarian cancer risks due to inherited mutations in BRCA1 and BRCA2. Science. 2003;302:643–6.
31. Risch HA, McLaughlin JR, Cole DE, et al. Population BRCA1 and BRCA2 mutation frequencies and cancer penetrances: a kin-cohort study in Ontario, Canada. J Natl Cancer Inst. 2006;98: 1694–706.
32. Ford D, Easton DF, Stratton M, et al. Genetic heterogeneity and penetrance analysis of the BRCA1 and BRCA2 genes in breast cancer families. The Breast Cancer Linkage Consortium. Am J Hum Genet. 1998;62:676–89.
33. Whittemore AS, Gong G, Itnyre J. Prevalence and contribution of BRCA1 mutations in breast cancer and ovarian cancer: results from three U.S. population-based case–control studies of ovarian cancer. Am J Hum Genet. 1997;60:496–504.
34. Casey MJ, Synder C, Bewtra C, Narod SA, Watson P, Lynch HT. Intra-abdominal carcinomatosis after prophylactic oophorectomy in women of hereditary breast ovarian cancer syndrome kindreds associated with BRCA1 and BRCA2 mutations. Gynecol Oncol. 2005;97:457–67.
35. Finch A, Beiner M, Lubinski J, et al. Salpingo-oophorectomy and the risk of ovarian, fallopian tube, and peritoneal cancers in women with a BRCA1 or BRCA2 Mutation. JAMA. 2006;296: 185–92.
36. Medeiros F, Muto MG, Lee Y, et al. The tubal fimbria is a preferred site for early adenocarcinoma in women with familial ovarian cancer syndrome. Am J Surg Pathol. 2006;30:230–6.
37. Consortium TBCL. Cancer risks in BRCA2 mutation carriers. J Natl Cancer Inst. 1999;91:1310–6.
38. Metcalfe K, Lynch HT, Ghadirian P, et al. Contralateral breast cancer in BRCA1 and BRCA2 mutation carriers. J Clin Oncol. 2004;22:2328–35.
39. Graeser MK, Engel C, Rhiem K, et al. Contralateral breast cancer risk in BRCA1 and BRCA2 mutation carriers. J Clin Oncol. 2009;27:5887–92.
40. Malone KE, Begg CB, Haile RW, et al. Population-based study of the risk of second primary contralateral breast cancer associated with carrying a mutation in BRCA1 or BRCA2. J Clin Oncol. 2010; 28:2404–10.
41. van Asperen CJ, Brohet RM, Meijers-Heijboer EJ, et al. Cancer risks in BRCA2 families: estimates for sites other than breast and ovary. J Med Genet. 2005;42:711–9.
42. Klein AP, Brune KA, Petersen GM, et al. Prospective risk of pancreatic cancer in familial pancreatic cancer kindreds. Cancer Res. 2004;64:2634–8.
43. Thompson D, Easton DF. Cancer Incidence in BRCA1 mutation carriers. J Natl Cancer Inst. 2002;94:1358–65.
44. Liede A, Karlan BY, Narod SA. Cancer risks for male carriers of germline mutations in BRCA1 or BRCA2: a review of the literature. J Clin Oncol. 2004;22:735–42.
45. Myriad Genetic Laboratories, Inc. Professional practice guidelines. 2011. http://www.myriadpro.com/guidelines. Accessed 30 Aug 2011.
46. Hartmann LC, Sellers TA, Schaid DJ, et al. Efficacy of bilateral prophylactic mastectomy in BRCA1 and BRCA2 gene mutation carriers. J Natl Cancer Inst. 2001;93:1633–7.
47. Heemskerk-Gerritsen BA, Brekelmans CT, Menke-Pluymers MB, et al. Prophylactic mastectomy in BRCA1/2 mutation carriers and women at risk of hereditary breast cancer: long-term experiences at the Rotterdam Family Cancer Clinic. Ann Surg Oncol. 2007;14:3335–44.
48. Kauff ND, Domchek SM, Friebel TM, et al. Risk-reducing salpingo-oophorectomy for the prevention of BRCA1- and BRCA2-associated breast and gynecologic cancer: a multicenter, prospective study. J Clin Oncol. 2008;26:1331–7.
49. Kauff ND, Satagopan JM, Robson ME, et al. Risk-reducing salpingo-oophorectomy in women with a BRCA1 or BRCA2 mutation. N Engl J Med. 2002;346:1609–15.
50. Rebbeck TR, Friebel T, Wagner T, et al. Effect of short-term hormone replacement therapy on breast cancer risk reduction after bilateral prophylactic oophorectomy in BRCA1 and BRCA2 mutation carriers: the PROSE Study Group. J Clin Oncol. 2005;23:7804–10.
51. Rebbeck TR, Kauff ND, Domchek SM. Meta-analysis of risk reduction estimates associated with risk-reducing salpingo-oophorectomy in BRCA1 or BRCA2 mutation carriers. J Natl Cancer Inst. 2009; 101:80–7.
52. Rebbeck TR, Lynch HT, Neuhausen SL, et al. Prophylactic oophorectomy in carriers of BRCA1 or BRCA2 mutations. N Engl J Med. 2002;346: 1616–22.
53. van Sprundel TC, Schmidt MK, Rookus MA, et al. Risk reduction of contralateral breast cancer and survival after contralateral prophylactic mastectomy in BRCA1 or BRCA2 mutation carriers. Br J Cancer. 2005;93:287–92.
54. King MC, Wieand S, Hale K, et al. Tamoxifen and breast cancer incidence among women with inherited mutations in BRCA1 and BRCA2: National Surgical Adjuvant Breast and Bowel Project

(NSABP-P1) Breast Cancer Prevention Trial. JAMA. 2001;286:2251–6.
55. Robson M. Tamoxifen for primary breast cancer prevention in BRCA heterozygotes. Eur J Cancer. 2002;38 Suppl 6:S18–9.
56. Beral V, Doll R, Hermon C, Peto R, Reeves G. Ovarian cancer and oral contraceptives: collaborative reanalysis of data from 45 epidemiological studies including 23,257 women with ovarian cancer and 87,303 controls. Lancet. 2008;371:303–14.
57. McLaughlin JR, Risch HA, Lubinski J, et al. Reproductive risk factors for ovarian cancer in carriers of BRCA1 or BRCA2 mutations: a case–control study. Lancet Oncol. 2007;8:26–34.
58. Saslow D, Boetes C, Burke W, et al. American Cancer Society guidelines for breast screening with MRI as an adjunct to mammography. CA Cancer J Clin. 2007;57:75–89.
59. Warner E, Plewes DB, Hill KA, et al. Surveillance of BRCA1 and BRCA2 mutation carriers with magnetic resonance imaging, ultrasound, mammography, and clinical breast examination. JAMA. 2004; 292:1317–25.
60. Julian-Reynier C, Mancini J, Mouret-Fourme E, et al. Cancer risk management strategies and perceptions of unaffected women 5 years after predictive genetic testing for BRCA1/2 mutations. Eur J Hum Genet. 2011;19:500–6.
61. Metcalfe KA, Birenbaum-Carmeli D, Lubinski J, et al. International variation in rates of uptake of preventive options in BRCA1 and BRCA2 mutation carriers. Int J Cancer. 2008;122:2017–22.
62. Schwartz MD, Isaacs C, Graves KD, et al. Long-term outcomes of BRCA1/BRCA2 testing: risk reduction and surveillance. Cancer. 2012;118(2): 510–7.
63. National Cancer Institute. Breast cancer prevention (PDQ). 2011. http://www.cancer.gov/cancertopics/pdq/prevention/breast/HealthProfessional/page2. Accessed 30 Aug 2011.
64. Bissonauth V, Shatenstein B, Fafard E, et al. Weight history, smoking, physical activity and breast cancer risk among French-Canadian women non-carriers of more frequent BRCA1/2 mutations. J Cancer Epidemiol. 2009;2009:748367.
65. Lecarpentier J, Nogues C, Mouret-Fourme E, et al. Variation in breast cancer risk with mutation position, smoking, alcohol, and chest X-ray history, in the French National BRCA1/2 carrier cohort (GENEPSO). Breast Cancer Res Treat. 2011;130(3): 927–38.
66. Pijpe A, Manders P, Brohet RM, et al. Physical activity and the risk of breast cancer in BRCA1/2 mutation carriers. Breast Cancer Res Treat. 2010;120: 235–44.
67. Schwartz MD, Lerman C, Brogan B, et al. Impact of BRCA1/BRCA2 counseling and testing on newly diagnosed breast cancer patients. J Clin Oncol. 2004;22:1823–9.
68. Schwartz MD, Lerman C, Brogan B, et al. Utilization of BRCA1/BRCA2 mutation testing in newly diagnosed breast cancer patients. Cancer Epidemiol Biomarkers Prev. 2005;14:1003–7.
69. Tai YC, Domchek S, Parmigiani G, Chen S. Breast cancer risk among male BRCA1 and BRCA2 mutation carriers. J Natl Cancer Inst. 2007;99:1811–4.
70. NCCN recommendations for BRCA1/2 mutation carriers. 2011. http://www.nccn.org/professionals/physician_gls/PDF/genetics_screening.pdf.
71. Canto MI. Screening and surveillance approaches in familial pancreatic cancer. Gastrointest Endosc Clin N Am. 2008;18:535–53; x.
72. Byrski T, Gronwald J, Huzarski T, et al. Pathologic complete response rates in young women with BRCA1-positive breast cancers after neoadjuvant chemotherapy. J Clin Oncol. 2010;28:375–9.
73. Byrski T, Huzarski T, Dent R, et al. Response to neoadjuvant therapy with cisplatin in BRCA1-positive breast cancer patients. Breast Cancer Res Treat. 2009;115:359–63.
74. Bryant HE, Schultz N, Thomas HD, et al. Specific killing of BRCA2-deficient tumours with inhibitors of poly(ADP-ribose) polymerase. Nature. 2005;434: 913–7.
75. Farmer H, McCabe N, Lord CJ, et al. Targeting the DNA repair defect in BRCA mutant cells as a therapeutic strategy. Nature. 2005;434:917–21.
76. Fong PC, Boss DS, Yap TA, et al. Inhibition of poly(ADP-ribose) polymerase in tumors from BRCA mutation carriers. N Engl J Med. 2009;361: 123–34.
77. Judkins T, Rosenthal E, Arnell C, et al. Clinical significance of large rearrangements in BRCA1 and BRCA2. Cancer. 2012;118:5210–6.
78. Saiki RK, Gelfand DH, Stoffel S, et al. Primer-directed enzymatic amplification of DNA with a thermostable DNA polymerase. Science. 1988;239:487–91.
79. Wilson RK, Chen C, Avdalovic N, Burns J, Hood L. Development of an automated procedure for fluorescent DNA sequencing. Genomics. 1990;6:626–34.
80. Brzovic PS, Meza J, King MC, Klevit RE. The cancer-predisposing mutation C61G disrupts homodimer formation in the NH2-terminal BRCA1 RING finger domain. J Biol Chem. 1998;273:7795–9.
81. Struewing JP, Abeliovich D, Peretz T, et al. The carrier frequency of the BRCA1 185delAG mutation is approximately 1 percent in Ashkenazi Jewish individuals. Nat Genet. 1995;11:198–200.
82. MRC-Holland. 2011. http://www.mlpa.com/WebForms/WebFormMain.aspx. Accessed 2 Nov 2011.
83. Kauff ND, Mitra N, Robson ME, et al. Risk of ovarian cancer in BRCA1 and BRCA2 mutation-negative hereditary breast cancer families. J Natl Cancer Inst. 2005;97:1382–4.
84. Richards CS, Bale S, Bellissimo DB, et al. ACMG recommendations for standards for interpretation and reporting of sequence variations: revisions 2007. Genet Med. 2008;10:294–300.

85. Plon SE, Eccles DM, Easton D, et al. Sequence variant classification and reporting: recommendations for improving the interpretation of cancer susceptibility genetic test results. Hum Mutat. 2008; 29:1282–91.
86. Mazoyer S, Dunning AM, Serova O, et al. A polymorphic stop codon in BRCA2. Nat Genet. 1996;14: 253–4.
87. Chapman MS, Verma IM. Transcriptional activation by BRCA1. Nature. 1996;382:678–9.
88. Haile DT, Parvin JD. Activation of transcription in vitro by the BRCA1 carboxyl-terminal domain. J Biol Chem. 1999;274:2113–7.
89. Kais Z, Chiba N, Ishioka C, Parvin JD. Functional differences among BRCA1 missense mutations in the control of centrosome duplication. Oncogene. 2012;31(6):799–804.
90. MacLachlan TK, Somasundaram K, Sgagias M, et al. BRCA1 effects on the cell cycle and the DNA damage response are linked to altered gene expression. J Biol Chem. 2000;275:2777–85.
91. Monteiro AN, August A, Hanafusa H. Evidence for a transcriptional activation function of BRCA1 C-terminal region. Proc Natl Acad Sci USA. 1996;93:13595–9.
92. Moynahan ME, Chiu JW, Koller BH, Jasin M. Brca1 controls homology-directed DNA repair. Mol Cell. 1999;4:511–8.
93. Parvin J, Chiba N, Ransburgh D. Identifying the effects of BRCA1 mutations on homologous recombination using cells that express endogenous wild-type BRCA1. J Vis Exp. 2011;48. doi: 10.3791/2468.
94. Lee MS, Green R, Marsillac SM, et al. Comprehensive analysis of missense variations in the BRCT domain of BRCA1 by structural and functional assays. Cancer Res. 2010;70:4880–90.
95. Farrugia DJ, Agarwal MK, Pankratz VS, et al. Functional assays for classification of BRCA2 variants of uncertain significance. Cancer Res. 2008;68: 3523–31.
96. Adzhubei IA, Schmidt S, Peshkin L, et al. A method and server for predicting damaging missense mutations. Nat Methods. 2010;7:248–9.
97. Ng PC, Henikoff S. Predicting deleterious amino acid substitutions. Genome Res. 2001;11:863–74.
98. Sunyaev S, Ramensky V, Koch I, Lathe 3rd W, Kondrashov AS, Bork P. Prediction of deleterious human alleles. Hum Mol Genet. 2001;10:591–7.
99. Gowen LC, Johnson BL, Latour AM, Sulik KK, Koller BH. Brca1 deficiency results in early embryonic lethality characterized by neuroepithelial abnormalities. Nat Genet. 1996;12:191–4.
100. Hakem R, de la Pompa JL, Sirard C, et al. The tumor suppressor gene Brca1 is required for embryonic cellular proliferation in the mouse. Cell. 1996;85: 1009–23.
101. Hohenstein P, Kielman MF, Breukel C, et al. A targeted mouse Brca1 mutation removing the last BRCT repeat results in apoptosis and embryonic lethality at the headfold stage. Oncogene. 2001;20:2544–50.
102. Liu CY, Flesken-Nikitin A, Li S, Zeng Y, Lee WH. Inactivation of the mouse Brca1 gene leads to failure in the morphogenesis of the egg cylinder in early postimplantation development. Genes Dev. 1996;10: 1835–43.
103. Ludwig T, Chapman DL, Papaioannou VE, Efstratiadis A. Targeted mutations of breast cancer susceptibility gene homologs in mice: lethal phenotypes of Brca1, Brca2, Brca1/Brca2, Brca1/p53, and Brca2/p53 nullizygous embryos. Genes Dev. 1997; 11:1226–41.
104. Frank TS, Deffenbaugh AM, Reid JE, et al. Clinical characteristics of individuals with germline mutations in BRCA1 and BRCA2: analysis of 10,000 individuals. J Clin Oncol. 2002;20:1480–90.
105. Tavtigian SV, Byrnes GB, Goldgar DE, Thomas A. Classification of rare missense substitutions, using risk surfaces, with genetic- and molecular-epidemiology applications. Hum Mutat. 2008;29:1342–54.
106. Tavtigian SV, Samollow PB, de Silva D, Thomas A. An analysis of unclassified missense substitutions in human BRCA1. Fam Cancer. 2006;5:77–88.
107. Easton DF, Deffenbaugh AM, Pruss D, et al. A systematic genetic assessment of 1,433 sequence variants of unknown clinical significance in the BRCA1 and BRCA2 breast cancer-predisposition genes. Am J Hum Genet. 2007;81:873–83.
108. Goldgar DE, Easton DF, Byrnes GB, Spurdle AB, Iversen ES, Greenblatt MS. Genetic evidence and integration of various data sources for classifying uncertain variants into a single model. Hum Mutat. 2008;29:1265–72.
109. Ambry Genetics. XLMR testing options. 2011. http://www.ambrygen.com/X-Linked-Intellectual-Disabilities.html. Accessed 30 Aug 2011.
110. Emory Genetics Laboratory. Congenital muscular dystrophy comprehensive next generation sequencing panel. 2011. http://genetics.emory.edu/egl/tests/?testid=440. Accessed 30 Aug 2011.
111. Walsh T, Lee MK, Casadei S, et al. Detection of inherited mutations for breast and ovarian cancer using genomic capture and massively parallel sequencing. Proc Natl Acad Sci USA. 2010;107: 12629–33.

11 Cystic Fibrosis: Carrier Testing, Newborn Screening, and Diagnostic Testing

W. Edward Highsmith Jr.

Introduction

Cystic fibrosis (CF) is the most common life-shortening autosomal recessive genetic disorder in the Caucasian population. CF is due to mutations in the cystic fibrosis transmembrane regulator (CFTR) gene, located on chromosome 7 at 7q31.2, which encodes a cyclic AMP-activated chloride channel [1, 2]. The disorder has a broad range of severity, but classical CF is manifested by chronic pulmonary disease, exocrine pancreatic insufficiency, and elevated concentrations of chloride in sweat. Approximately 85 % of individuals with CF do not retain sufficient exocrine pancreatic function to adequately digest food. Thus, without oral pancreatic enzyme supplementation, severe malnutrition and growth failure can occur within the first years of life. The major cause of morbidity and mortality in CF is the chronic, suppurative pulmonary disease. The CF lung is extremely susceptible to infection, particularly with the mucoid form of the gram negative bacterium *Pseudomonas aeruginosa* and the gram-positive *Staphylococcus aureus* [3]. Although the details are still unclear, the mechanism of the lung disease is thought to originate in the relative lack of airway surface hydration due to abnormal sodium and chloride transport and the associated movement of water across the apical epithelia. The dehydrated mucus lining the airways becomes difficult for the cilia to move and clear trapped particulate matter, including inhaled bacteria. Subsequent bacterial growth stimulates inflammation and mucus hypersecretion, which in turn becomes dehydrated and difficult to expel. Thus, there is cycle of increasing pulmonary obstruction and inflammation that leads, without treatment, and in some cases, in spite of treatment, to bronchiectasis and end-stage lung disease [4].

The ion transport abnormalities are not limited to the lining of the lung; rather, they affect many secretory epithelia, including those lining the pancreatic ducts, the biliary tree, and the sweat glands. Indeed, one of the early milestones in CF research occurred during a historic heat wave in the summer of 1948 in New York City when Dr. di Sant' Agnese and coworkers noted that a large number of the babies that presented with heat prostration has cystic fibrosis and that they had an excessive amount of salt in their sweat [5]. This observation lead to the development of a diagnostic test for CF, the measurement of the chloride ion concentration is sweat, which remains a cornerstone of CF diagnostics today. In addition to the epithelial dysfunctions, approximately 97 % of males with CF are infertile due to the absence of the vas deferens [3].

W.E. Highsmith Jr., Ph.D. (✉)
Molecular Genetics Laboratory, Department of Laboratory Medicine and Pathology, Mayo Clinic College of Medicine, Rochester, MN, USA
e-mail: Highsmith.W@mayo.edu

W.E. Highsmith Jr. (ed.), *Molecular Diagnostics: 12 Tests That Changed Everything*, Molecular and Translational Medicine, DOI 10.1007/978-1-4614-8127-0_11,

Over 1,800 mutations have been reported in the CFTR gene (http://www.genet.sickkids.on.ca/cftr/app), but only 10 % or fewer have high enough frequencies to have been well characterized (http://www.cftr2.org). Of the characterized mutations, one is by far the most common, with only approximately 23 having frequencies of greater than 0.1 % of CF chromosomes in North America. The most common mutation, deltaF508, a three base-pair (bp) deletion that leads to the deletion of a single phenylalanine residue at codon 508 of the protein, accounts for approximately 70 % of CF mutation in North American CF patients [6].

The clinical heterogeneity of CF had long been a puzzle, specifically; it was unclear why the majority of CF patients had severe exocrine pancreatic insufficiency, yet approximately 15 % of patients retained sufficient exocrine pancreatic function to digest food. As a consequence, these children are better nourished and typically (but not always) have milder pulmonary disease. With the identification of the CFTR gene and the most common mutation, studies of genotype/phenotype correlation quickly began. In 1990, a study appeared showing that CF patients with the pancreatic insufficient (PI) form of the disease were frequently found to be homozygous for the deltaF508 mutation. In contrast, patients with pancreatic sufficiency (PS) and milder lung disease were very rarely homozygous for the deltaF508 mutation [7]. The hypothesis that was generated was that there were two fundamental types of CFTR mutation—those associated with PI disease and those associated with PS disease; with the PS form being dominant, such that individuals who were compound heterozygotes with one PI and one PS mutation had the pancreatic sufficient form of the disease. This was soon shown to be correct.

There are multiple molecular mechanisms of CFTR dysfunction that have been identified. These are summarized in Table 11.1. Of these classes of mutation Types I–III have been identified as being associated with more severe disease (typically PI CF), while Types IV and V are often associated with less severe disease (often the PS form of the disease) [8]. Although genotype/phenotype correlations have been established for groups of CF patients, due to the contributions of other factors that affect disease severity, such as other genetic modifiers or environmental insults (secondhand smoke or smoking, for example), it is not recommended to try and predict the course of any given patient's disease using just the genotype.

Table 11.1 Categories of CFTR mutations

Mutation type	Molecular mechanism	Examples [3]
I	No protein production	W1282X, R553X
II	Defective processing	DeltaF508, N3103K
III	Defective regulation	G551D
IV	Defective conduction	R117H, R347P
V	Reduced protein production	3849+10 kb C>T, 2789+5 G>A

The diagnosis of CF is often straightforward using sweat chloride and/or DNA testing after, historically, presentation with characteristic symptoms or, today, most often (but not always) after a positive newborn screening test result. However, a minority of diagnostic cases can be very challenging. A Cystic Fibrosis Foundation Consensus Conference agreed that the sweat chloride was the primary test for confirming the diagnosis of CF. However, they noted that it was well known that a small percentage of CF patients can have sweat chloride values in the intermediate, or even normal, range. In addition, they noted that DNA mutation analysis had a very high predictive value when two known CF mutations were identified, but molecular testing was less useful when a known mutation and a variant of uncertain significance were identified. Further, they stated that an infant with an intermediate sweat chloride value and one or no CFTR mutations identified cannot be positively diagnosed with CF, but should be followed as they are at risk of developing symptoms at a later age [9].

The diagnostic conundrums are exacerbated by the realization that CF can present with a broad range of disease severities, not just the classical presentation of PI and severe, early onset pulmonary disease. Since the original observation in 1992, multiple studies have confirmed that isolated male infertility due to congenital bilateral absence of the vas deferens (CBAVD) was associated with one or two sequence variation in the CFTR gene [10]. Similarly, isolated chronic idiopathic pancreatitis, without elevated sweat chlorides or pulmonary disease, can be the result of CFTR mutations [11]. In order to distinguish these milder, single organ disorders from classical PI or PS CF, the term CFRD or CF-Related Disorder is often recommended [12].

Although CF is still associated with a decreased lifespan, the mean age of survival has increased markedly since the disease was first described in 1938 [13]. At that time, the typical age of death of children with CF was 2–3 years of age. Currently, the Cystic Fibrosis Foundation estimates that the median age of survival of a child born with CF in 2010 is 37 years [14]. Current CF treatment requires a specially trained team of healthcare providers, including physicians, nurses, genetic counselors, and respiratory and physical therapists. Therapy involves pancreatic enzyme supplementation, high calorie diets, both physical and medicinal methods to help clear inspissated mucus, and antibiotic regimens. Very recently, a molecularly targeted drug, Kalydeco™ (ivacaftor, Vertex Pharmaceuticals) has been cleared by the FDA for use in CF patients with a specific mutation (Gly551Asp) [15, 16]. The introduction of drugs targeting not the disease symptoms, but the root cause of the genetic disorder, is an extremely exciting development in CF therapeutics.

Cystic Fibrosis: Carrier Screening

Carrier Screening: Background

The identification of markers that were in linkage disequilibrium with the CF gene [17], and the inference that there would only be one CF mutation, or only a few, gave strength to the notion that population-based carrier testing could be reasonably accomplished. The principle driver behind the idea of population-based carrier screening was the desire to provide couples with the information needed for them to make informed decisions about their reproductive lives. However, there were significant concerns as well. One of the major concerns was the possibility of loss of insurance coverage after an individual was identified as a carrier of CF. In addition, the effects of revealed carrier status on families and marriages, particularly when one member of a couple was found to be a carrier while the other tested negative, was unknown. After the identification of the CFTR gene in 1989, it became clear that that, although one mutation accounted for the majority of CF alleles, the sensitivity of testing would be substantially less than 100 %.

In the early 1990s, with only a handful of CF mutations having been identified, testing was able to identify approximately 70 % of carriers (in the US population). Thus, only about half ($0.7 \times 0.7 = 0.49$) of couples at a one in four risk, i.e., both members of the couple test positive for carrier status, could be identified. This difficulty, along with issues of how to educate the population (and physicians) in the use of imperfect tests and the differing frequency of disease and mutational spectrum in different ethnic groups, lead, first the NIH and then the American College of Obstetrics and Gynecology (ACOG) and the American Association for Human Genetics (ASHG) to issue opinions that population-based testing was not yet appropriate in 1990, 1991, and 1992, respectively [18–20].

In 1991, using the new Ethical, Legal, and Social Issues (ELSI) program, the new National Human Genome Research Institute (NHGRI) funded the NIH Cystic Fibrosis Studies Consortium (CFSC), which supported eight RO1 grants that were designed to address the various concerns surrounding CF carrier testing [21]. Further, during the early 1990s, many investigators worldwide were sequencing CFTR genes from many different patient populations and a large number of new and novel mutations were identified. However, the majority of the identified mutations were very rare, probably even family specific, and the overall sensitivity of detection remained disappointing low. For example, in a widely cited review by Zielenski and Tsui from 1995, even though over 550 mutations had been reported, only 13 were recurrent in the general population, with a combined detection rate of 75.7 % [22].

After the ELSI studies were completed and the results published, the NIH called a consensus conference to, once again, address the question of whether the USA was ready for population-based carrier screening. As the ELSI studies were uniform in their conclusions that risk of harm was low, and, as the sensitivity of detection continued to slowly increase, the 1997 consensus conference recommended offering CF carrier testing not only to individuals with a family history of CF but also to the prenatal population and to couples planning a pregnancy [23].

Although there was a modest increase in obstetricians discussing CF carrier testing with their patients after the NIH Consensus Conference recommendations [24], it was not until the endorsement of population carrier testing by both the ACOG and ACMG in 2001 that testing volumes in the USA started to grow in earnest.

The 2001 ACOG and ACMG recommendations called for offering testing to all Ashkenazi Jews and non-Jewish Caucasians who were pregnant or planning a pregnancy and making testing available on request to individuals of other ethnic groups [25]. The test would consist of a panel of mutations comprised of those mutations which had a frequency of greater than or equal to 0.1 % of CF alleles in the general American population.

In 2004, ACOG modified their recommendations [26]. The differences between offering testing to individuals of some ethnic groups while "making it available" to others created significant confusion in the already busy obstetrics community. Accordingly, the 2004 recommendations removed this distinction and called for offering testing to all, regardless of ethnicity. In addition, two mutations from the original list of 25 were removed. Several years of testing large numbers of individuals revealed that the 1078delT mutation was not as common as previously thought. As its frequency did not rise to the level of 0.1 % on CF chromosomes, it was dropped from the panel. I148T was removed from the panel because it was shown by investigators at Genzyme Genetics and the University of North Carolina not to be a mutation at all, but a benign polymorphism that was linked to a disease causing mutation (3199del6) on approximately 1 in 50 I148T-bearing chromosomes [27].

The sensitivity of the 23 mutation panel for the detection of mutations in the Northern European Caucasian population is relatively high. It is, however, difficult to determine exactly what the sensitivity of a given panel is. The only way to accomplish this is to study a population of individuals with diagnosed CF and determine the fraction of alleles that are identified. The mutations for the panel were selected from the over 15,000 cases with molecular results in the Cystic Fibrosis Foundation registry; however, a figure for the sensitivity of the selected panel could not be determined as many of the patients were only tested with a number of different small panels of mutations.

The decision to limit the standard panel to 23 mutations was not without controversy and is not without drawbacks. Even though the sensitivity of detection is high in the Northern European population, estimated at 80.2 % in a 1997 paper from the Cystic Fibrosis Mutation Analysis Consortium, the detection rates were known to be significantly reduced in other populations, specifically Southern Europeans, Hispanics, and African Americans [28]. Even though the ACMG recommendation specifically did not recommend offering panels with additional mutations, one commercial laboratory, Genzyme Genetics, marketed a 64 mutation panel, claiming increased sensitivity in the North American population. Indeed, in the next issue after the publication of the ACMG recommendations in Genetics in Medicine, Genzyme Genetics published a study of 5,840 CF chromosomes from individuals with clinical diagnoses using panels with 64, 70, or 86 mutations. In this study, the sensitivity of detection in the CF patients of Northern European ancestry rose modestly as the number of mutations tested increased from 23 (81.5 % detected) to 70 (84.3 % detected) to 86 (85.7 % detected). The increase in detection rate for individuals of Hispanic ancestry also increased modestly from 56 % detected with 23 mutations to 58.3 % with 86 mutations. However, the gain in sensitivity in the African-American patients was more impressive, rising from only 47 % detected with 23

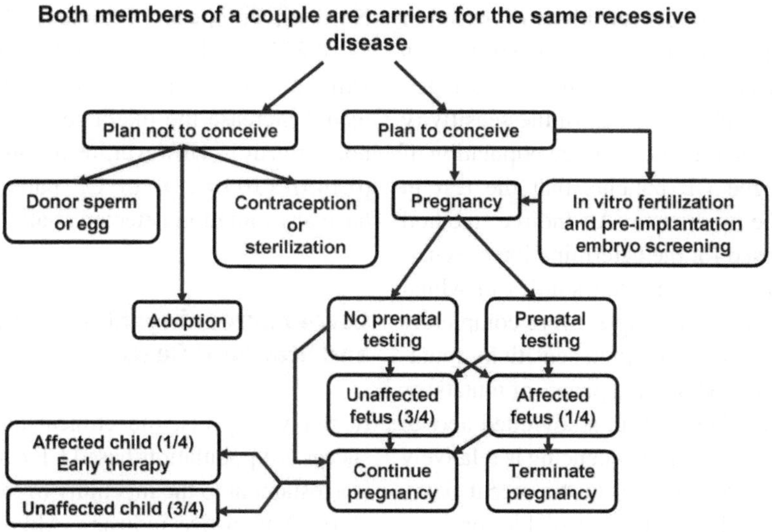

Fig. 11.1 Carrier screening yields options. Couples who know that they are both carriers for the same recessive disorder have numerous options available to them. Whether they take advantage of these options or not is a decision that is entirely left to the couple. The profession of genetic counseling has arisen, in part, to assist individuals and couples navigate through technically difficult and personally challenging decisions. When the couple knows of their carrier status prior to pregnancy, options include those centered on whether to take the known risk of an affected child or not. When the information is only available after pregnancy, the decisions available center on whether or not to seek prenatal testing or not and decisions of what to do in the case that an affected fetus is identified

mutations to 61.9 % with 86 [29]. The authors concluded that, particularly given the racial mixture and ethnic heterogeneity in the USA, a pan-ethnic, expanded panel had value for population screening.

The question of what is the optimal number of mutations to include in screening assays is, somewhat surprisingly, still an open question. The debate over whether "less is more" or "more is better" continues and is further explored in the Standard Reagents section.

Carrier Screening: Clinical Applications and Test Interpretation

The purpose of CF carrier testing, reiterated in numerous articles and reviews, is the empowerment of individual couples to better plan their reproductive lives [30]. For couples who know that both partners are carriers of the same autosomal recessive disorder, there are numerous actions and alternatives available to them (Fig. 11.1). As most carriers of autosomal recessive diseases, in particular, carriers of CF, are asymptomatic, the typical way that a couple finds out that they are both carriers is by having an affected child. The purpose of carrier screening is to provide couples with the information that they are at a one in four risk *before* the birth of the first affected child.

A key concept for the use of tests with less than perfect sensitivity is that of residual risk. An individual who tests negative for carrier status with a test that is, for example, 90 % sensitive, has had their chances of being a carrier reduced, but not eliminated.

In order to fulfill the goals of the carrier-screening program, to inform the patient, it is necessary to calculate the residual risk that an individual with a negative test result is still a carrier. This can be a complex task, given a family history of CF (if any); the variation of carrier risks in different populations and ethnic groups; and, the variation in the distribution of mutations in different groups, which results in different levels of clinical sensitivity when using the same test in different populations.

First, an estimate of the sensitivity of detection for each ethnic group that the laboratory is expecting to serve needs to be made. As noted previously, it is difficult to determine sensitivity experimentally as it requires a large population of well-characterized CF patients that the test in question can be applied to. An indirect method that is widely used for the determination of sensitivity is to examine published studies in which either all of the patient samples were completely sequenced or tested with a high sensitivity mutation scanning method or large panels of mutations (for example, the Heim et al. study cited above) were used. As whole gene sequencing is relatively expensive (and was more so in the recent past), the number of studies that are available for comparison are relatively few.

Given an estimate of sensitivity, and knowing the a priori carrier rate in the population, the residual risk is calculated using Baysean analysis. For example, the carrier rate is 1 in 25 the Northern European Caucasian population. Using a panel of mutations with a sensitivity of 91 % in that population, a Baysean analysis yields a posttest risk of 1 in 267 of being a CF carrier for an individual with a negative test result.

A secondary, but still important clinical application of multi-mutation panel testing is in the conformation of clinical diagnoses. However, the use of specific mutation panels to confirm a clinical diagnosis should be approached with caution. As noted above, even expanded panels have much less than perfect sensitivity for the detection of CF carriers. The sensitivity for the detection of two CF mutations, required to make or confirm a diagnosis, is significantly less. Using the Hardy–Weinberg equation

$$p^2 + 2pq + q^2 = 1,$$

where p is the fraction of CF mutations that are detectable in a population with a given test, and q is the fraction that is not detected, then the fraction of cases in which both mutations are detected is the square of the fraction detectable. For example, using the Genzyme 86 mutation panel in the Northern European Caucasian population, with a sensitivity of 85.7 %, both mutations would be detected in $(0.857 \times 0.857) \times 100 = 73.4$ % of Northern European CF patients. Similarly, $2pq$, $(2 \times 0.857 \times 0.143) \times 100 = 24.5$ %, of CF patients will only have one mutation identified, which would increase the likelihood of CF, but would not confirm it. However, using this test, only q^2, $(0.143)^2 \times 100 = 2$ % of CF patients would not have any mutation detected at all.

Carrier Screening: Methodology and Standard Reagents

In many respects, the clinical and commercial success of population-based CF carrier screening is a testament to the ingenuity of the American In Vitro Diagnostics industry. Although multiplex PCR for a genetic disease was first developed in 1988 for the detection of deletions in Duchenne muscular dystrophy [31], prior to 2001, there were few publications using multiplex analysis, and no commercial products were available which utilized it.

The opening of a large market, approximately four million births per year in the USA, about three million of them being Caucasian, stimulated multiple companies to develop robust multiplex amplification and mutation detection strategies. A cursory examination of the commercially available methods reveals something remarkable—how few of them only offer the 23 mutation panel recommended by the ACMG and ACOG. Although somewhat speculative, it is very likely that the choices of numbers of mutations offered by each company are driven by thoughts of competitive advantage. Why would a physician order one test versus another, and why would a laboratory choose to implement one system over another? One driver could certainly be price. However, from a corporate point of view, it often is considered best not to compete on price, but on some other feature of a product that distinguishes it from its competition. In the case of CF carrier-screening tests, that differentiator was very likely to have been number of mutations. Shouldn't a 32 mutation test be better than a 23 mutation test? Shouldn't 60, 96, or 106 mutation tests be even better?

The escalation of numbers of mutations tested for by commercial panels was the subject of an editorial in the journal Genetics in Medicine in 2007. The coauthors, all of whom were coauthors on the 2001 and 2004 ACMG recommendations, called this development "a rather unseemly arms race" and emphasized that the reasons that expanded panels "should not be offered routinely" were just as valid in 2007 as they were in 2001. The authors argue against the upsurge in expanded panels citing: since the increase in sensitivity is so small, their use gives a false sense of security; there is substantial uncertainty regarding allele frequency and genotype–phenotype correlations with the rarer mutations; the futility of targeting ethnicity-specific mutations in such diverse populations as Hispanics or African Americans; and the added costs and diminishing returns for testing rarer and rarer mutations [32].

However, multiple studies have shown that there is an approximately 10–15 % increase in detection rate in Hispanic and African-American populations with expanded panels. Heim et al., cited previously, increased the numbers of mutations identified by 15 % using the 86 mutation Genzyme panel. A follow-up manuscript, published in 2004, specifically addressed the increase in sensitivity in Hispanic and African-American populations seen with the Genzyme 86 mutation panel. Compared to the recommended 23 mutation panel, the investigators observed an additional 9.7 and 7.4 % mutation in the Hispanic and African-American population, respectively [33]. They noted that some of the most common of the additional mutations were ones that were associated with a mild or variable clinical phenotype, D1152H and L206W [34, 35]. This is consistent with our experience with the 70 mutation Luminex Tag-IT assay. We found a similar increase in mutation detection in the Hispanic and African Americans, respectively, who submitted samples for CF testing to the Mayo Clinic Molecular Genetics laboratory from 2007 to 2009, with the most common non-ACMG panel mutations being D1152H and L206W (unpublished data).

Genzyme added additional mutations to their panel in 2005, bringing the total to 98. In a recent analysis of over 370,000 samples submitted for carrier testing over 33 months, the Genzyme group found that 27 % and 23 % of mutations detected in their Hispanic and African-American patients, respectively, were non-ACMG panel mutations [36]. Together, these reports clearly indicate that the sensitivity of detection of CF carrier status in minority populations can be increased with expanded panels; however, fairly large panels are required to affect a significant increase. (Our experience with a 106 mutation laboratory developed test is shown in Fig. 11.2.)

On the other hand, in another recent publication, Quest Diagnostics published its experience with 23–32 mutation panels (depending on the time when the samples were analyzed). They reported data on almost three million samples analyzed between 2002 and 2010. Overall, the observed carrier rate was 1 in 37.6, which, after adjusting to a figure of 1 in 25, yields an overall sensitivity of 77 %. After extensive analysis of their data, the Quest group concluded that the ACMG/ACOG panel was performing as it was designed to do and that they found no compelling reason to recommend that the recommendations be changed in favor of expanded panels [37].

Thus, the controversy over the use of expanded panels continues. However, the market is speaking to this issue. With over 350,000 tests done over 2.5 years, there are clearly physicians and patients who prefer the expanded panel approach of Genzyme. On the other hand, many more samples were analyzed with the Quest panels, which are much closer to the recommended panel. The complete reasoning for this is not clear, but may, in part, be due to lower costs of smaller panels. Intriguing is the observation that in the Quest series approximately 60 % of the samples tested were from individuals who self reported as Caucasian, whereas that fraction was about 40 % in the 2011 Genzyme series. Perhaps clinicians are sorting this out themselves and are tending to send samples from minority populations for expanded panels and reserving the standard panel for Caucasians.

Carrier Screening: Regulatory Issues

Between 2001 and 2005, none of the CF mutation detection kits on the market were cleared for

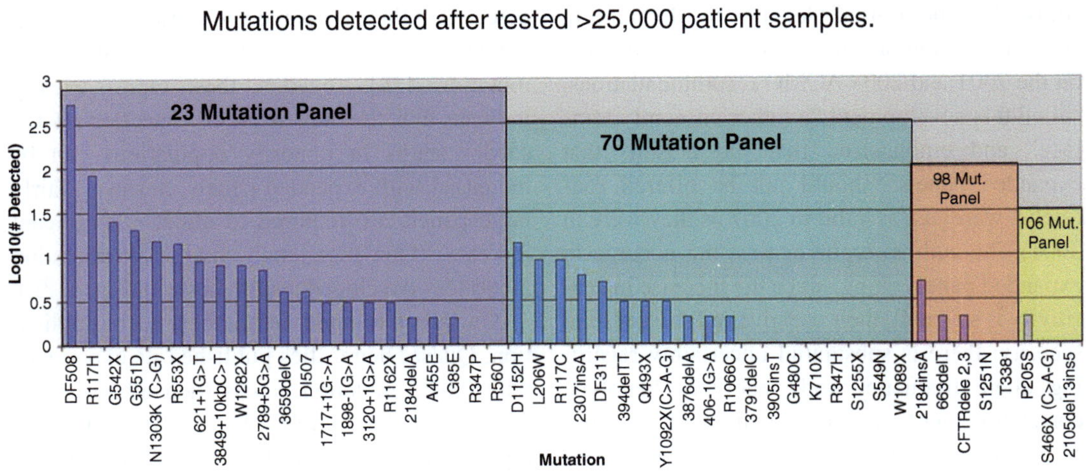

Fig. 11.2 Mayo Clinic experience with a 106 mutation cystic fibrosis-screening panel. Shown are the 819 mutations identified after testing 27,339 samples. As the range of number of mutations detected range from 521 (for deltaF508) to 1, the data is displayed on a log scale for convenience. The mutations are grouped according to commercially available testing panels. Shown is the distribution of mutations detectable with: the ACMG 23 mutation panel; a 70 mutation panel; a 98 mutation panel; and the Mayo 106 mutation panel. Note that more mutations are detected as the number of mutations tested for increases; however, the number of positive cases identified decreases fairly quickly after testing for the most common ~50 mutations

use as in vitro diagnostic tests by the FDA. Rather, they were marketed as analyte-specific reagents, something of a stretch for the original meaning of the term. In 2005, the Tm Biosciences 40+4 Tag-IT assay, which used the Luminex flow cytometer for detection, became the first CF kit to be FDA approved (since then, Luminex Inc. purchased Tm Bioscience. It continues to market the CF assay, and has received FDA approval for a 60-mutation Version 2 of the test). Since 2005, several other companies have taken their CF tests through the FDA and have received approval. At this writing, in addition to Luminex, Celera Diagnostics, GenMark Diagnostics, Hologic, Inc., and Nanosphere Inc. all have FDA cleared CF carrier-screening kits on the market. Companies that have not are likely in the process of doing so. Shortly, it is very likely that all CF carrier screening done in the USA will be done using FDA-approved kits.

It is interesting to note that when the ACMG/ACOG recommendations were published, control material, required for test validation under the CLIA regulations, for all of the 23 mutations were, in the words of Grody et al., "were not to be had for love or money" [32]. Indeed, it was not until 2005, when a conference was called by the CDC, that this problem was addressed [38]. Currently, genomic DNA samples heterozygous for all 23 ACMG panel mutations (and additional mutations) are available from the Coriell Cell Repository [39]. In addition, several companies are marketing so-called super-controls, samples with synthetic constructs corresponding to mutant and wild-type sequences for multiple mutations that can be analyzed simultaneously.

Carrier Screening: How CF Carrier Screening Has Changed Medical Practice

As previously noted, the purpose of population-based CF carrier screening programs is to provide individuals and couples the information that they may use to plan their reproductive lives. The purpose of screening was never eugenic. That is, the purpose of carrier testing was never to "wipe out CF." Nevertheless, evidence is emerging that the birth rates of CF is declining in areas of the world where screening is commonplace. Whether this is due primarily to carrier screening is debatable, as areas with robust carrier-screening programs also typically have newborn-screening (NBS) programs as well. Indeed, it is from NBS programs that the trends in incidence figures are derived. As both programs result in the referral of couples to genetic counseling and access to prenatal diagnostics, it is likely that both are having an effect.

Using data from the Canadian CF Foundation, Dupus et al. found that although the birth incidence of CF had remained stable from 1971 to 1987, after the cloning of the gene in 1989, the birth rate had fallen from 1 in 2,714 to 1 in 3,608 in 2000. The author speculated that the decline was due to the availability of carrier testing and prenatal diagnosis [40]. The State of Massachusetts has seen a fall in the frequency of CF births after 2003. Interestingly, the decrease in the number of babies with a homozygous dF508 genotype was almost halved. Again the authors speculated that the increase in numbers of individuals screened for CF carrier status was the reason for the fall [41]. An interesting study from Italy was published in which it was possible to compare the CF birth rates in two adjacent regions, one of which has widely available carrier testing and one that limits testing to individuals with a family history of CF. The region with the carrier screening had a threefold fewer CF births in 2006 and 2007 than the region with the more conservative approach to screening [42]. Thus, CF carrier screening, along with newborn screening, appears to be decreasing the incidence of CF in countries and regions that offer these services. As importantly, millions of women and likely tens of thousands of couples have been screened for CF carrier status at this point worldwide. The great majority of these individuals and couples tested negative and thus were relieved of at least one worry about the birth of their child that that child would have CF. The individuals and couples who tested positive had options available to them that they otherwise would not have had. Thus, screening can be said to be accomplishing the goals that it set out to meet.

Carrier Screening: Future Directions

The controversy over how many mutations comprise an optimal carrier test is likely to continue. At this writing, there are discussions of greatly expanded panels, consisting of 150–300 mutations that could have sensitivities as high as 95+% in all ethnic groups in the USA. It will be very interesting to see if this strategy comes to fruition and how such a highly multiplexed panel could be achieved technically.

However, it is worth asking whether, given the recent success of ivacaftor for one specific CFTR mutation [15, 16] and the aggressive investigation and development of molecularly targeted therapeutics for other mutations, particularly the deltaF508 mutation, will CF soon become a chronic disease that is well managed by medication? If so, what would the role of carrier screening be?

Cystic Fibrosis Newborn Screening

Newborn Screening: Background

Newborn Screening (NBS) was first demonstrated as an effective public health program when Robert Guthrie showed that phenylketonuria, a devastating genetic disorder characterized by profound mental retardation, could be detected well in advance of symptoms by testing a small blood sample collected onto filter paper and that symptoms could be essentially eliminated by dietary intervention [43]. Other disorders such as congenital hypothyroidism and medium chain acyl dehydrogenase deficiency were soon identified and added to state sponsored NBS programs in the USA and Europe. NBS for CF was first demonstrated in 1979 when it was shown that CF babies had high levels of trypsinogen detectable by immunoassay in dried blood spots [44]. Pilot studies began almost immediately in Australasia,

Europe, and the USA. The cloning of the CFTR gene in 1989 and the identification of the most common mutation allowed a substantial increase in specificity by introducing a molecular second tier test. Following up a positive IRT (immunoreactive trypsinogen) result with molecular analysis for CFTR mutations has been further developed and refined on the past two decades and is in use in many areas of the world.

In the USA, NBS programs are administered by state public health agencies and, historically, there has been substantial variation in how many and which conditions were tested for in each state. An expert panel convened by the ACMG in response to a request by the Health Resources and Services Administration, an agency of the US Department of Health and Human Services, and charged with recommending a standardized panel of NBS target disorders and tests in the US. Results of the group's deliberations were published as a special issue of the Journal Genetics in Medicine in May of 2006 [45]. As part of their work, this Newborn Screening Expert Group established guiding principles as a framework for defining criteria for the evaluation of conditions and making recommendations. These principles included a statement that NBS is an essential public health responsibility that is critical to improve the health of affected children. For a disorder or condition to be included in an NBS program, they had to meet certain minimal criteria: it can be detected in the early newborn period, at a phase in the natural history of the disease that it would not ordinarily be clinically detected; that an analytical test with appropriate sensitivity and specificity is available for it; and, there are demonstrated benefits of early therapeutic intervention which is only made possible by early detection. The group reviewed the published literature on over 80 disorders and conducted surveys of stakeholders and experts to identify those conditions that by consensus best met the criteria for inclusion in a recommended standard NBS panel. Cystic fibrosis was included in the final set of disorders that the expert group felt had sufficient objective evidence for inclusion. At this time, all 50 states in the USA, over 25 regions of Europe, Australia, and New Zealand include CF in their NBS programs.

Newborn Screening: Clinical Applications and Test Interpretation

The devastating consequences of some of the disorders screened for in NBS programs, such as profound mental retardation in PKU or the high likelihood of sudden infant death in MCAD deficiency, can be all but eliminated by the early intervention afforded by presymptomatic detection. Unfortunately, this is not the case with CF. The improvement in outcomes in CF are more modest, but are significant nonetheless.

The improvements in outcome for children with CF as a result of NBS have been extensively studied and documented [46, 47]. There have been two large, randomized controlled trials, one in the USA and one in the UK [48, 49]. In addition, there have been numerous reports of the experiences of individual programs in the Western world. Recently, the Clinical and Laboratory Standard Institute published Approved Guidelines for laboratories engaged in CF NBS [50]. Overall, benefits in nutritional status, growth, pulmonary function have been observed, as well as a decrease in frequency of antibiotic usage and hospitalizations for children who were identified in NBS programs versus cohorts who were diagnosed clinically later in life (reviewed in [51, 52]). Increased survival has been less well demonstrated, but evidence to this effect is emerging [53]. That there are potential hazards to CF NBS has also been widely acknowledged. The parental anxiety caused by false positive or inconclusive NBS tests is a challenge not restricted to CF testing. The disclosure of CF carrier status of infants who test positive for one mutation but have a negative sweat chloride test is an unwanted consequence of CF NBS. The hazard that this represents is unknown, and has been the subject of study, but may impact parental interactions with the child and influence views of self-worth later in life [54]. One hazard that was identified early in the history of CF newborn screening was the possibility of cross-infection from older children with established pulmonary infections to infants who were newly diagnosed via NBS programs [55, 56]. This observation leads quickly to implementation of screening days in CF clinics where only infants without *P. aeruginosa* were seen. However, whether the infections were person-to-person or artifacts of older, more crowded facilities have recently been studied [57]. Prevention of respiratory colonization is a topic of ongoing research and keen interest. A CDC workshop reviewed the evidence for CF NBS and concluded that the health benefits to children with CF outweigh the risks and justify screening [58].

A European consensus conference on CF NBS was convened in 2008. This group reviewed the evidence supporting CF NBS and presented a set of recommendations for best practices in European programs. This group noted that there were many different protocol types across Europe, reflecting differences in ethnic group makeup of different populations; variations in resources and healthcare provision; and, the structure of existing NBS protocols, particularly with respect to infrastructure for obtaining follow-up specimens. Due to these differences, which are also at play in the USA, development of a single method for carrying out CF NBS was not realistic and probably not desirable. Some harmonization was thought to be useful, however. The panel of experts reviewed the use of IRT and mutation analysis, as well as sweat chloride testing, still regarded as the "gold standard" of a CF diagnosis. They made a number of recommendations regarding the counseling before NBS, after a positive NBS result, after a positive diagnosis of CF, and when CF NBS identifies a carrier infant [59].

Newborn Screening: Methodology

There are four general strategies for CF NBS: IRT/IRT, IRT/DNA, IRT/IRT/DNA, and IRT/DNA-whole gene analysis. The choice of what strategy and method to use in any given state or province is complex and depends upon multiple factors, including cost of the testing, the ethnic makeup of the population to be screened, and whether the NBS program takes only one blood spot during the first few days of life, or whether it takes a second one at 2–3 weeks of age.

One strategy which does not involve molecular test is the IRT/IRT method. Here, the first bloodspot is tested for IRT concentration, and babies who have levels greater than the cutoff, typically the top 0.5–1 % of values, will have IRT done on a second blood spot after 2–33 weeks. Babies who have a second result greater than the cutoff are referred for sweat chloride testing. The advantage of this method is the simplicity and low cost. In addition, since carriers are not identified with a molecular technique, there is no need for parental genetic counseling in this situation. The disadvantages are the need for a second sample, difficulties in setting appropriate cutoff values, and possible false positives due to IRT elevation in low birth weight and African-American babies. The state of Colorado has used the IRT/IRT method for many years with an estimated sensitivity for the detection of CF of approximately 95 % [60]. The recent European CF Society best practices guidelines found little evidence to support the use of IRT alone as a second tier test, although it acknowledged that such a strategy may be appropriate in some circumstances [11].

Soon after the identification of the deltaF508 mutation, its detection was applied to NBS, with positive results. In the IRT/DNA strategy for screening, the first test is still the IRT. Those samples with results higher than the cutoff are reflexed, not to a second IRT test, but to a molecular test for the common CFTR mutation. Trials in large screening programs demonstrated that testing for detaF508 decreased the number of false-positive cases, babies referred for sweat chloride test, versus the IRT/IRT strategy [61, 62]. As the number of mutations identified continued to grow, so did the number tested in NBS programs. Currently, the majority of NBS programs utilize commercial kits that were developed for carrier screening. Several retrospective analyses have been carried out using data from 14 to 20 years of screening demonstrating that here is an increased sensitivity using an IRT/DNA strategy when the DNA portion of the test consists of (at least) the 23 mutation panel versus IRT/deltaF508 or IRT/IRT approaches [46, 63]. The disadvantage is that a number of heterozygote carriers will be identified. A CF carrier with an elevated IRT will be referred for sweat chloride testing, which, if the infant is only a carrier, will be negative. Although these children are not identified as having CF, they are identified as being carriers. As noted above, the actual hazard that this represents is unknown. Currently, the IRT/DNA method is the most commonly used strategy worldwide.

A combination strategy, termed IRT/IRT/DNA, has been proposed for programs that collect two NBS blood spots [64]. The main difference between this method and the IRT/IRT method is that the IRT cutoff value is lowered in the second tier test to increase sensitivity. Infants with one or two mutations identified will be referred for sweat chloride testing. An advantage of this method is that it identified fewer heterozygote carriers.

A disadvantage of any DNA-based NBS strategy that relies on testing specific mutations, no matter how large the number, will have less than perfect sensitivity because the square of (1 – detection frequency) (q^2) will not have a mutation identified and $2(pq)$ will have only one mutation identified. As the number of CF patients with one identified mutation is significantly smaller than the number of carriers in any given population, a relatively large fraction of infants referred for sweat chloride testing will be carriers. For example, as noted above, for a test that detects 85 % of CF alleles in a given population, 2(85 % × 15 %), or 25.5 % will have one mutation and $(15\ \%)^2$, or 2.25 % of CF patients will not have a mutation identified and will be missed. For populations that are ethnically diverse, the problem is greater because the overall detection rate decreases. One such population is found in the state of California, which has a particularly large Hispanic population and significant numbers of other minority groups such as African or Asian Americans. To address this problem, California has adopted a three-tier strategy termed IRT/DNA/whole gene analysis. In this method, the top 1.5 % of IRT samples is forwarded to DNA testing using a commercial 30–40 mutations panel. Infants with two mutations are referred for sweat chloride testing and early therapy at a CF Center. Infants with no mutations identified are reported as screen negative. Samples with one mutation are forwarded for whole gene analysis, which consists of a mutation scanning/sequencing method plus deletion/duplication testing (Ambry Test®:CF, Ambry Genetics, Aliso Viejo, CA) [65]. Samples that do not have another mutation identified are reported as screen negative, while infants with a second mutation are referred to a CF Center. Although per case the cost is much higher than a typical NBS test, as only a small percentage of samples are sent for expanded testing, the additional cost to the entire program is minimal. The advantage of this method is increased sensitivity; the disadvantages are the increased cost and the detection of variants of uncertain significance in the whole gene analysis.

Newborn Screening: Regulatory Issues

In the USA, the FDA does not currently regulate NBS, which is almost uniformly carried out in state-operated public health laboratories (which are CAP or CLIA certified). Although many state NBS laboratories utilize molecular methods and kits that have been cleared by the FDA for carrier screening, none of these kits have been approved for use in diagnostic testing or NBS.

Newborn Screening: How CF NBS Has Changed Medical Practice

It would be difficult to overstate the impact that NBS has had on public health. By identifying infants before genetic disease would be clinically apparent and instituting appropriate therapy, many of the identified children will go on to lead normal, productive lives. Thus, NBS is viewed by many as a model for public health practice. For babies with CF, the institution of therapy yields significantly better outcomes. Coupled with better therapies and molecularly targeted pharmaceuticals, CF NBS is helping reduce the burden of this common, life-shortening genetic disorder.

Newborn Screening: Future Directions

Research into optimizing CF NBS continues worldwide. When whole genome sequencing is sufficiently sophisticated and low cost, it is difficult to believe that it will not be applied to NBS, at least in wealthier Western countries. In principle, this would allow, not only the identification of babies with CF and other genetic disorders with very high sensitivity and specificity, it could also identify drug targets and genetic modifiers. However, there is a significant amount of work to do before NextGeneration sequencing technology is prepared to take on this challenge.

Diagnostic Testing of Cystic Fibrosis Using Exon Sequencing and Deletion/Duplication Analysis

Diagnostic Testing: Background

Panel tests, as described above, are often used to confirm clinical diagnoses as well as for their intended use in carrier screening. Although there is little disadvantage to this use, some caveats are worth noting. When a homozygous result is observed, it is wise to confirm with another method, as an unsuspected variant maybe interfering with detection of the wild-type allele. When the purpose of testing is to rule-out CF, the use of panel tests may be more problematic. If the clinical diagnosis is not clear cut, the likelihood that there is at least one non-panel mutation increases. The reason is that the standard panel was developed for classical CF (pancreatic sufficient as well as pancreatic insufficient), not variant presentations.

Even in the best case, when a panel test is used to confirm the diagnosis in a classical case of CF that has been established with an elevated sweat chloride tests, the sensitivity for detecting both mutations is limited. It should be remembered that $2pq\%$ of cases, where p is the fraction of CF alleles that is detectable with the test, and q is the fraction that is not, will only have one mutation identified. For example, for a test with a sensitivity of 85 %, the percentage of classical CF cases that will only have one mutation detected is: $2(0.85)(0.15)\times 100 = 25.5\ \%$. For non-Caucasian ethnic groups and variant presentations, where the sensitivity of the panel tests will be lower, the fraction of cases with one or zero mutations identifiable increases. The identification of a single mutation increases the likelihood of CF, but does not confirm it.

Exon-by-exon sequencing from genomic DNA, coupled with a robust deletion/duplication detection method such as Southern blot or Multiplex Ligation dependent Probe Amplification (MLPA) [66], is often termed whole gene analysis. This combined approach detects all mutations in the coding regions of the gene and is considered the reference method, or gold standard method, for mutation detection in virtually all genes, including CFTR.

Diagnostic Testing: Clinical Applications and Interpretation

In the USA, the CF Foundation recommends characterization of each CF case by mutation analysis. This commitment began early, with the identification of the dF508 mutation in 1989. It was the accumulation of a large database of mutations with associated clinical information, which provided the data for research on genotype–phenotype correlation [8] and the design of the standard 23 mutation panel. Thus, characterization of each patient by genotyping is typically done in the USA, Europe, and Australia, exceptions being cases where this relatively expensive test would pose a financial hardship for the family. It is up to the clinician and the family (and third-party payer) how far they want to go in pursuit of a genotype result. In $q^2\%$ of cases, both mutations will be identified with a panel test, with homozygous dF508 being the most common genotype.

The clinical utility of whole gene analysis is in characterizing and confirming, not only clinical diagnoses but also variant presentation such as late onset disease, pancreatitis, or CBAVD. Another utility, infrequently, but not rarely, used is for carrier screening for the spouse of an individual who has tested positive with a panel test.

When a well-characterized mutation, such as one of the standard panel mutations, is identified, the interpretation is straightforward. Similarly, when a variant that results in a truncated protein is detected, such as a frame-shifting insertion or deletion, or, a nonsense mutation, an interpretation that the variant is pathogenic has a very high probability of being correct. However, when a novel missense mutation, one where the wild-type amino acid is replaced by another, is detected, it is impossible to determine whether the variant is a benign polymorphism or a disease-causing mutation. These events, which are reported as Variants of Uncertain Significance (VUS) are a source of frustration for the clinician and laboratory alike. Although there is a substantial body of literature describing a variety of statistical approaches to the prediction of pathogenicity, none have been sufficiently validated for clinical use. The value of the use of such commonly used prediction tools as SIFT (http://sift.jcvi.org/) and PolyPhen (http://genetics.bwh.harvard.edu/pph/) for CFTR in particular is uncertain.

That over 1,500 mutations have been identified in the CFTR gene is a widely quoted statistic. However, the overwhelming majority of these variants have not been proven to affect CFTR function. Indeed, a recent analysis of the variants list in the CFTR Mutation Database maintained at Sick Kids Hospital in Toronto revealed that only 43 had either functional studies done or at least ten examples in the published literature (unpublished data).

The ongoing CFTR2 project is designed to address the uncertainty of the clinical significance in the reported missense CFTR mutations. The investigators are compiling the literature on individual mutations, as well as doing functional studies. When completed, this is expected to be an extremely useful resource for CF testing laboratories and clinicians.

However, novel sequence variants continue to be detected and the number of VUSs is certain to stay well ahead of any attempts to characterize them. The interpretation of a VUS in CFTR, or any other gene, is that the results of the test are uninformative. Indeed, such a result should be interpreted as if the test had not been done.

Diagnostic Testing: Methodology and Standard Reagents

Gene sequencing is the gold standard to detect aberrations such as substitutions and small deletions and insertions at the nucleotide level. Sequencing is particularly useful when allelic heterogeneity is high in a disease, as with CF.

The first step in any DNA sequencing is the extraction, or purification, of DNA, typically from a peripheral blood sample. Many platforms are commercially available for DNA extraction; the author's laboratory uses the M96 (Roche Diagnostics). Following DNA extraction, the samples are prepared for PCR with primers specific to the gene of interest and the usual PCR constituents (Taq polymerase, buffer, magnesium chloride, and sterile PCR-grade water). The authors perform a gel electrophoresis step to confirm the PCR reaction prior to proceeding with the sequencing assay. Next, the PCR product is treated or "cleaned" to remove unincorporated primers and nucleotides. Again, there are multiple ways that this can be accomplished. One widely used method utilizes shrimp alkaline phosphatase [to convert unincorporated deoxynucleotide triphosphates (dNTP's) into dephosphorylated products that will not interfere with the downstream sequencing reaction] and exonuclease (to digest unextended PCR primers into nucleotides to prevent unwanted extension during the sequencing reaction). The cleaned PCR product is next combined with a mixture of fluorescently labeled di-deoxynucleotide triphosphates and dNTP's (ex: BigDye® terminators [Applied Biosystems]), sequencing buffer, and a thermostabile DNA polymerase. After carrying out the sequencing reaction by thermal cycling and another purification step, this time removing unincorporated fluorescent material, the sample is analyzed by capillary electrophoresis. There are multiple software programs commercially available for base calling, alignments, and mutation detection. The authors use Mutation Surveyor® (Soft Genetics, College Station, PA).

Diagnostic Testing: Regulatory Issues

Currently, there are no FDA-approved tests or instruments for the sequence analysis of any human gene for diagnostic purposes. There are over 2,000 genetic diseases for which clinical diagnostic testing availability is listed at GeneTests.org. Although not all of these tests are whole gene analysis tests, a sizable fraction are. All of these are currently available as Laboratory Developed Tests (LDTs). As such, all of them that are offered by US CAP or CLIA certified laboratories validated their sequencing and deletion testing according to CLIA guidelines.

The performance characteristics that are required by CLIA to be validated are: accuracy, precision, reference range, reportable range, and analytic sensitivity and specificity. Although the meanings of reference range and reportable range as applied to DNA sequencing is debatable, the need for a rigorous validation of the analytical characteristics of sequencing assays is not.

How Has CFTR Diagnostic Testing Changed Medical Practice?

Although not as transformative as either population-based carrier screening or newborn screening, the broad availability of extended CFTR analysis has proven useful for affected individuals whose mutations are not detected using the standard screening panels. In particular, the availability of extended gene analysis has helped define a new category of disease—the CFTR-related disorder (CFRD) [12].

Diagnostic Testing: Future Directions

Sequencing and deletion detection technology are in the early phases of revolutionary changes. The availability of the so-called Next Generation sequencing technology will transform how we approach virtually all diseases, but genetic disorders in particular. With respect to CF, it will soon be possible (and economically feasible) to not only obtain the completed CFTR gene sequence of every CF patient but also the sequence of all known gene modifiers. Ultimately, knowledge about CF patients at the genomic level, not only the sequences of CFTR and gene modifiers, but genes involved in drug metabolism and immune responses, will allow for more finely nuanced therapeutic regimens and truly personalized medical care.

References

1. Kerem B, Rommens JM, Buchanan JA, Markiewicz D, Cox TK, Chakravarti A, Buchwald M, Tsui LC. Identification of the cystic fibrosis gene: genetic analysis. Science. 1989;245:1073–80.
2. Anderson MP, Gregory RJ, Thompson S, Souza DW, Paul S, Mulligan RC, Smith AE, Welsh MJ. Demonstration that CFTR is a chloride channel by alteration of its anion selectivity. Science. 1991;253: 202–5.
3. Cutting GR, Accurso F, Ramsey BW, and Welsh MJ. Cystic fibrosis. In: Valle D, Beaudet A, Vogelstein B, Kinzler K, Antonarakis S, Ballabio, editors. The online metabolic and molecular basis of inherited disease. http://www.ommbid.com/
4. Boucher RC. Airway surface dehydration in cystic fibrosis: pathogenesis and therapy. Annu Rev Med. 2007;58:157–70.
5. di Sant' Agnese PA, Darling RC, Perera GA, Shea E. Abnormal electrolyte composition of sweat in cystic fibrosis of the pancreas. Pediatrics. 1953;12:549.
6. Cystic Fibrosis Genetic Analysis Consortium. Worldwide survey of the deltaF508 mutation – report from the cystic fibrosis genetic analysis consortium (CFGAC). Am J Hum Genet. 1990;47:354–9.
7. Kerem E, Corey M, Kerem BS, Rommens J, Markiewicz D, Levison H, Tsui LC, Durie P. The relation between genotype and phenotype in cystic fibrosis–analysis of the most common mutation (delta F508). N Engl J Med. 1990;323:1517–22.
8. McKone EF, Emerson SS, Edwards KL, Aitken ML. Effect of genotype on phenotype and mortality in cystic fibrosis: a retrospective cohort study. Lancet. 2003;361:1671–6.
9. Farrell PM, Rosenstein BJ, White TB, Accurso FJ, Castellani C, Cutting GR, Durie PR, Legrys VA, Massie J, Parad RB, Rock MJ, Campbell III PW, Cystic Fibrosis Foundation. Guidelines for diagnosis of cystic fibrosis in newborns through older adults: cystic fibrosis foundation consensus report. J Pediatr. 2008;153:S4–14.
10. Anguiano A, Oates RD, Amos JA, Dean M, Gerrard B, Stewart C, Maher TA, White MB, Milunsky A. Congenital bilateral absence of the vas deferens. A primarily genital form of cystic fibrosis. JAMA. 1992;267(13):1794–7.

11. Cohn JA, Friedman KJ, Noone PG, Knowles MR, Silverman LM, Jowell PS. Relation between mutations of the cystic fibrosis gene and idiopathic pancreatitis. N Engl J Med. 1998;339:653–8.
12. Bombieri C, Claustres M, De Boeck K, Derichs N, Dodge J, Girodon E, Sermet I, Schwarz M, Tzetis M, Wilschanski M, Bareil C, Bilton D, Castellani C, Cuppens H, Cutting GR, Drevínek P, Farrell P, Elborn JS, Jarvi K, Kerem B, Kerem E, Knowles M, Macek Jr M, Munck A, Radojkovic D, Seia M, Sheppard DN, Southern KW, Stuhrmann M, Tullis E, Zielenski J, Pignatti PF, Ferec C. Recommendations for the classification of diseases as CFTR-related disorders. J Cyst Fibros. 2011;10 Suppl 2:S86–102.
13. Anderson D. Cystic fibrosis of the pancreas and its relationship to celiac disease Clinical and pathologic study. Am J Dis Child. 1938;56:344.
14. Cystic Fibrosis Foundation. Annual report, p. 8. http://www.CFF.org (2010). Accessed 11 Feb 2012.
15. Van Goor F, Hadida S, Grootenhuis PD, Burton B, Cao D, Neuberger T, Turnbull A, Singh A, Joubran J, Hazlewood A, Zhou J, McCartney J, Arumugam V, Decker C, Yang J, Young C, Olson ER, Wine JJ, Frizzell RA, Ashlock M, Negulescu P. Rescue of CF airway epithelial cell function in vitro by a CFTR potentiator, VX-770. Proc Natl Acad Sci USA. 2009;106:18825–30.
16. Ramsey BW, Davies J, McElvaney NG, Tullis E, Bell SC, Dřevínek P, Griese M, McKone EF, Wainwright CE, Konstan MW, Moss R, Ratjen F, Sermet-Gaudelus I, Rowe SM, Dong Q, Rodriguez S, Yen K, Ordoñez C, Elborn JS. VX08-770-102 Study Group. A CFTR potentiator in patients with cystic fibrosis and the G551D mutation. N Engl J Med. 2011;365:1663–72.
17. Estivill X, McLean C, Nunes V, Casals T, Gallano P, Scambler P, Williamson R. Isolation of a new DNA marker in linkage disequilibrium with cystic fibrosis, situated between J3.11 (D7S8) and IRP. Am J Hum Genet. 1989;44:704–10.
18. No Authors Listed. Statement from the National Institutes of Health workshop on population screening for the cystic fibrosis gene. N Engl J Med. 1990; 323(1):70–1.
19. American College of Obstetricians and Gynecologists. Committee on Obstetrics: Maternal and Fetal Medicine. Current status of cystic fibrosis carrier screening. ACOG Committee Opinion No. 101. ACOG Comm Opin. 1991;101:1–2.
20. No Authors Listed. Statement of the American Society of Human Genetics on cystic fibrosis carrier screening. Am J Hum Genet. 1992;51(6):1443–4.
21. Grody WW. Cystic fibrosis: molecular diagnosis, population screening, and public policy. Arch Pathol Lab Med. 1999;123(11):1041–6.
22. Zielenski J, Tsui LC. Cystic fibrosis: genotypic and phenotypic variations. Annu Rev Genet. 1995;29:777–807.
23. No Authors Listed. Genetic testing for cystic fibrosis. National Institutes of Health Consensus Development Conference Statement on genetic testing for cystic fibrosis. Arch Intern Med. 1999;159:1529–39.
24. Doksum T, Bernhardt BA, Holtzman NA. Carrier screening for cystic fibrosis among Maryland obstetricians before and after the 1997 NIH Consensus Conference. Genet Test. 2001;5:111–6.
25. Grody WW, Cutting GR, Klinger KW, Richards CS, Watson MS, Desnick RJ, Subcommittee on Cystic Fibrosis Screening, Accreditation of Genetic Services Committee, ACMG. Laboratory standards and guidelines for population-based cystic fibrosis carrier screening. Genet Med. 2001;3:149–54.
26. Watson MS, Cutting GR, Desnick RJ, Driscoll DA, Klinger K, Mennuti M, Palomaki GE, Popovich BW, Pratt VM, Rohlfs EM, Strom CM, Richards CS, Witt DR, Grody WW. Cystic fibrosis population carrier screening: 2004 revision of American College of Medical Genetics mutation panel. Genet Med. 2001; 3(2):149–54.
27. Rohlfs EM, Zhou Z, Sugarman EA, Heim RA, Pace RG, Knowles MR, Silverman LM, Allitto BA. The I148T CFTR allele occurs on multiple haplotypes: a complex allele is associated with cystic fibrosis. Genet Med. 2002;4:319–23.
28. Estivill X, Bancells C, Ramos C. Geographic distribution and regional origin of 272 cystic fibrosis mutations in European populations. The Biomed CF Mutation Analysis Consortium. Hum Mutat. 1997;10: 135–54.
29. Heim RA, Sugarman EA, Allitto BA. Improved detection of cystic fibrosis mutations in the heterogeneous U.S. population using an expanded, pan-ethnic mutation panel. Genet Med. 2001;3:168–76.
30. Wilfond BS, Nolan K. National policy development for the clinical application of genetic diagnostic technologies. Lessons from cystic fibrosis. JAMA. 1993; 270:2948–54.
31. Chamberlain JS, Gibbs RA, Ranier JE, Nguyen PN, Caskey CT. Deletion screening of the Duchenne muscular dystrophy locus via multiplex DNA amplification. Nucleic Acids Res. 1988;16(23): 11141–56.
32. Grody WW, Cutting GR, Watson MS. The cystic fibrosis mutation "arms race": when less is more. Genet Med. 2007;9:739–44.
33. Sugarman EA, Rohlfs EM, Silverman LM, Allitto BA. CFTR mutation distribution among U.S. Hispanic and African American individuals: evaluation in cystic fibrosis patient and carrier screening populations. Genet Med. 2004;6:392–9.
34. Highsmith WE, Friedman KJ, Burch LH, Spock A, Silverman LM, Boucher RC, Knowles MR. A CFTR mutation (D1152H) in a family with mild lung disease and normal sweat chlorides. Clin Genet. 2005;68: 88–90.
35. Rozen R, Ferreira-Rajabi L, Robb L, Colman N. L206W mutation of the cystic fibrosis gene, relatively frequent in French Canadians, is associated with atypical presentations of cystic fibrosis. Am J Med Genet. 1995;57:437–9.
36. Rohlfs EM, Zhou Z, Heim RA, Nagan N, Rosenblum LS, Flynn K, Scholl T, Akmaev VR, Sirko-Osadsa

DA, Allitto BA, Sugarman EA. Cystic fibrosis carrier testing in an ethnically diverse US population. Clin Chem. 2011;57:841–8.
37. Strom CM, Crossley B, Buller-Buerkle A, Jarvis M, Quan F, Peng M, Muralidharan K, Pratt V, Redman JB, Sun W. Cystic fibrosis testing 8 years on: lessons learned from carrier screening and sequencing analysis. Genet Med. 2011;13:166–72.
38. The Quality Control Materials for Genetic Testing Group. Developing a sustainable process to provide quality control materials for genetic testing. Genet Med. 2005;7(8):534–49.
39. Pratt VM, Caggana M, Bridges C, Buller AM, DiAntonio L, Highsmith WE, Holtegaard LM, Muralidharan K, Rohlfs EM, Tarleton J, Toji L, Barker SD, Kalman LV. Development of genomic reference materials for cystic fibrosis genetic testing. J Mol Diagn. 2009;11:186–93.
40. Dupuis A, Hamilton D, Cole DE, Corey M. Cystic fibrosis birth rates in Canada: a decreasing trend since the onset of genetic testing. J Pediatr. 2005;147(3): 312–5.
41. Hale JE, Parad RB, Comeau AM. Newborn screening showing decreasing incidence of cystic fibrosis. N Engl J Med. 2008;358:973–4.
42. Castellani C, Picci L, Tamanini A, Girardi P, Rizzotti P, Assael BM. Association between carrier screening and incidence of cystic fibrosis. JAMA. 2009;302: 2573–9.
43. Guthrie R. The introduction of newborn screening for phenylketonuria. A personal history. Eur J Pediatr. 1996;155 Suppl 1:S4–5.
44. Crossley JR, Elliott RB, Smith PA. Dried-blood spot screening for cystic fibrosis in the newborn. Lancet. 1979;1:472–4.
45. Watson MS, Lloyd-Puryear MA, Mann MY, Rinaldo P, Howell RR. Newborn screening: toward a uniform screening panel and system [main report]. Genet Med. 2006;8:12S–252S.
46. Massie RJ, Curnow L, Glazner J, Armstrong DS, Francis I. Lessons learned from 20 years of newborn screening for cystic fibrosis. Med J Aust. 2012;196(1): 67–70.
47. Balfour-Lynn IM. Newborn screening for cystic fibrosis: evidence for benefit. Arch Dis Child. 2008;93(1): 7–10.
48. Farrell PM, Lai HJ, Li Z, Kosorok MR, Laxova A, Green CG, Collins J, Hoffman G, Laessig R, Rock MJ, Splaingard ML. Evidence on improved outcomes with early diagnosis of cystic fibrosis through neonatal screening: enough is enough! J Pediatr. 2005;147(3 Suppl):S30–6.
49. Chatfield S, Owen G, Ryley HC, Williams J, Alfaham M, Goodchild MC, Weller P. Neonatal screening for cystic fibrosis in Wales and the West Midlands: clinical assessment after five years of screening. Arch Dis Child. 1991;66:29–33.
50. CLSI. Newborn screening for cystic fibrosis: approved guideline. CLSI Document I/LA35-A. Wayne, PA. Clinical and Laboratory Standards Institute.
51. Castellani C. Evidence for newborn screening for cystic fibrosis. Paediatr Respir Rev. 2003;4:278–84.
52. Southern KW, Mérelle MM, Dankert-Roelse JE, Nagelkerke AD. Newborn screening for cystic fibrosis. Cochrane Database Syst Rev. 2009;1, CD001402.
53. Salvatore D, Buzzetti R, Baldo E, Forneris MP, Lucidi V, Manunza D, Marinelli I, Messore B, Neri AS, Raia V, Furnari ML, Mastella G. An overview of international literature from cystic fibrosis registries 2. Neonatal screening and nutrition/growth. J Cyst Fibros. 2010;9(2):75–83.
54. Castellani C, Southern KW, Brownlee K, Dankert Roelse J, Duff A, Farrell M, Mehta A, Munck A, Pollitt R, Sermet-Gaudelus I, Wilcken B, Ballmann M, Corbetta C, de Monestrol I, Farrell P, Feilcke M, Férec C, Gartner S, Gaskin K, Hammermann J, Kashirskaya N, Loeber G, Macek Jr M, Mehta G, Reiman A, Rizzotti P, Sammon A, Sands D, Smyth A, Sommerburg O, Torresani T, Travert G, Vernooij A, Elborn S. European best practice guidelines for cystic fibrosis neonatal screening. J Cyst Fibros. 2009;8(3): 153–73.
55. Collins JL, La Pean A, O'Tool F, Eskra KL, Roedl SJ, Tluczek A, Farrell MH. Factors that influence parents' experiences with results disclosure after newborn screening identifies genetic carrier status for cystic fibrosis or sickle cell hemoglobinopathy. Patient Educ Couns. 2013;90:378–85.
56. Farrell PM, Shen G, Splaingard M, Colby CE, Laxova A, Kosorok MR, Rock MJ, Mischler EH. Acquisition of *Pseudomonas aeruginosa* in children with cystic fibrosis. Pediatrics. 1997;100:E2.
57. Kosorok MR, Jalaluddin M, Farrell PM, Shen G, Colby CE, Laxova A, Rock MJ, Splaingard M. Comprehensive analysis of risk factors for acquisition of *Pseudomonas aeruginosa* in young children with cystic fibrosis. Pediatr Pulmonol. 1998;26:81–8.
58. Hayes Jr D, West SE, Rock MJ, Li Z, Splaingard ML, Farrell PM. *Pseudomonas aeruginosa* in children with cystic fibrosis diagnosed through newborn screening: assessment of clinic exposures and microbial genotypes. Pediatr Pulmonol. 2010;45:708–16.
59. Grosse SD, Boyle CA, Botkin JR, Comeau AM, Kharrazi M, Rosenfeld M, Wilfond BS, CDC. Newborn screening for cystic fibrosis: evaluation of benefits and risks and recommendations for state newborn screening programs. MMWR Recomm Rep. 2004;53:1–36.
60. Sontag MK, Hammond KB, Zielenski J, Wagener JS, Accurso FJ. Two-tiered immunoreactive trypsinogen-based newborn screening for cystic fibrosis in Colorado: screening efficacy and diagnostic outcomes. J Pediatr. 2005;147(3 Suppl):S83–8.
61. Gregg RG, Wilfond BS, Farrell PM, Laxova A, Hassemer D, Mischler EH. Application of DNA analysis in a population-screening program for neonatal diagnosis of cystic fibrosis (CF): comparison of screening protocols. Am J Hum Genet. 1993;52:616–26.
62. Larsen J, Campbell S, Faragher EB, Götz M, Eichler I, Waldherr S, Dobianer K, Spona J. Cystic fibrosis screening in neonates–measurement of immunoreactive

trypsin and direct genotype analysis for delta F508 mutation. Eur J Pediatr. 1994;153:569–73.
63. Baker MW, Groose M, Hoffman G, Rock M, Levy H, Farrell PM. Optimal DNA tier for the IRT/DNA algorithm determined by CFTR mutation results over 14 years of newborn screening. J Cyst Fibros. 2011; 10:278–81.
64. Sontag MK, Wright D, Beebe J, Accurso FJ, Sagel SD. A new cystic fibrosis newborn screening algorithm: IRT/IRT1 upward arrow/DNA. J Pediatr. 2009; 155(5):618–22.
65. Keiles S, Koepke R, Parad R, Kharrazi M, California Cystic Fibrosis Newborn Screening Consortium. Impact of IVS8-(TG)m(T)n on IRT and sweat chloride levels in newborns identified by California CF newborn screening. J Cyst Fibros. 2012;11:257–60.
66. Schouten JP, McElgunn CJ, Waaijer R, Zwijnenburg D, Diepvens F, Pals G. Relative quantification of 40 nucleic acid sequences by multiplex ligation-dependent probe amplification. Nucleic Acids Res. 2002;30(12):e57.

Newborn Screening by Tandem Mass Spectrometry and Molecular Confirmation

12

Sean Hofherr and Devin Oglesbee

Over the last several of decades, newborn screening (NBS) has rapidly expanded from the application of a single test to identify a severe but treatable disorder in presymptomatic newborns in order to provide therapy and prevent disease, to a complex and important health program.

Background and Clinical Applications of NBS

History of NBS

Newborn screening for genetic conditions was first applied to the autosomal recessive disorder phenylketonuria (PKU). PKU was, and still is, an ideal candidate for newborn screening as PKU infants can be fed a diet with a reduced concentration of phenylalanine and remain asymptomatic [1]. Originally, PKU was screened postnatally in urine by a colorimetric ferric chloride assay [2]. Although this assay was effective, it was often difficult to collect the urine required and was prone to false-positive results due to interfering substances. This issue was addressed by Dr. Robert Guthrie, often referred to as "the father of newborn screening" when he developed and championed a specific bacterial inhibition assay (BIA) [3]. The BIA test was successfully applied to dried blood spots on filter paper, which could be easily collected, shipped, and stored at ambient conditions, but it was impeded by the fact that the dried blood spots had to be sterilized by autoclaving prior to analysis. In the immediately following years, BIA tests for other metabolic disorders (e.g., maple syrup urine disease, orotic aciduria, and argininosuccinic aciduria) were developed for newborn screening, although not as widely accepted as the original PKU screen [4, 5]. In following decades, screens for several alternative technologies (radioimmunoassays, fluorometric enzyme assays, electrophoresis, etc.) were developed and utilized to screen newborns for other disorders including congenital adrenal hyperplasia (CAH), congenital hypothyroidism (CH), and hemoglobinopathies [6–8]. As with the additional BIA tests, these were not as widely adopted by public health laboratories as the "PKU test" leading to a disparity in the number, ranging from 1 to 9, of disorders that a newborn is screened for depending on the baby's birth state.

S. Hofherr, Ph.D. (✉)
Laboratory Medicine, Children's National Medical Center, 111 Michigan Avenue, NW, Washington, DC, USA
e-mail: Hofherr.Sean@Mayo.edu

D. Oglesbee, Ph.D.
Laboratory Genetics, Mayo Clinic, 200 First Street SW, Rochester, MN, USA

Department of Laboratory Medicine and Pathology, Mayo Clinic, 200 First Street SW, Rochester, MN, USA

Department of Medical Genetics, Mayo, Clinic 200 First Street SW, Rochester, MN, USA
e-mail: Oglesbee.devin@mayo.edu

W.E. Highsmith Jr. (ed.), *Molecular Diagnostics: 12 Tests That Changed Everything*, Molecular and Translational Medicine, DOI 10.1007/978-1-4614-8127-0_12,

Tandem Mass Spectrometry in NBS

Newborn screening had a quantum leap in the late 1980s when tandem mass spectrometry (MS/MS) was introduced for the diagnosis of inborn errors of metabolism, and in particular, fatty acid metabolism. This technology was initially described for the detection of acylcarnitine species in urine, plasma, and tissue by Millington et al. [9]. The usefulness of this technique to NBS was quickly realized, and in 1990, its application to this topic was demonstrated [10]. By 1993, a complementary MS/MS method for the detection of amino acids was developed and its application to the diagnosis of aminoacidopathies in the newborn period was also shown [11]. Robert Guthrie's successful campaign decades earlier convinced states to collect dried blood spot samples from newborns, thereby the combination of these two MS/MS analyses for the detection of acylcarnitines and amino acids in dried blood spots significantly increased the number of screenable disorders from 9 to greater than 60 without disrupting previously established infrastructure.

As a single new technology, MS/MS, allowed state newborn screening laboratories to screen for over 60 disorders with only one additional punch of the NBS card (Guthrie card). This completely shattered the paradigm of 1 punch/1 test/1 disorder, which would have forced the number of tests possible to quickly reach a maximum based on the amount of blood spotted on the card.

Uniform Panel of Disorders

With this huge jump came an even larger disparity in the number of disorders for which state newborn screening laboratories across the USA were testing (4–49). This meant that the detection of crippling disorders was entirely dependent on location of an infant's birth state. To address this serious issue, in 2002 the Department of Health and Human Services commissioned the American College of Human Genetics (ACMG) to form an expert group and generate a consensus-recommended panel of disorders to be screened by state newborn screening laboratories.

This ACMG expert group adapted the World Health Organization's "Principles and Practice of Screening for Disease" written by Wilson and Jungner originally for infectious and chronic disease screening in 1968 [12]. In the WHO document, ten criteria highlighted the need for establishing a definitive benefit to the patient and society as well as for demonstrating cost-effectiveness that benefits society. The ACMG ranking adapted these ten Wilson and Jungner criteria yielding several weighted categories including the following: the availability of a screening test; the availability and complexity of diagnostic services; and the availability and effectiveness of treatments related to targeted genetic conditions.

Eighty-four conditions were ranked and the top 29 were classified as the minimum recommended panel of disorders that each state NBS laboratory should screen. An additional 25 disorders were classified as secondary targets due to the fact that these conditions would be identified using the available technologies for the core panel of disorders, but had either incomplete disease characterization or an unclear benefit of detection in the newborn period. In an impressively short time span, the ACMG-recommended core disorders were integrated into almost all of the state NBS programs. In 2003, the Secretary's Advisory Committee on Heritable Disorders in Newborns and Children (SACHDNC) was chartered to advise the Secretary regarding NBS and eventually the Newborn Screening Saves Lives Act of 2008 was passed. In May of 2010, the Secretary agreed to the SACHDNC recommendation to adopt the ACMG panel (screen for the 29 core conditions and report on the 25 secondary conditions) as a national standard for state newborn screening labs. The SACHDNC also established guidelines for adding and removing disorders from the core and secondary conditions, and formed seven Regional Genetics and Newborn Screening Service Collaboratives and a National Coordinating Center groups to aid in the advancement of NBS.

Increasing the Effectiveness of NBS

Since the adoption of MS/MS for newborn screening, most advancement in the field has been directed at increasing the positive predictive value of newborn screening by decreasing the number of false-positive and false-negative results. Several simple innovations have guided NBS programs in this direction and these are discussed below.

Evidence-Based Disease Ranges

Evidence-based approaches to diagnostic testing utilize the most scientifically sound information (evidence) to determine the most effective way to test for a specific disorder. Historically, the reference ranges used in most clinical laboratories come from single reports or small studies using "normal controls" that were either selected at random or arose from patients tested for a completely different assay, and therefore considered "normal". Often, laboratory reference range are formulated using the 5th and 95th percentiles as cutoffs. This may work for some diagnostic assays, but with NBS, the subtle differences between a "normal" newborn and an affected newborn may be too small to confidently trigger a true positive result. In addition, using traditional reference ranges may lead to a significant number of false positives and false negatives results. An innovative way to avoid the problems associated with normal control reference ranges is to collect enough data (evidence) on patients with true positive NBS results in order to generate disease-specific ranges.

Regional Collaboratives

One of the four original Regional Genetics Collaboratives, Region 4 (encompassing US states IL, IN, KY, MI, MN, OH, and WI), has taken up the challenge of creating a system to facilitate data collection and analysis for the evidence-based determination of disease ranges for NBS conditions. Initially, this effort was focused on the states included in the regional collaborative, but it was quickly realized that a more global effort would be required to compensate for the low prevalence of true positive cases for a large number of the NBS conditions. Currently there are over 47 states and 42 countries that have submitted their newborn screening data on over 15,000 positive cases and contributed to the effort. Having such a large number of true positives and true negatives, the Region 4 Collaborative has designed disease-specific cutoff ranges for each analyte [13] and has developed post-analytical tools that permit newborn screening labs to determine the likelihood that a particular analyte flag (high or low) will be indicative of a genetic condition and a positive newborn screen. In addition, the Newborn Screening Clearinghouse (NBSC) was generated to provide families and providers with information on NBS, condition-specific information, state-specific NBS program information, and nationwide NBS statistics.

Second-Tier Testing and the Reduction of False Positives

The development of second-tier testing has greatly reduced the number of false positives in newborn screening programs that have adopted this methodology [14]. Since newborn screening is based on the use of MS/MS for acylcarnitine (AC) and amino acid (AA) analyses, oftentimes the marker for a specific disease or the specific reference range is not ideal, but is used because it is available. An example of such a marker is the measurement of tyrosine to detect tyrosinemia type 1 [15]. By developing a test for a specific analyte not measured in the initial MS/MS analysis, specimens with preliminary positive AC or AA result can be reflexed for a second-tier test prior to determining whether an initial result is positive or negative, and thereby significantly reducing the number of false-positive patients. For the example of tyrosinemia type 1, instead of using a nonspecific marker like tyrosine, a second-tier test for the disease-specific metabolite, succinylacetone, was developed, which is pathognomonic for that specific disorder, and therefore, dramatically reducing the false-positive rate [15]. These second-tier tests are run at no additional cost to the patient and only insignificantly increase the turnaround time of a final result. The reasons these tests are not added to the primary screen of all newborns are that the increased cost can be prohibitive and separate analyses are be needed for each specific analyte, which will increase the turnround time. Currently available second-tier testing includes the following: elevation of propionylcarnitine (C3)—measurement of methylmalonic acid (MMA), methylcitrate, and homocysteine; elevation of branched chain amino acids—measurement of alloisoleucine; and elevation of tyrosine—measurement of succinylacetone. The latter has been incorporated directly into the Minnesota primary newborn screen methodology and other states will likely follow suit to more precisely screen for tyrosinemia type 1 [16]

Methodology

NBS by MS/MS

An electrospray ionization triple quadrupole tandem mass spectrometry system (ESI-MS/MS) is the workhorse of the modern newborn screening laboratories and biochemical genetics laboratories. The system gains its specificity from its three quadrupoles; the Q1, which measures the parent ion mass; the q2, which is the collision cell that fragments the parent molecule; and the Q3, which measures the mass of the daughter ions produced (Fig. 12.1a). This instrument typically uses two different scans for newborn screening: a precursor ion scan for acylcarnitine analysis and a neutral loss scan for amino acid analysis (Fig. 12.1b, c).

Acylcarnitine Analysis by Precursor Ion Scan

Acylcarnitine analysis by MS/MS detects and quantitates acylcarnitines of various chain lengths taking advantage of the common fragmentation that all acylcarnitines share, the splitting off of a positively charged 85 mass unit (mu) following fragmentation in the collision cell. Initially the parent compound is measured and recorded by the first quadrupole. Then the compound enters into the collision cell and is broken apart. The fragments are detected in the third quadrupole, and if one of the daughter ions is 85 mu, the information is correlated to the measurement taken at the first quadrupole corresponding to the respective parent ion. In this sense, all compounds in the specimen are detected in the first quadrupole, but only parent ions leading to an 85 mu daughter ion are measured; i.e., all other compounds are ignored. Dueterated internal standards are added to each sample before analysis and at a known concentration against which the resulting acylcarnitine species are quantified. The quantitative values for each acylcarnitine species are compared to an age-matched reference range and disease-specific range, and high and/or low flags are interpreted in the context of other acylcarnitine levels as positive or negative.

Amino Acid Analysis by Neutral Loss

Similar to the fragmentation of acylcarnitine species resulting in an 85 mu daughter ion, the analysis for most amino acids in a dried blood spot is based on a common fragmentation pattern. In contrast to the acylcarnitine analysis, the common daughter ion that is produced following the fragmentation in the collision cell (q2) is a neutral 102 mu species, which cannot be detected by the Q3. Therefore, the loss of this 102 mu neutral fragment is the defining characteristic that is utilized to measure the relative abundance of the amino acid parent ion detected in Q1. Dueterated amino acids are used as internal standards at a known concentrations. The resulting abundances of each amino acid (parent ion detected in Q1) are quantitated against these internal standards.

Fig. 12.1 (continued) 85 mu (m/z). The instrument correlates and quantitates the parent ion detected in Q1 for each 85 mu daughter ion detected in Q3 (*filled circles*), which represents the different acylcarnitine species. (**c**) For amino acid analysis, the tandem mass spectrometer is programmed to perform a neutral loss scan. In this setup, the Q1 measures the parent ions within a predetermined range, and the Q3 measures only daughter ions created by a loss of a neutral mass fragment of 102 mu and correlates and quantitates the parent ion detected in Q1 for each daughter ion detected in Q3 (*open circles*), representing the specific amino acids. An exemplary group of amino acids and acylcarnitine species were used to simplify the schematics in (**b**) and (**c**)

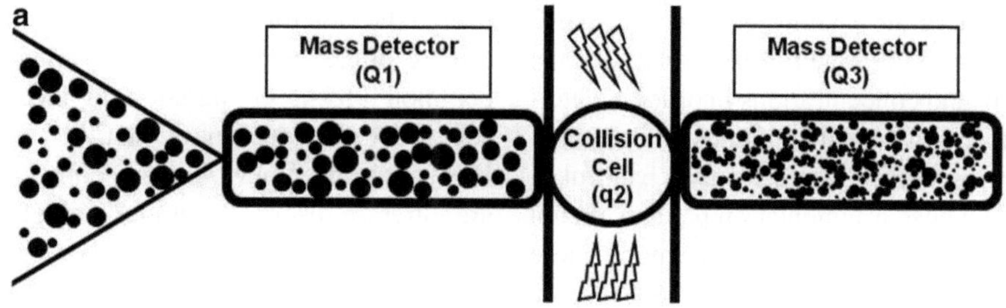

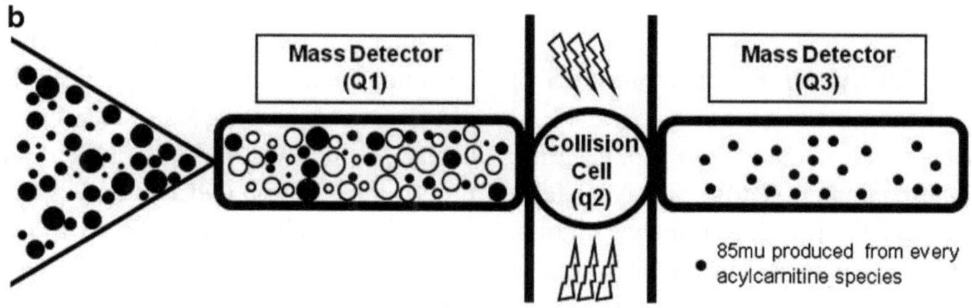

Parent Ion Mass (m/z)	Corresponding Acylcarnitine Species	Representation of Quantitation
260	C2	• • •
288	C4	● ● ● ● ●
344	C8	● ●
372	C10	● ● ● ● ● ●
426	C14:1	● ●
456	C16	● ● ● ●
498	C18:1-OH	●

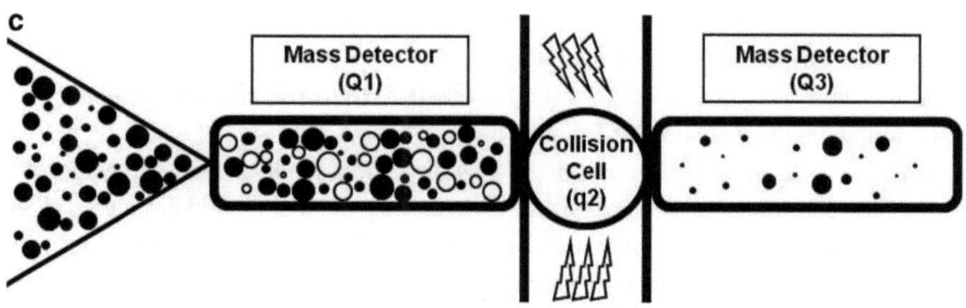

Parent Ion Mass (m/z)	Corresponding Amino Acid	Representation of Quantitation
146	Alanine	○ ○
174	Valine	○ ○
222	Phenylalanine	○ ○ ○ ○ ○
238	Tyrosine	○ ○
261	Tryptophan	○ ○ ○ ○
459	Argininosuccinic acid	○ ○

Fig. 12.1 Schematic of tandem mass spectrometer. (**a**) All ions that are sprayed into the first quadrupole (Q1) within a specific mass range are measured (parent ions). These ions are broken apart in the collision cell (q2) forming daughter ions, which are measured in the third quadrupole, (Q3), where their masses are recorded. (**b**) For acylcarnitine analysis, the tandem mass spectrometer is programmed to perform a precursor scan. In this setup, the Q1 measures the parent ions within a predetermined range, and the Q3 measures only daughter ions with a mass of

Values outside of the established reference range are flagged and interpreted in the context of the other amino acid concentrations in order to determine whether a test results in a positive or negative newborn screen. There are only a handful of amino acids whose fragmentation patterns do not elicit a 102 mu neutral fragment; among these compounds is citrulline, which provides 103 mu and 119 mu daughter ions for quantification.

Laboratory Follow-Up of Positive NBS

With any screening test, the trade-off for ensuring that the highest number of true positives (false negative) are detected is to lower analyte cutoffs, which inadvertently increases the number of false positives. The high number of false positives leads to the need for adequate follow-up testing typically performed in biochemical genetics laboratories and molecular genetics laboratories.

Biochemical Genetics Follow-Up of Positive NBS

The three often used diagnostic tests to follow up an abnormal newborn screen include plasma acylcarnitine analysis, urine organic acid analysis, and plasma amino acid analysis. Specific testing algorithms are found in the ACMG ACT Sheets available at (http://www.acmg.net). The additional testing of urine acylcarnitines, plasma total and free carnitine, and urine amino acids may also be required depending on the specific elevations found on the NBS. These biochemical genetics assays are often conclusive and diagnostic. However, for a few target conditions this is not the case, or for the purpose of counseling the parents for future pregnancies and testing siblings, molecular analyses for confirmation is needed (Fig. 12.2).

Molecular Follow-Up of Positive NBS

In the few disorders caused by common mutations, allele-specific hybridization methods have been utilized as a first-tier molecular test. This is mainly the case for the five common galactosemia disease alleles and the Duarte variant, and the common 985A>G mutation in medium-chain acyl CoA dehydrogenase (MCAD) deficiency. However, many newborn screening conditions are ultrarare disorders without a single common mutation, and thus, full gene sequencing analyses are necessary for confirmation. Most molecular analyses can be performed directly from the NBS blood spot card, but fresh EDTA blood is often the specimen of choice. More recently, deletion detection, which has always been limited in direct exon sequencing assays, has become a necessary practice via multiplex ligation-dependent probe amplification (MLPA) and/or comparative genomic hybridization (CGH-Array) due to the increased recognition of exonic deletions for some of these conditions.

Regulatory Issues of NBS

Newborn screening is not currently regulated by the FDA, but this may change in the future. The regulation of NBS can be split into two distinct areas: regulation of NBS programs and regulation of laboratories performing NBS.

Regulation of NBS Programs

As previously discussed, in May of 2010, the Secretary of Health and Human Services agreed to the SACHDNC recommendation to adopt the ACMG panel (screen for the 29 core conditions and report on the 25 secondary conditions) as a national standard for state newborn screening labs. However, the specific state NBS programs are controlled by each individual state. Each state regulates their respective NBS programs and determines where the testing will occur, which disorders are screened in addition to the 29 core conditions, how the residual dried blood spots will be stored, and how consent from parents is obtained.

Oftentimes, an appointed group is responsible to consult with state legislators and provide insight into the disorders that should be added or removed from a state's newborn screening

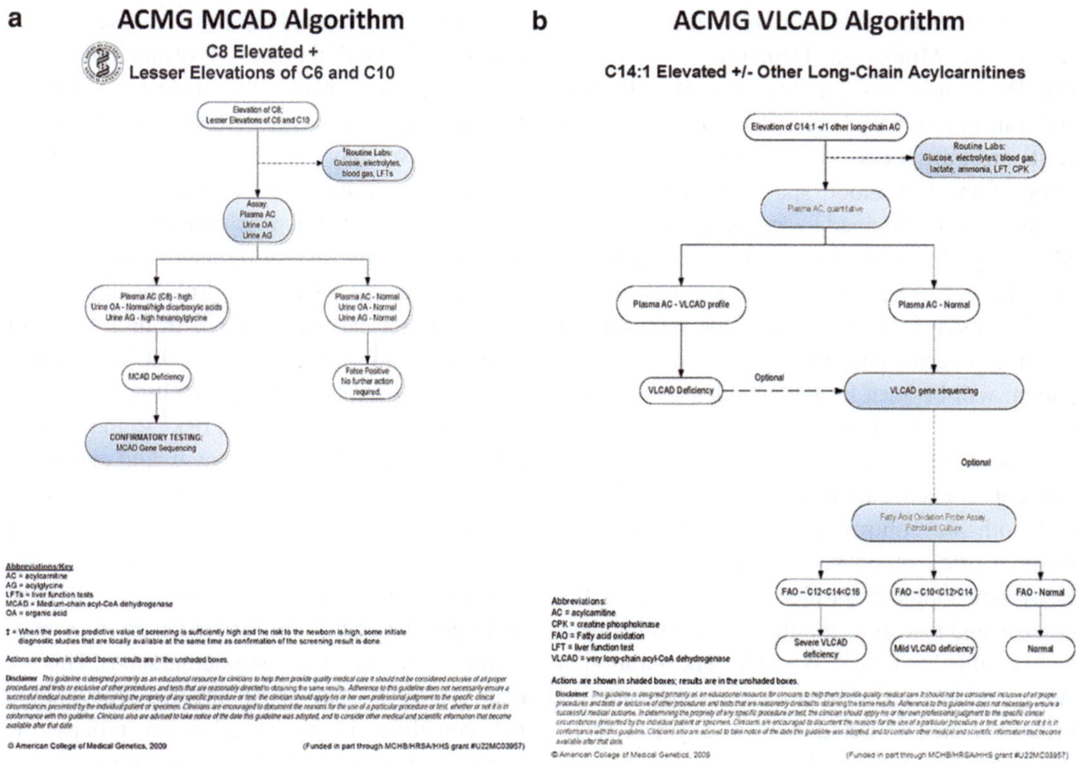

Fig. 12.2 ACMG testing algorithms for medium-chain acyl-CoA dehydrogenase (MCAD) deficiency and very long-chain acyl-CoA dehydrogenase (VLCAD) deficiency. (**A**) The testing algorithm for the follow-up of an abnormal newborn screen consistent with MCAD deficiency almost exclusively involves biochemical testing to determine the legitimacy of the abnormal call. The use of molecular sequencing is only utilized once the biochemical follow-up testing is consistent with MCAD deficiency. The purpose of molecular sequencing confirmation is to aid in the counseling of the family and testing other family member including future pregnancies. (**B**) In contrast, the algorithm for VLCAD deficiency relies heavily on the molecular sequencing because patients with VLCAD deficiency have been reported to have normal biochemical follow-up testing of an abnormal newborn screen consistent with this disorder

program, but this group is not always filled with clinicians and scientists, and it may not be as influential as a strong lobbyist or lobbying group. The respective state's Health Department has central role in regulating the logistics of screening and compliance throughout the state. The Health Department also is in charge of ensuring that a positive newborn screen is followed up in a reasonable time, and this may include sending law enforcement authorities to insure that a newborn who is screened positive is taken to a clinical geneticist to initiate treatment.

There are several different models utilized in the USA for each NBS programs' design involving the relationships between the State's Department of Health, the testing laboratory, and the physicians who perform newborn screening follow-up. The first of these models involves an all-inclusive system where the State's Department of Health coordinates the collection and transport of blood spots, performs each test in a government laboratory, and provides referrals to physicians and nurses the patients with abnormal newborn screening results. This all-inclusive model exists in Florida. The second model involves the State's Department of Health performing all the aforementioned tasks with the exception of the testing. In this model, the testing might be performed by a commercial lab, as in Washington, DC, or by another state's NBS laboratory, as is the case for New Mexico, whose newborn screening is performed by Oregon's NBS laboratory.

In Minnesota, there exists a third system, where the Minnesota Department of Health (MDH) coordinates the logistics of collection and transport of blood spots. Once the blood spot cards are transported to a central MDH facility, three of the five blood spots on each card are catalogued and retained to screen for all non-MS/MS assays. The other two spots are couriered to the Mayo Clinic, where they are run for all MS/MS assays. MDH handles the reporting of positive screens and ensures that the positive patient will be seen by the genetics clinic at the University of Minnesota.

How residual dried blood spots are stored and how consent is acquired differ between each state and both are controversial topics. In the past, residual dried blood spots were often used for assay development, proficiency testing, quality control, and research, and the residual specimens were retained as long as possible. The duration of storage widely varied between each state and was usually related to the amount of physical space that a specific program had for sample storage. In recent years, the retention of dried blood spots is limited and tightly controlled because of the risk to potentially disclose genetic information that can now be obtained from DNA, which can readily be isolated from blood spots. This was exemplified when Texas was accused of shipping NBS residual blood spots to the military for the generation of a forensic database [17].

There have been two recent court cases, one in Texas and the other in Minnesota, which centered on the issue of informed consent and retention and use of residual dried blood spots. Up to this point, every state had an opt-out policy, where the parents must explicitly state that they do not consent to their child to be screened. This differs from most medical procedures, which are based on an opt-in system, whereby the parents must consent that they want a procedure performed on their child before the procedure can be done. The Texas Department of Health lost and the result was the mandatory destruction of all stored dried blood spots and the requirement to obtain informed consent for each newborn screen. A Minnesota Supreme Court case was ruled against the Minnesota Department of Health, and it has prohibited the use of residual newborn screening specimens for research without informed consent. Other states like Michigan chose to avoid any potential conflicts and altered their process from opt-out to opt-in.

The opt-out method is considered the gold standard by most state programs because it is in the best interest of a newborn's health, and if informed consent was required from a parent or guardian, some newborns may not be screened due to their parent's inability to fully comprehend the screening process and its risks to the infant's privacy. While a balanced view would claim that each side has a basis for concerns, the best manner to address these legal conflicts is by educating the public about the importance and outcomes from newborn screening. The education needs to be widespread with the ability to reach an entire population regardless of socioeconomic status. This is a daunting task that must involve cooperation between different patient advocacy groups, the American College of Obstetrics and Gynecology, the American College of Medical Genetics, the American Medical Association, and the American Society of Genetic Counseling.

Regulation of Laboratories Performing the Newborn Screening and Follow-Up Testing

Many laboratories performing the newborn screening tests as well as those performing most follow-up testing of positive screens are regulated by the Centers for Medicare and Medicaid Services (CMS) and are guided by the Clinical Laboratories Institutional Act of 1988 (CLIA). CMS contracts third-party groups to administer programs to help enforce CLIA, such as College of American Pathologists (CAP), the Joint Commission, JASCO, and others. These groups perform on-site visits, inspections, proficiency testing, and certification of diagnostic laboratories in the USA. This ensures that each laboratory continues to function with the highest quality standards needed for complex genetic and diagnostic testing.

Interpretation of Newborn Screening Testing

Positive or Negative

The result of any newborn screen should be reported as either a positive or a negative result. There is no room for ambiguity or inconclusiveness. It must be recognized that a screen is not a diagnostic test, but is designed to avoid as many false negatives, and to collect as many true positives, as possible. For the genetic conditions detected by MS/MS, the request for a second blood spot collection should be limited as there are laboratory procedures available that can delineate as possible diagnosis in a timely manner, and the alternative would delay the initiation of treatment prior to the onset of irreversible damage.

A positive newborn screen report should list the relevant elevated markers along with corresponding reference ranges, the differential diagnosis of the particular analyte elevations detected in the sample, and a recommendation of appropriate follow-up tests in order to help sort out a final diagnosis. A possible differential diagnosis can include one to five or more possible disorders that are associated with a particular elevation(s). Follow-up guidelines and recommendations should also be listed with an emphasis on a mandatory emergency follow-up procedure.

ACMG ACTion Sheets

Each state has a different protocol for reporting a positive test, but all states have a protocol that involves either contacting the ordering physician to coordinate follow-up testing, or where required, providing a referral to a genetic specialist. Due to the rarity, severity, and complexity of the targeted genetic disorders, the patient is often referred to an experienced geneticist. The American College of Medical Genetics (ACMG) developed *ACTion Sheets* accessible on the web through the ACMG website (http://www.acmg.net) that have simplified instructions for the follow-up of an abnormal newborn screen by the primary health professional. These ACT Sheets have confirmatory testing guidelines and guidance on when referral is required. In addition, the ACMG formed confirmatory algorithms, which guide physicians through the tests to be ordered and reach the diagnosis and confirmation of a positive screen.

Post-analytical Tools

Similarly, post-analytical tools generated by the large amount of data accumulated by the Region 4 Collaborative have allowed screening labs to reliably use ratios of markers not necessarily expected to be informative for a particular disorder to differential true positives. These post-analytical tools can be accessed by all participants at the Region 4 Collaborative website (http://www.region4genetics.org), (personal communication with Piero Rinaldo) [18].

Confirmation of NBS by Molecular Analyses

Following up a positive NBS with molecular analyses previously described in this chapter has become the standard of care in most states. There are three main purposes for the use of molecular diagnostic testing in this capacity.

The first rationale is to provide accurate genetic counseling to an infant's family and to have the ability to screen future pregnancies for the specific mutation detected in the proband. This is the most frequent reason for referral in the clinical molecular genetics laboratories offering these assays. Although not all disorders on the ACMG-recommended panel would qualify, the ability to use preimplantation genetic diagnosis (PGD) to screen fertilized embryos prior to implantation would require the genetic abnormality to be defined in the proband.

The second rationale is for the confirmation of a positive newborn screening result. This is important due to the fact that some disorders can have an abnormal newborn screen result with normal biochemical genetics follow-up testing even though the newborn may have the respective disorder. This is the case with very long-chain acyl-CoA dehydrogenase (VLCAD) deficiency (Fig. 12.2b), where patients have been reported to screen positive by the MS/MS method, but follow-up plasma acylcarnitine analysis is completely normal [19]. The options for clinicians to confirm or dispute the putative positive screen for VLCAD deficiency include molecular analysis, fibroblast culture fatty acid oxidation probe assay, or an enzyme-specific assay in fibroblasts or leukocytes. Considering the time required for culturing cells, and the invasive nature of obtaining a fibroblast biopsy from the patient, molecular analysis is frequently the desired method to confirm a newborn screening result. Additionally, it is possible that some biochemical tests may lead to an equivocal result indicating possible carrier or affected status and cannot be informative without the additional molecular analysis. However, considering the current high cost and low reimbursability of molecular genetics testing in the USA, biochemical genetic testing should be the first line of follow-up testing of an abnormal newborn screen.

The third rationale is to assess the specific genotype of the patient in order to guide therapy. This practice is in its infancy, but as more targeted therapies come into the marketplace, its relevance will increase dramatically. An example of the current use of molecular analysis to guide therapy is in the BH4 responsiveness of PKU. Different genotypes are more amenable to BH4 treatment and therefore this is useful when determining the treatment plan [20].

Unfortunately, these three purposes are frequently bypassed and molecular genetic testing is performed regardless of the usefulness to the patient. This practice is oftentimes unnecessary when the follow-up biochemical genetic testing is confirmatory and diagnostic for a particular disorder. Given the type of analysis and reduced costs associated with biochemical genetic testing, follow-up biochemical assays are more likely to be reimbursed by insurance companies in the USA and usually have faster turnaround times than molecular testing. Therefore, while molecular genetics testing has its utility in the follow-up of an abnormal newborn screen, it should not be used indiscriminately to each situation because of the limitations and pitfalls to molecular analyses.

The limitations of molecular genetics in the current practice of newborn screening are centered on obtaining an equivocal molecular genetic result. The issue that frequently comes up in practice is the occurrences of familial variants of uncertain significance (VUS) and the corresponding poor genotype–phenotype correlation. This is especially problematic in the follow-up of an abnormal newborn screen because it leaves the clinician unable to definitively call the newborn screen a true positive or false positive. This can result in additional and unnecessary follow-up testing and cause undue psychological stress to a family.

Similarly, when a patient has a positive newborn screen and biochemical genetic follow-up testing results disagree with the molecular genetics testing results, irreparable harm can occur to the patient and their family. This often manifests as a positive newborn screening result with confirmatory biochemical genetic testing results but with a subsequent molecular analysis that detects only a single mutation, or one VUS, or one mutation and one VUS. It would be a grave mistake to attempt to negate the positive screen and positive biochemical genetic testing with such a finding, but the molecular testing can also not be ignored. One possibility leading to this scenario could be that both the NBS and the biochemical genetics follow-up testing were incorrect due to an interfering substance, which could be the result of a medication or specific gestational or nutritional factor. Another possibility is that the NBS and the biochemical genetics follow-up testing were correct, but the molecular testing was a false negative. This occurrence is not too infrequent, as with all gene-specific sequencing reactions, large exonic deletions are often missed and rare polymorphisms under a primer's binding site will lead to allele dropout during PCR. These issues can often be delineated with further testing, such as a specific enzyme assay, but this type of testing is typically invasive and increases costs and the turnaround time to a final diagnosis. This period when a NBS-positive infant is neither positive nor negative for a disorder has recently been described as a "patient in waiting," and may have an impact on the psychology of parents [21].

How Newborn Screening Changed the Medical Practice

Newborn screening by MS/MS has dramatically changed the fields of public health, clinical genetics, biochemical genetics, molecular genetics, genetic counseling, and many others. Each newborn in the USA is screened for 29 to 60+ disorders (depending on the state), and approximately 1:700 to 1:800 newborns are now presymtomatically diagnosed and treated, leading to a reduction in harm to the patient and providing an irreplaceable benefit to society. In addition, the financial advantage of screening newborns over the chronic long-term care of individuals diagnosed symptomatically after irreversible damage has been calculated and is consistently demonstrated to be cost-effective from condition to condition [22, 23].

Newborn screening by MS/MS has revolutionized the perception of these rare disorders amongst members of the medical community. In fact, many physicians have never heard of some of the conditions included on the ACMG NBS panel. With the work of the regional collaboratives, the public health community, and the ACMG, there are now freely available follow-up guidelines and algorithms for the diagnosis of each disorder as well as clinical descriptions of their symptoms for the educational benefit of primary care physicians and parents. Universal newborn screening in the USA has pushed these disorders to the forefront of everyone involved in neonatal care. Unfortunately, more education is still needed to inform the public about the benefits of newborn screening, and until this can occur there will continue to be deficiencies in the system.

NBS by MS/MS has also led to an evolution in the characterization of many of the rare disorders selected for inclusion in the ACMG-recommended panel. For instance, disorders that were once thought to be only severe, like isovaleric acidemia (IVA), are now realized to be a spectrum of phenotypes, ranging from very severe to essentially benign. Disorders that were once thought to be pathogenic, like short-chain acyl CoA dehydrogenase (SCAD) deficiency and 2-methylbutyryl CoA dehydrogenase (SBCAD) deficiency, are now classified as benign conditions by most biochemical geneticists and clinical geneticists. Conditions that were once thought to be caused by one common mutation in most cases, like medium-chain acyl-CoA dehydrogenase (MCAD) deficiency with its frequent Northern European 985A>G mutation, are now known to be more often caused by compound heterozygosity with a rare mutation, and less than 50 % of cases are caused by homozygosity of the common allele. And finally, disorders that were once thought to be only present in the newborn period with severe and debilitating disease, like glutaric aciduria, type 1, and VLCAD deficiency, have now been even detected in relatively asymptomatic adult women identified by an abnormal screen on their newborn offspring.

Future Directions

The future of NBS is one of expansion and increased specificity. First, disorders that were excluded from the ACMG-recommended NBS panel due to the lack of an available treatment or an available assay at the time of nomination would be elected for inclusion as these deficiencies are corrected. Lysosomal storage disorders (LSDs) are a great example of this expansion in play. Since the ACMG-recommended NBS panel was made, therapeutics for several of the LSDs have been FDA approved. In addition, among testing modalities, a multiplex-enzyme assay for these disorders using an MS/MS platform has been reported and more recently improved [24, 25].

Diagnostic platforms other than MS/MS are more frequently being used for newborn screening and could rapidly alter the field of NBS. Flow cytometry-based bead array systems, like those available from Luminex, have been shown to have utility in the diagnostic setting for molecular alterations common to cystic fibrosis and can be used to multiplex analytes much like MS/MS methods [26]. Microfluidics- or "Lab-on-a-Chip"-based assays, like those from Advanced Liquid Logics, are starting to be found in diagnostic labs, and they may demonstrate an enhanced potential in regard to multiplexing enzyme assays [27]. Any new technology that has the ability to reduce sample volume will become a necessity as new disorders are added piecemeal to screening panels, as the amount of blood spot surface area on a NBS "Guthrie" card will become a limiting factor the expansion to new conditions. In fact, another attractive outcome of reducing reagent volume is the added benefit of reducing reagent cost as price is another driver of technological advancement.

Finally, we anticipate that in the future some manifestation of DNA sequencing will become an integral part of newborn screening. In order for DNA sequencing to be adopted as a frontline screening methodology, the time of analysis and the cost must be significantly reduced, as well as its sensitivity and specificity must be markedly increased. If current estimates are correct, this should occur not too far in the future. In addition to cost, we anticipate that the bioinformatics needed for whole-genome analysis will eventually be refined to the point that very few de novo alterations will be detected. Indeed, person-to-person variation at the genomic level will likely be the biggest technical challenge facing DNA sequencing as a NBS methodology.

From a technical applications standpoint, there are several key program modifications that must be made in order to exploit the most from a Next-Generation DNA Sequencing (NGS) methodology for newborn screening. The first of which is the need to change the specimen requirements for screening each newborn. The current system's use of filter paper cards, and dried blood spots, is currently insufficient to perform a whole-genome DNA analysis. However, at first glance, cord blood is likely ethically one of the best sample types since a peripheral blood draw on a newborn could be easily avoided and circulating fetal DNA analysis would be socially unacceptable. Another possible, but less desirable option, would be a blood draw within the first year of life. Nevertheless, following up all babies outside of the immediate postpartum period could prove to be difficult and it would fail to aid in the diagnosis and treatment of conditions that appear in the immediate neonatal period.

The next issue facing NGS for newborn screening is the task of deciding what to analyze and what to report. There are currently three options. The first is to perform a targeted gene panel looking only for specific mutations that are known to cause disorders that fall within the Wilson and Jungner criteria. A good starting point would be looking for known mutations that lead to the disorders included in the ACMG-recommended NBS panel. A targeted approach would have the lowest involvement of bioinformatics and could potentially be the most cost-effective, but if the lessons learned from MCAD deficiency have anything to teach, a targeted approach would have the disadvantage of providing a relatively higher false negative outcome over current MS/MS technology. Another viable option would be to perform whole-exome sequencing. With a minimal increase in cost, this approach could potentially have less false negatives, but the bioinformatics involved would be significantly increased as would the time needed to complete each exome analysis. This option has the benefit of potentially detecting a larger number of Mendelian disorders caused by missense mutations, but it also has the potential to uncover a larger number of VUSs present in each patient, and the interpretation of such findings in an asymptomatic newborn could prove to be a daunting task at the start of a program. We also anticipate that a NBS program using this methodology would benefit from a tiered inform-consent process, thereby enabling a parent to select only the disorders for which they wish their child to be screened. Evidence supporting this consent approach is found in the literature surrounding the molecular analysis of Huntington's disease. Many people may not want to know their status for conditions such as Huntington's disease, and a substantial number of parents would be unprepared to deal with this information in the neonatal period. The third option, which is whole-genome sequencing, has potentially the greatest benefit, because it would be all-inclusive, but it is also the most problematic. This large amount of genetic information would enable the detection of known gene mutations and variants of unknown significance, as well as signal nucleotide polymorphisms and copy number variants associated with multifactorial diseases among other genetic changes. While such knowledge is not hard to imagine lying just beyond one's fingertips, it is difficult to anticipate the time it will take to accumulate the necessary bioinformatics to make sense of such information and apply it with the best ethical standards during the newborn period.

References

1. Bickel H. The effects of a phenylalanine-free and phenylalanine-poor diet in phenylpyruvic oligophrenis. Exp Med Surg. 1954;12(1):114–7.
2. Cunningham GC. Phenylketonuria testing—its role in pediatrics and public health. CRC Crit Rev Clin Lab Sci. 1971;2(1):45–101.
3. Guthrie R, Susi A. A simple phenylalanine method for detecting phenylketonuria in large populations of newborn infants. Pediatrics. 1963;32:338–43.
4. Naylor EW, Guthrie R. Newborn screening for maple syrup urine disease (branched-chain ketoaciduria). Pediatrics. 1978;61(2):262–6.
5. Murphey WH, Patchen L, Guthrie R. Screening tests for argininosuccinic aciduria, orotic aciduria, and other inherited enzyme deficiencies using dried blood specimens. Biochem Genet. 1972;6(1):51–9.
6. Dussault JH, Coulombe P, Laberge C, Letarte J, Guyda H, Khoury K. Preliminary report on a mass screening program for neonatal hypothyroidism. J Pediatr. 1975;86(5):670–4.
7. Pang S, Hotchkiss J, Drash AL, Levine LS, New MI. Microfilter paper method for 17 alpha-hydroxyprogesterone radioimmunoassay: its application for rapid screening for congenital adrenal hyperplasia. J Clin Endocrinol Metab. 1977;45(5):1003–8.
8. Thielmann K, Moreira Aquino A. Whole blood samples dried and stored on filter paper as substrate for the electrophoretic separation on hemoglobin S from hemoglobin A. A screening procedure. Clin Chim Acta. 1971;35(1):237–8.
9. Millington DS, Norwood DL, Kodo N, Roe CR, Inoue F. Application of fast atom bombardment with tandem mass spectrometry and liquid chromatography/mass spectrometry to the analysis of acylcarnitines in human urine, blood, and tissue. Anal Biochem. 1989; 180(2):331–9.
10. Millington DS, Kodo N, Norwood DL, Roe CR. Tandem mass spectrometry: a new method for acylcarnitine profiling with potential for neonatal screening for inborn errors of metabolism. J Inherit Metab Dis. 1990;13(3):321–4.
11. Chace DH, Millington DS, Terada N, Kahler SG, Roe CR, Hofman LF. Rapid diagnosis of phenylketonuria by quantitative analysis for phenylalanine and tyrosine in neonatal blood spots by tandem mass spectrometry. Clin Chem. 1993;39(1):66–71.
12. Wilson JM, Junger G. Principles and practice of screening for disease. Geneva: World Health Organization; 1968.
13. McHugh DM, Cameron CA, Abdenur JE, et al. Clinical validation of cutoff target ranges in newborn screening of metabolic disorders by tandem mass spectrometry: a worldwide collaborative project. Genet Med. 2011;13(3):230–54.
14. Matern D, Tortorelli S, Oglesbee D, Gavrilov D, Rinaldo P. Reduction of the false-positive rate in newborn screening by implementation of MS/MS-based second-tier tests: the Mayo Clinic experience (2004–2007). J Inherit Metab Dis. 2007;30(4):585–92.
15. Pass KA, Morrissey M. Enhancing newborn screening for tyrosinemia type I. Clin Chem. 2008;54(4):627–9.
16. Turgeon C, Magera MJ, Allard P, et al. Combined newborn screening for succinylacetone, amino acids, and acylcarnitines in dried blood spots. Clin Chem. 2008;54(4):657–64.
17. Texas Supplied Newborn Blood Samples to Forensic Database. AAAS, 2010. http://news.sciencemag.org/scienceinsider/2010/02/texas-supplied-newborn-blood-sam.html (2010). Accessed 23 Nov 2011.
18. Marquardt G, et al. Enhanced interpretation of newborn screening results without analyte cutoff values. Genet Med. 2012;14(7):648–55.
19. Boneh A, Andresen BS, Gregersen N, et al. VLCAD deficiency: pitfalls in newborn screening and confirmation of diagnosis by mutation analysis. Mol Genet Metab. 2006;88(2):166–70.
20. Desviat LR, Perez B, Belanger-Quintana A, et al. Tetrahydrobiopterin responsiveness: results of the BH4 loading test in 31 Spanish PKU patients and correlation with their genotype. Mol Genet Metab. 2004;83(1–2):157–62.
21. Timmermans S, Buchbinder M. Patients-in-waiting: living between sickness and health in the genomics era. J Health Soc Behav. 2010;51(4):408–23.
22. Venditti LN, Venditti CP, Berry GT, et al. Newborn screening by tandem mass spectrometry for medium-chain Acyl-CoA dehydrogenase deficiency: a cost-effectiveness analysis. Pediatrics. 2003;112(5):1005–15.
23. Norman R, Haas M, Chaplin M, Joy P, Wilcken B. Economic evaluation of tandem mass spectrometry newborn screening in Australia. Pediatrics. 2009; 123(2):451–7.
24. Li Y, Scott CR, Chamoles NA, et al. Direct multiplex assay of lysosomal enzymes in dried blood spots for newborn screening. Clin Chem. 2004;50(10):1785–96.

25. Metz TF, Mechtler TP, Orsini JJ, et al. Simplified newborn screening protocol for lysosomal storage disorders. Clin Chem. 2011;57(9):1286–94.
26. Strom CM, Janeszco R, Quan F, et al. Technical validation of a TM Biosciences Luminex-based multiplex assay for detecting the American College of Medical Genetics recommended cystic fibrosis mutation panel. J Mol Diagn. 2006;8(3):371–5.
27. Sista RS, Eckhardt AE, Wang T, et al. Digital microfluidic platform for multiplexing enzyme assays: implications for lysosomal storage disease screening in newborns. Clin Chem. 2011;57(10):1444–51.

Part IV

Future Directions: The Test That Will Change Everything—Again

Next Generation Clinical Diagnostics: The Sequence of Events

13

Nicole Hoppman, David I. Smith, Eric W. Klee, and Matthew J. Ferber

Introduction

The development of automated sequencing platforms based upon capillary electrophoresis and fluorescently labeled terminator bases made it possible to generate the first draft sequence of the human genome. However, what started as an effort to develop new technologies to sequence entire human genomes cheaper and faster than capillary electrophoresis-based technologies has engendered a sequencing revolution that has resulted in tremendous increases in sequence output capacity. Since the introduction of these so-called next-generation sequencing technologies in 2006, the sequencing output of various platforms has been increasing greater than fivefold every year. This has led to dramatic increases in sequencing output and correspondingly decreased costs for DNA sequencing. These sequencing platforms will quickly make whole genome sequencing so affordable that it will inevitably become a routine part of clinical practice. In this chapter we will review the sequencing revolution and discuss the potential clinical applications of this transformative technology.

History of DNA Sequencing

Technologies to Develop a Draft Sequence of the Human Genome

The human genome is comprised of 6.6 gigabases (Gb, billion bases) of genomic sequence, 3.3 Gb of which is inherited from our mothers and 3.3 Gb from our fathers [1]. Developing the technology to sequence this quantity of DNA has spanned several decades, starting with cumbersome chemical cleavage and manual di-deoxy terminator (Sanger sequencing) methods that utilized gel electrophoresis [2, 3]. The sequencing strategy that was utilized to develop the first draft sequence of the human genome was a semiautomated form of Sanger sequencing, which utilized labeled di-deoxy nucleotides as chain terminators on a large number of identical molecules that were cloned into bacterial plasmids carrying inserts from random locations in the human genome [4]. When this technology

N. Hoppman, Ph.D. (✉)
Clinical Cytogenetics Laboratory, Department of Laboratory Medicine and Pathology, Mayo Clinic College of Medicine, Rochester, MN, USA
e-mail: hoppman.nicole@mayo.edu

D.I. Smith, Ph.D.
Division of Experimental Pathology, Department of Laboratory Medicine and Pathology, Mayo Clinic College of Medicine, Rochester, MN, USA

E.W. Klee, Ph.D.
Division of Biomedical Informatics, Department of Health Sciences Research, Mayo Clinic College of Medicine, Rochester, MN, USA

M.J. Ferber, Ph.D.
Molecular Genetics Laboratory, Department of Laboratory Medicine and Pathology, Mayo Clinic College of Medicine, Rochester, MN, USA

W.E. Highsmith Jr. (ed.), *Molecular Diagnostics: 12 Tests That Changed Everything*, Molecular and Translational Medicine, DOI 10.1007/978-1-4614-8127-0_13,

was first developed, the di-deoxy nucleotides were radioactively labeled; hence, four separate reactions were necessary to terminate the growing chains for each of the four different nucleotides. Each separate reaction was then run on a polyacrylamide gel to separate the different size fragments generated [5].

A significant advance with Sanger sequencing was the utilization of four differently colored, fluorescently labeled di-deoxy nucleotides, which made it possible to run the sequencing reaction for all four nucleotide bases in a single sequencing reaction and gel lane [4]. Another important advance was to develop long, polymer-filled, reusable capillaries to resolve different sized DNA fragments in place of the nonreusable polyacrylamide gels [6]. This was termed capillary electrophoresis (CE). By combining these two advances in a single machine capable of performing up to 96 simultaneous sequencing reactions in approximately 3 hours, such as the ABI3700 (Applied Biosystems, Foster City, CA), it became technically feasible to set up large sequencing facilities with many CE machines in order to sequence hundreds of thousands of independently cloned DNA fragments, which could then be assembled into a draft human genome sequence [7]. This technology has also been leveraged extensively in current clinical diagnostic laboratories, allowing for the development of numerous single gene sequencing assays. In fact, there are currently over 2,300 different genetic tests that are clinically available in the USA, the majority of which are sequencing assays that utilize this technology (GeneTests.org).

Public Versus Private Sequencing Efforts

The development of the first draft sequence of a human genome was done by two competing groups. The first was a public genome sequencing effort based upon two tenets. Tenet one was that the developed sequence would be freely available to everyone as soon as the data was generated [8]. Tenet two was a sequencing strategy based upon a top-down approach where the genome was first fractionated into individual chromosomes, and then the chromosomes themselves were further fractionated into smaller and smaller regions [9]. Eventually, an entire genome contig of physically mapped large insert clones could be sequenced by sub-cloning the large insert pieces into even smaller, overlapping inserts, followed by sequencing on a CE machine [10]. This public genome sequencing effort also utilized a number of orthogonal strategies including the generation of both physical and genetic maps of the human genome, which provided a genomic framework to string together the resulting sequences into a coherent integrated genome sequence [11].

The alternative sequencing strategy was a private effort pioneered by Craig Venter and his colleagues at Celera. Their hope was to develop a draft sequence of the human genome to be made commercially available to the scientific community. The Celera effort utilized a bottom-up sequencing strategy based upon shot-gun cloning of the entire genome into small, overlapping cloned fragments, which could then be sequenced randomly and assembled together into a first draft sequence using powerful bioinformatics [12].

There was considerable competition between the public and private genome sequencing efforts, as well as much discussion about which of these two strategies was superior. Much of the discussion was regarding whether or not the necessary raw computing power existed to assemble the gargantuan numbers of sequencing reads without a framework to reference them to. Eventually, due to advances in bioinformatics and computer hardware, it became clear that the shot-gun sequencing strategy was the easier and more straightforward method to generate a draft sequence. However, the efforts of Craig Venter and his Celera colleagues were reportedly facilitated by utilizing some of the framework mapping performed by the public genome effort [12]. In 2000, both the public and the private sequencing efforts published their first draft sequences [11, 12].

The combined scientific contribution of these two efforts towards the development of Next Generation DNA sequencing should not be underappreciated. The presence of a physical reference map of the human genome allowed for the development of unguided approaches where a priori knowledge of the sequence generated was no longer a requirement for successful DNA sequencing. This allowed scientists to propose systems that could generate massive amounts of DNA sequencing data without knowledge of its spatial relationship to any other sequence in the experiment. These random sequences were then placed into a meaningful context by utilizing powerful computers that could map them back to the reference sequence.

Lessons Learned from the Human Genome Project

The first draft sequences provided important answers to a number of questions about the future of genome sequencing. One of these was the cost for generating the first draft sequence, which was an astounding three billion dollars [13]. This was considerably less than it would have cost if not for the advances in CE fluorescent sequencing. However, in order to make routine genome sequencing feasible it would be necessary to further decrease this cost substantially, most probably with a completely distinct sequencing platform from CE.

The generation of these draft sequences coupled with the implementation of "genome browsers" such as the University of California Santa Cruz (UCSC) genome database made it very straightforward for researchers to design polymerase chain reaction (PCR) primers anywhere within the sequenced genome in order to amplify that specific region of any individual. This greatly facilitated efforts to more quickly identify underlying mutations that were responsible for many Mendelian disorders as well as identify important mutational targets during the development of different cancers.

Next Generation Sequencing

Putting together a sequencing factory based upon many CE machines with each generating 96 simultaneous sequences every 3 hours made it possible to generate the first draft sequences. However, the cost of the first genome sequences was over three billion dollars and took several years. While it would certainly be less expensive to generate subsequent human genome sequences, especially since the genome assembly would no longer be de novo but instead based upon the existing draft sequences, considerable advances in sequencing technology were still necessary such that the cost and turnaround time for an individual genome sequence could decrease adequately to be useful for basic, scientific research. Ultimately, the hope was that the costs would eventually decrease sufficiently to be useful for routine clinical testing. With the development of next-generation sequencing (NGS) platforms, this hope is now becoming a reality.

The unifying feature of all NGS platforms is the ability to perform massively parallel DNA sequencing in a non-relational format. While the ABI 3,700 generates 96 simultaneous sequences using CE, the first NGS sequencer could generate hundreds of thousands of sequencing reactions simultaneously, and current high-throughput machines are capable of generating billions of fragments simultaneously. The major similarities between Next Generation sequencing platforms and Sanger sequencing are the need to isolate individual fragments from a genome, and to produce sufficiently large amounts such that the signal generated by the sequencer is detectable. Early applications of Sanger sequencing, up to and including the Human Genome Project, utilized bacterial cloning for the first step and expanded each bacterial colony that harbored an insert bearing plasmid in liquid culture on a milliliter scale for the second step. Current clinical sequencing assays accomplish this using PCR. The individual fragment is isolated by amplifying the DNA between the two PCR primers. Sufficient quantities for analysis are produced by choosing the appropriate number of thermal cycling steps. Both the bacterial cloning and PCR strategies are easily automatable for production on a reasonably large scale (hundreds to thousands of reactions per day). Indeed, the PCR-based strategy is used routinely by both clinical and research laboratories daily. However, for truly massive throughput (hundreds of thousands

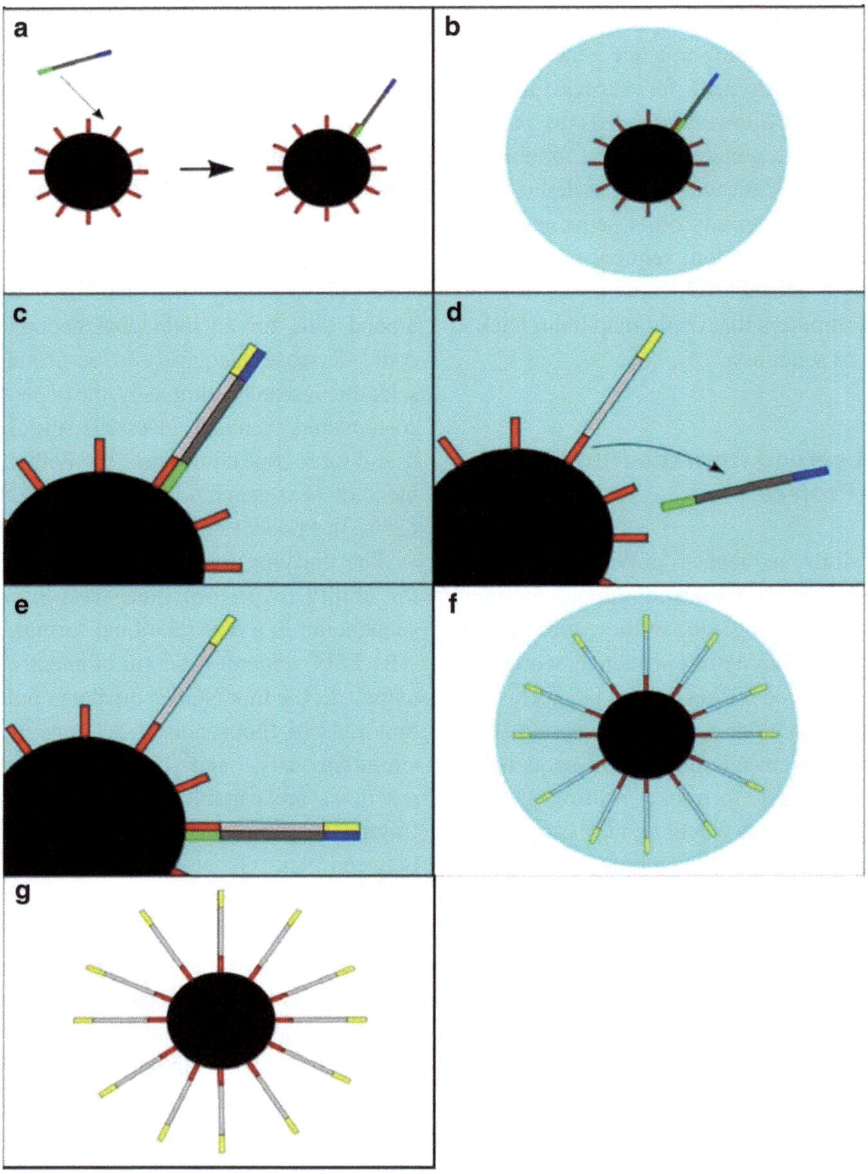

Fig. 13.1 Emulsion PCR. (**a**) Template with ligated adapters is mixed with beads containing complementary adapters. (**b**) Beads with attached template are emulsified in droplets containing PCR reaction components. (**c–f**) Standard PCR reaction amplifies product attached to beads. (**g**) Droplet lysed, amplified product is ready for sequencing

to millions of reactions per day), these methodologies are insufficient. However, recently two key amplification strategies were developed that enabled massively parallel NGS methodologies: emulsion PCR and bridge amplification.

Emulsion PCR utilizes very small water droplets in a lipid solution, creating individual PCR reaction vessels that amplify specific DNA fragments onto small beads (Fig. 13.1) [14]. Key to this approach is balancing the concentrations of DNA and beads in the reaction such that, on average, each emulsion droplet contains a single copy of the DNA starting material. If this is the case, then the product produced by the PCR amplification within the droplet is pure, representing only a single allele. Furthermore, as one of the PCR

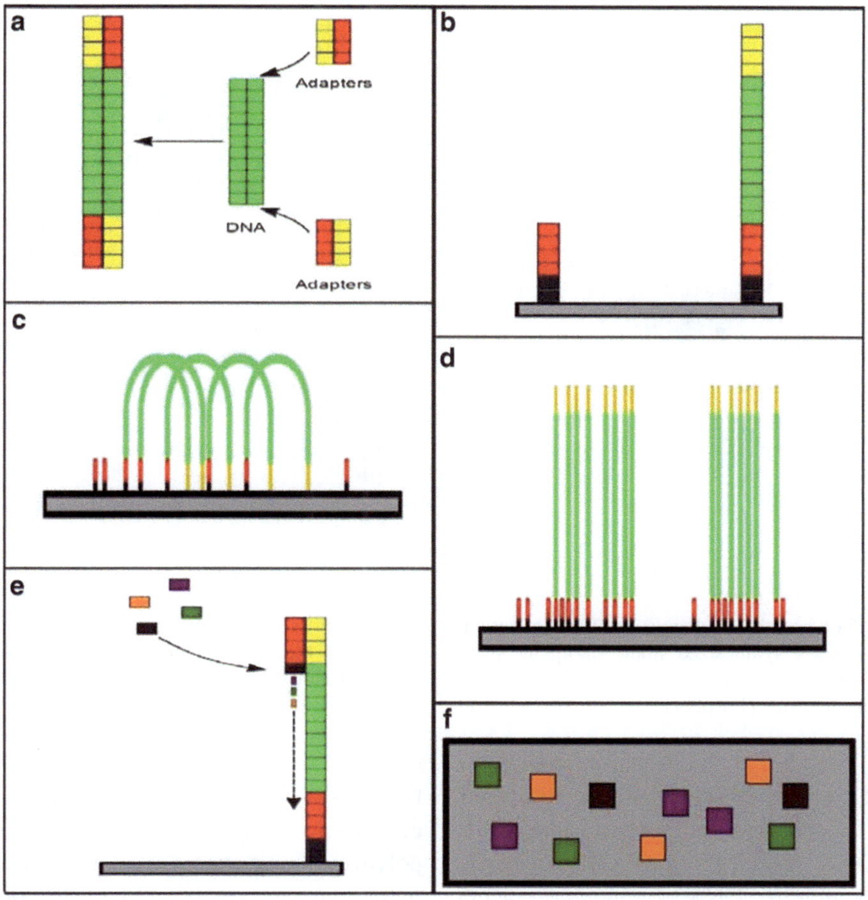

Fig. 13.2 Bridge amplification and Illumina sequencing chemistry. (**a**) Adapters ligated to randomly fragmented DNA. (**b**) Fragments attach to flow cell randomly. (**c–d**) Bridge amplification generates multiple copies of DNA fragment, resulting in clusters of DNA fragments containing universal sequencing primer sequences. (**e**) Fluorescent reversible terminator nucleotides wash over flow cell, extending sequencing by one base per cycle. (**f**) Image of flow cell captured, after which fluorescent molecular and block removed. New sequencing cycle begins

primers is chemically tethered to the surface of the beads, the resulting pure, amplified product is bound to the bead surface. Depending upon the size of the beads, each bead will carry a unique DNA fragment with 50,000 to 1 million copies bound per bead. The beads containing amplified DNA can then be used by one of several NGS sequencing platforms [15].

The alternative to emulsion PCR is bridge amplification. Instead of using emulsions and small beads, the actual amplification occurs on a slide surface coated with oligonucleotides complementary to those that have been ligated onto the ends of a sheared DNA sample [16]. If the DNA with the adapter oligonucleotides ligated to the ends (the library) is bound to the slide at sufficiently low concentration, individual molecules of DNA are physically isolated on the slide. Adding PCR reagents and thermal cycling of the slide gives a solid phase PCR reaction that can generate 30–50,000 copies of each individual fragment. Advances in slide design and reaction conditions now allow for the production of millions of clonally amplified DNA, which can then undergo the sequencing reactions (Fig. 13.2).

Once library preparation is completed using a methodology such as emulsion PCR or bridge amplification, the DNA is ready to be sequenced on an NGS machine. The first NGS platform to be commercialized was the 454 Genome Sequencer

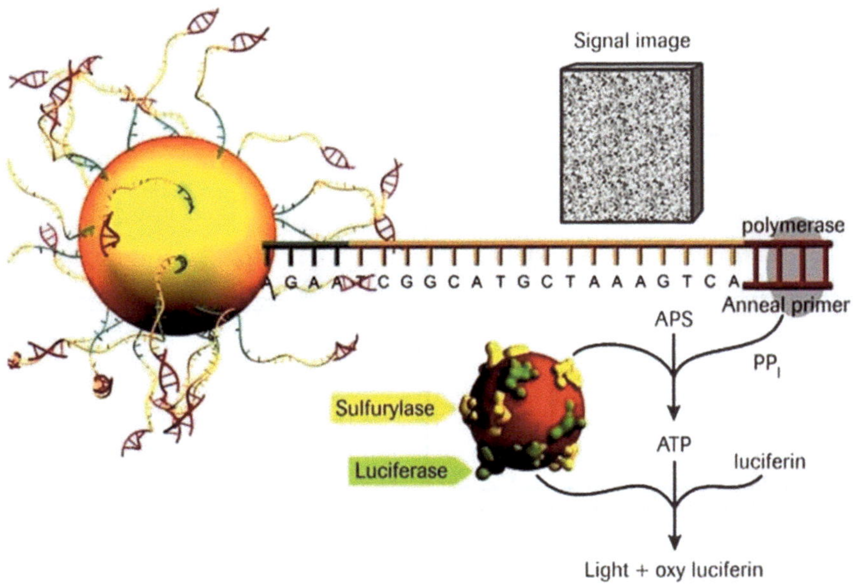

Fig. 13.3 454 sequencing chemistry. When a base is added to the newly synthesized strand, inorganic pyrophosphate (PPI) is released. ATP sulfurylase uses PPI in a reaction with adenosine phosphosulfate (APS) to generate ATP, which is in turn utilized by the enzyme luciferase along with the substrate luciferin to produce light. The light is detected by a camera and indicates incorporation of that base into the growing DNA strand

(454 Life Sciences, a Roche Company, Branford, CT) [17]. This platform utilizes emulsion PCR to amplify DNA fragments onto 28 μm beads. Beads with amplified DNA are spun into a picotiter plate constructed from fiber optic cables, and then hundreds of thousands of beads are simultaneously sequenced by pyrosequencing. The picotiter plate is first flooded with dATP, and those beads that incorporate adenosine at their first position generate light via the pyrosequencing reaction that is detected by a CCD camera. The machine then repeats the same process with the remaining three bases, one at a time. By continuing this process 454 instrument is able to generate hundreds of bases of sequence from each bead in the experiment (Fig. 13.3).

The strength of this platform was how it dramatically increased sequence output from CE sequencing. The first 454 machines could generate 20 megabases (Mb, millions of bases) of sequence data in a 12-h run, and this quickly increased to over 500 Mb in just a few years. Other advantages included sequence read length (which was comparable to CE sequencing) and overall sequence accuracy. However, there were several key disadvantages to this platform. The first was problems in distinguishing the number of bases in a sequence while sequencing homopolymers (long stretches of a single base). In pyrosequencing reactions, the incorporation of a nucleotide into a growing strand of newly synthesized DNA is coupled to a luciferase reaction such that each incorporation event yields a photon of light. For example, when a single A occurs in a sequencing reaction, the pyrosequencing instrument will record a "flash" of light from a bead located at a particular place on the plate when the plate is flooded with dATP. When two A's occur in a sequence, two photons of light are generated. However, due to inefficiencies in the chemistry and in optical geometry, the intensity of the two photons observed is not quite double that seen from one. Nevertheless, it is straightforward to distinguish one A from two, two from three, and three from four A's in a row. However, when there are approximately eight nucleotides or more in a stretch of homopolymer sequence, it becomes increasingly difficult to accurately assess the correct number of bases. A second problem was that the emulsion PCR steps are clumsy, messy, and cumbersome, although automation of the process could solve this problem.

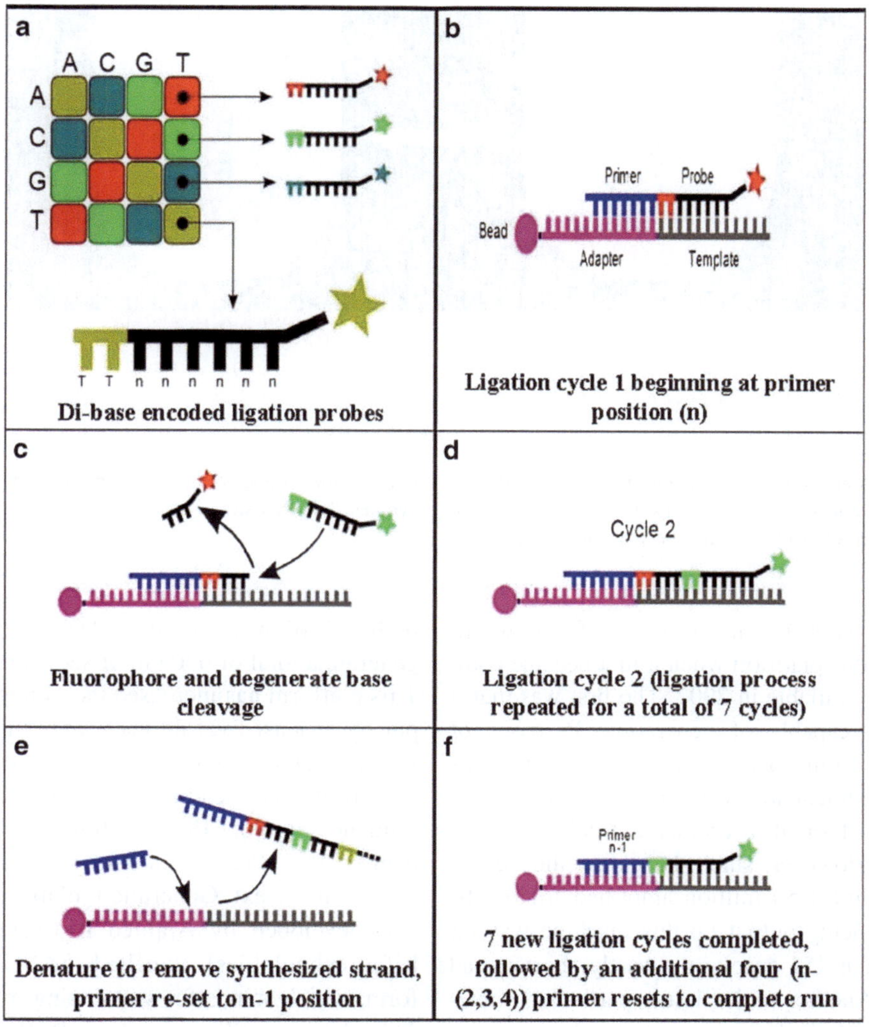

Fig. 13.4 SOLiD sequencing chemistry. (**a**) Sequencing probes are fluorescently labeled di-base probes that interrogate two-base positions at a time. (**b**) During ligation cycle 1, a di-base probe anneals to the template strand and is ligated to the sequencing primer. Unbound probe is washed away, and the fluorescent signal is imaged. (**c**) The fluorophore and degenerate bases are cleaved, so that (**d**) the second ligation cycle can begin. This is repeated for a total of seven cycles. (**e**) The newly synthesized strand is denatured to remove, and a new sequencing primer is added that is one basepair off ($n - 1$). (**f**) Seven new ligation cycles are completed, and an additional four primer resets are then performed to complete the sequencing run

Ultimately, this platform was limited by its inability to compete with the volume of sequence output that other approaches were able to achieve.

A second platform, developed by Solexa Inc. and later purchased by Illumina Inc. (San Diego, CA), utilizes bridge amplification to generate many millions of DNA fragments, which are then sequenced with four different colored, blocked, and fluorescently labeled terminated nucleotides in a “sequencing by synthesis” strategy [18]. Briefly, all four nucleotides are washed over the glass slide (flow cell) simultaneously. Because the nucleotides are blocked at the 3′ position by the fluorescent tag, only one can be added per round of sequencing, effectively solving the homopolymer problem. After each base addition, a camera takes a picture of the colored nucleotides that are incorporated at each cluster. Then, the fluorescent and blocking tags are chemically removed, and the slide is flooded with fresh-labeled nucleotides for the next base addition (Fig. 13.4).

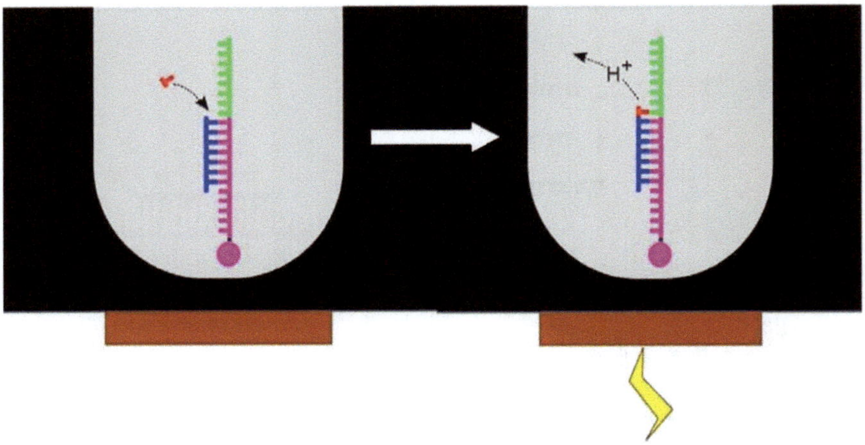

Fig. 13.5 Ion Torrent sequencing chemistry. Real-time base incorporation is monitored inside the wells of an Ion Torrent microchip by sensing the pH change upon H+ release when a nucleotide is incorporated into the newly synthesized DNA strand

There were a number of significant weaknesses to this platform when it first became commercially available in 2007. The first was that it was only capable of generating 36 bases of sequence from each amplified fragment. This made alignment to the reference sequence and detection of small insertions and deletions very difficult. However, since the entire slide could contain almost 50 million amplified fragments, the sequencing output on this machine was far greater than 454 despite the vastly shorter read lengths. Another major issue, particularly relevant to the clinical laboratory, is that this sequencing platform is quite slow, with a single run requiring 5–14 days of run time on the machine. A third problem is sequence accuracy, which was less than 454 and progressively decreases towards the end of the sequencing read.

Despite these disadvantages, there are a number of key strengths to this platform, such as the tremendous potential for greater sequence output. This has already been accomplished by the combination of improvements in the sequencing chemistry, which have now resulted in the capability of sequencing 150 base pair reads off both ends of the amplified fragments, and by dramatically increasing the number of amplified fragments that can be sequenced simultaneously on the flow cell. The current Illumina sequencing machines (the HiSeq 2000) can generate 150 bases of sequence from both ends of over two billion DNA fragments to generate a total of 600 Gb of sequence per run. This platform has increased its sequencing output by at least fivefold each year since it was first available in early 2007. Because of these improvements leading to its impressive sequence output, this machine has captured over 65 % of the NGS market.

A third Next Generation platform, which was developed by Applied Biosystems (now Life Technologies), is called the SOLiD platform, which stands for sequencing by ligation. This platform utilizes emulsion PCR to amplify fragments onto beads with a radius of 0.5 μm, which are then covalently attached to a slide surface. The actual sequencing is done by ligating oligonucleotides to the amplified DNA fragments on the beads (Fig. 13.5) [19]. The strength of this platform is that each base is actually analyzed twice (in a process called two-base encoding) for potentially greater sequence accuracy. However, this platform has a number of limitations that include the cumbersome emulsion PCR, shorter read-lengths (now maximizing around 50–60 bp), and the fact that the output from this sequencing platform is now lagging behind that currently obtained on the Illumina platform (the current output on the SOLiD platform is about 80 Gb, while the HiSeq 2000 can currently generate over 600 Gb per run).

One common theme among the first three NGS platforms that were commercially available is that all used an optical (fluorescent or pyrosequencing) method for the actual sequence detection. A fourth platform, The Ion Torrent, represents a different strategy for massively parallel sequencing. This instrument utilizes the same emulsion PCR and sequencing chemistry that the 454 does, but instead of using a CCD camera to detect the incorporation of nucleotides, the sequencing reaction is performed in tiny semiconductor-based chips [20]. This platform takes advantage of the hydrogen atom released following base addition and measures the pH changes in the small sequencing wells as a result (Fig. 13.6). There are a number of strengths to this sequencing platform. First, since it is based upon semiconductors, there is considerable headroom for improvements in sequence output. In fact, this platform has seen a tenfold increase in sequence output every 6 months over the past 18 months. A second strength is that the nucleotides utilized are non-modified; hence, they are much cheaper than the bases used in many other Next Generation sequencing platforms. However, there are weaknesses to this platform, including the need for emulsion PCR and the fact that the unmodified, and thus unblocked, bases have the same homopolymer problem as the 454 sequencing platform.

Single Molecule Sequencing

Each of the NGS platforms discussed above has amplification-related limitations affecting accuracy of the platform. In addition, the shorter read lengths of some NGS platforms create problems with sequence alignment when the generated sequence diverges significantly from the reference. Also, it is often important to know if a series of variants are linked to one another on the same or different chromosomes. Short read platforms do not allow for direct evaluation of "phase." An obvious solution to this problem is to sequence individual, large, unamplified molecules, as this circumvents many of the aforementioned problems inherent with short read, amplification-based strategies.

The first company to develop a single molecule sequencer was Helicos Inc. (Cambridge, MA) [21]. This machine has been commercially available for several years, but this platform has been plagued by two significant issues. The first is sequencing accuracy, largely due to the fact that there is no signal amplification strategy employed in most single molecule sequencing strategies. This makes it difficult for the detection devices to "recognize" when base incorporation actually happened. The second impediment has been the high cost of the instrument itself. Together, these have resulted in poor commercial adaption of this platform.

A potentially more viable single molecule sequencer was developed by Pacific Biosciences (Lacey, WA). Their platform tethers a single DNA polymerase molecule to the bottom of a sequencing chamber (a zero mode waveguide chamber) and then uses four different fluorescently labeled nucleotides [22]. The strength of this platform is that it generates sequence data very quickly (just a few minutes to generate hundreds of bases of sequence from a template) and that it generates relatively long reads (sometimes in excess of several kilobases). However, the sequence accuracy of this machine is quite poor (barely 86 %), and the current total output per run of this machine is very low. The output of this platform is, however, ideal for analyzing the genome sequence from organisms with small genomes such as bacteria. Another strength of this platform is its ability to discern unmethylated cytosines from methylated cytosines (as well as other base modifications); hence, it could have potential applications in analyzing genomic methylation patterns [23].

The next generation of single molecule sequencing machines currently being developed are those that use some type of nanopore device through which individual DNA molecules are pushed or pulled. The nanopores can be either biologically formed by a pore-forming protein in a membrane such as a lipid bilayer or solid state, formed in synthetic materials such as silicon nitride or grapheme. One company working on this type of system is Oxford Nanopore, which is developing a sequencer that works by passing intact DNA polymers through a protein nanopore [24]. They are currently commercializing machines that should be available by the end of 2012.

Obviously, the NGS field is incredibly dynamic and there are many different competing platforms. Unfortunately, these technologies are developing so rapidly that they are also highly disruptive; when a laboratory purchases one of these instruments, by the time they have it in place and generating data, it is nearly obsolete. In spite of this, the competition in this field has resulted in sequencing capabilities increasing at least fivefold every year over the past 5 years. This has decreased the cost of sequencing an entire human genome from three billion dollars (in 2000) to greater than one million dollars (in 2007) to the current cost of about $2,000 (in 2012) [25]. This decrease in cost is projected to continue further as sequence output continues to increase.

Genome Complexity Reduction

Next Generation sequencing can also be utilized to sequence only a portion of the genome. For example, one might only be interested in a small panel of genes involved in a specific disease process. There are a variety of technologies that can be employed to reduce genome complexity and isolate specific regions or genes of interest prior to sequencing. This enables clinical tests to be developed that target multiple genes at a cost point cheaper than current molecular genetic tests that only analyze a single gene, one exon at a time.

There are two distinct strategies that have been used to capture defined portions of the genome. The first utilizes a hybridization strategy with oligonucleotide probes either on a microarray surface or in solution [26, 27]. Of the various hybridization platforms available, one that works quite well is the Agilent SureSelect platform (Fig. 13.7). There are a number of advantages to this platform including low set-up costs and its inherent flexibility to enable efficient capture of either small numbers or very large numbers of targets. One powerful application of this technology is the capture of all 200,000 exons in the genome (the "exome"). SureSelect can be utilized to select for the 38 Mb of the exome that can be very readily sequenced at excellent depth on a fraction of an Illumina HiSeq 2000 flow cell lane.

The alternative to the hybridization strategy is a PCR-based method using microfluidic droplets [28]. One excellent example of this is RainDance, which performs PCR reactions in microfluid droplets. The advantage of this platform is the high efficiency and specificity with which it amplifies the desired targets. However, this system requires an expensive equipment purchase and is limited in the number of targets that you can enrich for in a single experiment.

Clinical Applications

Introduction

For several years after the first publication introduced next-generation sequencing (NGS) to the world [17], these technologies rapidly took the research realm by storm. Not only were entire genomes of multiple organisms, including humans, being sequenced in a matter of weeks or, later, days, but cancer genomes were also interrogated and compared to normal tissue in the same patient. NGS led to many important discoveries, many of which had potentially important clinical implications. However, in its beginnings, the error rates of next-generation sequencing technologies compared to the Sanger method were high, and the cost was not sufficiently low to consider it for clinical use. Over a short time, with improvements in chemistry, the error rate has dropped to near Sanger levels. At the same time, the cost has plummeted nearly 10,000-fold [29]. Because of these two key advances, NGS now promises to revolutionize clinical testing across the board, in areas including but not limited to testing for congenital Mendelian disorders, oncology, and infectious disease. However, this technology is not without its pitfalls. The potential uses, advantages, and disadvantages of NGS in a clinical setting will be discussed here, using congenital (Mendelian) disorders as a model.

Small Gene Sequencing Panels

DNA-based sequencing for congenital disorders utilizing the Sanger method typically consists of assays examining genes known to harbor mutations with known, well-characterized clinical phenotypes. However, to limit the cost of testing, most clinical laboratories performing this type of testing limit their assays to include only the exons, splice junctions, and, in some cases, the promoter and other regulatory regions. Since deep, intronic disease causing mutations are extremely rare, focusing on these regions not only dramatically decreases the cost of a sequencing assay, but it also decreases turnaround time and limits discovery of variants of unknown significance (VUS) while maintaining a sensitivity of up to 99 % in many cases.

From the clinicians' perspective, test ordering in the case of a symptomatic patient typically follows an algorithm in which the initial test(s) ordered depends on the phenotype of the patient. For example, in a case where a diagnosis of cystic fibrosis (CF) is suspected, *CFTR* gene sequencing would be ordered; since this is the only gene in which mutations have been identified that cause CF [30], it is the only gene that needs to be sequenced. In situations such as this, Sanger sequencing is generally an ideal method and is often accompanied by a separate assay to detect large deletions and duplications encompassing one or more exons. However, when several genes are known to cause a particular phenotype, gene panels can be utilized to sequence multiple genes either simultaneously or in a tiered approach where the most commonly mutated genes are sequenced first, and the remainder are sequenced only if a negative or inconclusive result is obtained. This concept is exemplified by the case of nonsyndromic hereditary hearing loss, for which multiple genes are known to harbor mutations that result in hearing loss; however, mutations in *GJB2* are responsible for up to half of all autosomal recessive cases. Therefore, the approach to genetic testing in a patient with hereditary hearing loss typically begins with sequencing of *GJB2*, and then, if pathogenic mutations are not identified, reflexing to sequencing of one or more other genes will likely be considered [31].

There is an obvious interpretive advantage to this approach, as the diagnostic value from sequencing one or a few well-characterized genes is relatively high, minimizing the likelihood that a variant of undermined significance (VUS) will be discovered. On the other hand, genes that are not well characterized with only a few known pathogenic mutations are unlikely to ever be added to a laboratory's test menu because the probability of detecting a pathogenic mutation does not justify the cost of developing, validating, and performing a clinical sequencing test for that mutation utilizing the Sanger method. However, by limiting the number of genes included in an assay, one also effectively lowers the overall sensitivity of the test. Therefore, patients in whom a specific diagnosis is being questioned are sometimes unable to obtain a positive mutation test result because additional testing is not available through a CLIA-certified laboratory. This is a major obstacle in conducting testing in at-risk relatives for carrier status, presymptomatic testing, prenatal diagnosis, and in some cases this may even prevent the correct diagnosis from being obtained.

Next generation sequencing overcomes these disadvantages by allowing low-cost, massively parallel sequencing of potentially hundreds or even thousands of potential gene targets. The concept of disease-centered sequencing panels is quite feasible using next-generation sequencing. One begins by utilizing one of the genome complexity reduction strategies mentioned earlier. These methods are customizable so that only the gene(s) of interest will be captured and isolated; hence, a laboratory could develop and offer several disease and/or phenotype-specific custom panels for physicians to choose from. This not only allows sequencing of only the target of interest but also eliminates the majority of unwanted genetic material from being sequenced. Therefore, most of the reads obtained will be of relevance. This helps the laboratory director focus his or her attention on only the genes of interest, and also physically decreases the amount of bases sequenced per patient. Therefore, multiple patients can be run in a single lane via multiplexing, dramatically decreasing both the cost and turnaround time of the test.

In addition, this technology allows both the most common and extremely rare disease genes to be screened in parallel for mutations, greatly increasing the sensitivity of the test, at lower cost than the Sanger method. However, one of the most obvious drawbacks to adding rare genes is that these genes are less likely to be well characterized in terms of both benign and disease-causing mutations. Therefore, the chance that the laboratory will identify a VUS increases with each additional gene sequenced. Furthermore, the current commercially available capture reagents typically do not include introns and regulatory regions, due to lack of mutations in these regions as well as physical difficulty with capturing such regions because they typically have more repetitive elements and higher G+C content than the coding regions. So, these sequencing panels are also likely to be limited to exons, splice junctions, and regulatory elements with known pathogenic mutations for the time being.

The majority of known pathogenic mutations described for most Mendelian disorders to date are point mutations or small insertion/deletion mutations that can be detected by either Sanger or next-generation technologies. However, the current algorithm of genome complexity reduction followed by NGS is not amenable to detection of large deletions and duplications. Therefore, as with the Sanger method, supplementary deletion/duplication analysis must also be performed to identify large deletions and duplications that traditional sequencing assays are not able to detect (i.e., whole exon, multi-exon, whole gene, etc.) in order to offer a complete, comprehensive test panel. Currently, several methodologies are utilized to detect deletions and duplications. Southern blot is a low-cost but low-throughput, time and labor intensive method for detecting large variants which is currently being phased out of many clinical laboratories. Quantitative polymerase chain reaction (qPCR) and multiplex ligation-dependent probe amplification (MLPA) [32] are faster, less laborious methods which have gained popularity over the last several years and are being increasingly utilized in clinical laboratories. Although methods such as qPCR and MLPA are useful in determining the presence and extent of large deletions and duplications, they are limited in the number of sites one can multiplex and interrogate within the same reaction.

While these techniques are suitable when analyzing a single or handful of genes, the addition of a large number of genes to a sequencing panel requires more high-throughput methods in order to decrease cost, effort, and turnaround time. Targeted array comparative genomic hybridization (array CGH) is currently the most suitable method to use as a complementary deletion/duplication analysis for large gene sequencing panels [33, 34]. Such arrays are commercially available in multiple formats and probe densities, and are customizable so that a laboratory can select probes to interrogate only the genes of interest at high density. Since the frequency of large deletions and duplications is quite low, one could perform the sequencing portion of the test first and reflex to the copy number analysis portion only if the sequencing result is negative; however, this potential cost savings is offset by the increased turnaround time. Furthermore, despite the hope that an expanded panel will increase sensitivity, the reality may be that the majority of patients tested will nevertheless be negative for a known disease-causing mutation for a variety of reasons. First, many patients will be tested even if they do not fit, or weakly satisfy, the criteria for a given phenotype, especially if the cost of sequencing continues to decline. Second, although an expanded panel will have increased sensitivity, a large proportion of variants will still not be identified either due to location in a gene not included in the panel or a region of a known gene that is not covered by the sequencing assays. Also, a significant proportion of variants identified will be of unknown significance, in which case copy number analysis will still be necessary to exclude the possibility of a known pathogenic deletion or duplication. Therefore, a tiered approach to testing would theoretically decrease costs for a limited set of patients, while leading to increased turnaround time for the majority of patients.

Expanded Panels

Disease-specific gene panels performed by NGS are already being utilized in clinical molecular diagnostics and will become more widespread over time. However, NGS easily has the potential to expand beyond these focused panels. Complexity-reduction techniques can be utilized to create more diffuse panels, which could have implications for the "healthy" population and revolutionize the public health sector. For example, an obvious extension of disease-specific panels would be a panel that includes every known autosomal recessive and X-linked disorder, which could be performed on an individual as a carrier screening panel. Presently, carrier screening panels are typically targeted towards populations with high carrier frequencies for certain Mendelian disorders. For example, due to a founder effect, the Ashkenazi Jewish population has a high carrier frequency for several disorders, including Tay–Sachs disease, Gaucher disease, Bloom Syndrome, and several others. Preconception carrier testing is encouraged in this population in order to identify couples who are carriers for the same autosomal recessive disorders and has resulted in a dramatic reduction in the incidence of these disorders in the Ashkenazi Jewish population [35]. This type of carrier testing is performed using a targeted mutation panel that tests only for mutations known to have a high frequency in the target population. Hence, the test has high sensitivity and specificity within this population.

For individuals not of Ashkenazi Jewish ancestry, unless an affected family member has been diagnosed with a particular disorder and has a documented mutation, carrier testing is not feasible, as there are hundreds of known autosomal recessive disorders for which any one person could be a carrier. Furthermore, with a few exceptions, the majority of mutations causing autosomal recessive disorders are private, familial mutations that can be found anywhere throughout a given gene. Therefore, for the general population, carrier screening for any such autosomal recessive disorder without a documented familial mutation currently would have to be performed by Sanger sequencing, which is too expensive and low throughput to be carried out on a large scale. Next-generation sequencing, on the other hand, has the potential to open the door for general population-based screening of autosomal recessive disorders.

Although technically feasible, this type of testing is not without its disadvantages. As with the small, disease-focused panels, as the number of genes sequenced increases, so does the number of variants of undetermined significance one will uncover. As clinical laboratories are able to increase their test menus and examine genes in which mutations have been described rarely, this will become an increasingly large issue.

Whole Exome/Whole Genome Sequencing

The decreasing cost of NGS is now enabling the sequencing of every exon at a cost comparable to that of some focused panels. Although the number of exons sequenced will increase, the cost will still be relatively low given that less than 1.5 % of the genome contains coding exons. Hence, exome sequencing is the next logical step after the panels mentioned above; the only difference being that instead of examining only known, clinically relevant exons, a laboratory instead utilizes a capture method to sequence every exon in the human genome. Exome sequencing has made headlines recently in the research realm as a useful tool for identifying causative mutations for patients in whom a genetic disorder is suspected but either no known gene has been identified, or all known genes have been tested with negative results. Recent examples of this include Kabuki Syndrome (mutations in *MLL2*), Fowler Syndrome (mutations in *FLVCR2*), and many others (reviewed in [36]). This technology has been particularly useful in cases of very rare

Mendelian disorders, for which linkage studies are impossible due to the lack of families available for testing, and sporadic disorders.

Whole genome sequencing is, then, the logical next step after whole exome sequencing. In fact, exome sequencing will likely be a short-lived bridge in-between targeted panels and whole genome sequencing, as it will rapidly be cheaper and faster to simply sequence genomic DNA directly rather than utilize capture methodologies as a sample preparation method, which adds time, money, and complexity to clinical testing. The other major advantage to whole genome sequencing is that by using modified protocols, such as paired-end or mate-pair sequencing, one is not limited to detection of point mutations and small insertions and deletions. With whole genome sequencing, one can also detect large deletions, duplications, and structural rearrangements (both balanced and unbalanced) such as translocations and inversions [37]. In a sense, whole genome sequencing is not merely "sequencing"; instead it provides much of the same information as sequencing, array CGH, and a chromosome study combined. That, combined with the ability to examine regulatory regions of any gene of interest and lack of exon dropout due to incomplete or suboptimal capture, makes whole genome sequencing a very powerful diagnostic tool. In addition, a clinical laboratory can still choose to apply the same filters as discussed previously in order to limit the data analyzed as per the clinical question.

Both whole exome and whole genome sequencing have the potential to revolutionize molecular medicine and help us enter the era of genomic medicine. However, the amount of data and variants generated by these methodologies can be overwhelming to the laboratory director, who must interpret the data, and the clinician and/or genetic counselor, who must relay this information to the patient in a meaningful manner. In fact, some estimates predict that each whole genome sequence may generate more than three million variants, all of which must be classified and potentially interpreted [38]. A small fraction of these variants will be known, clinically relevant detrimental mutations that are straightforward to interpret. However, the majority of variants (>99 %) will fall into one of several categories: variants of unknown significance in a clinically relevant gene, variants in genes with no known phenotypic effect, and known benign variants.

In order to interpret the overwhelming data in a meaningful way for the clinicians, identified variants will have to be filtered and classified to the best of the laboratory's ability. However, because neither whole exome sequencing nor whole genome sequencing is restricted to genes of known phenotypic significance, both will result not only in a huge number of variants of unknown significance, but also potentially a plethora of incidental findings such as variants resulting in infertility or carrier status for late-onset autosomal dominant disorders such as Huntington's disease that are both devastating and incurable. Because of issues such as these, even when whole exome sequencing becomes cost-effective as a clinical test, labs may choose to mask data and only analyze genes relevant to the patient's reason for testing or those with a known phenotype. For example, a laboratory may perform whole exome sequencing for every patient in order to simplify processes in the lab, and then apply different data "masks" in order to limit analysis to only the genes of interest given the reason for testing. In the case that additional sequence information was desired at a later time, either due to new information about a gene's pathogenicity or desire on the part of the patient, that data could theoretically be "unmasked" and analyzed at any time.

One publication addressed the issue of incidental findings in great depth [39]. Here, the authors describe a "binning" classification system. The first essential step of this process is determining, for each gene, which of the following bins it belongs: genes in which pathogenic variants are clinically actionable (bin 1); genes in which pathogenic variants have clinical relevance and pose high risk (bin 2C); genes in which variants have clinical significance and of moderate risk (bin 2B); genes in which variants have some clinical relevance but are of low risk (bin 2A); and finally, genes which currently have no known clinical significance (bin 3). Then, variants within each gene are classified by pathogenicity (known pathogenic, likely pathogenic, unknown significance, likely benign, etc.). For each patient, the authors propose, the variants found within these categorized genes may or may not be reported depending on their potential pathogenicity. This is only one of many potential ways to filter the enormous amount of data that will be generated for each patient using whole genome and whole exome sequencing; however, a clinical laboratory offering such testing must establish a similar system before commencing suchtesting.

Obviously, one laboratory alone cannot establish a comprehensive, accurate classification system for every gene in the human genome. The establishment of collaborations between multiple laboratories must occur to help classify genes and decide on reporting criteria. This will not only ensure consistency and standardization both within and between clinical laboratories but also will enable periodic review and, in the future, reclassification of genes and/or variants. The latter necessitates that multiple laboratories share deidentified patient sequence data, preferably including patient phenotype data, similar to that of the International Standards for Cytogenomic Arrays (ISCA) consortium [40].

Despite all of the benefits of next-generation sequencing's use in the world of molecular diagnostics, the Sanger method is likely to persist for the foreseeable future. Most laboratories will utilize Sanger sequencing to confirm variants identified by NGS, in fact this will likely be a regulatory requirement. In addition, there will also be situations in which there is a known genetic disorder in which the causative mutation has been identified segregating in a family. Individuals at risk of inheriting such a mutation may opt to have testing performed for only that specific mutation; since this would involve sequencing only a single exon or even just a portion, the most cost-effective way for a laboratory to perform such a test will likely be the Sanger method.

Other (Oncology and Infectious Disease)

Sequencing for Mendelian disorders exemplifies many of the potential abilities of NGS in the clinical laboratory. Obviously, its potential applications are much more far-reaching than merely congenital disorders. NGS has the potential to impart profound implications in the area of oncology and infectious disease.

Currently, a large battery of tests is utilized in order to provide diagnostic and prognostic information regarding solid tumors and especially hematologic malignancies. Patients with such neoplasms, depending on the type, may receive a series of tests that include one or more of the following: chromosome studies, molecular assays such as quantitative real-time PCR, and fluorescent in situ hybridization (FISH) using one or more probes specific for certain chromosomal rearrangements.

Next-generation sequencing could potentially replace most, or even all, of the battery of tests performed on oncology specimens while giving additional information that many of these tests cannot due to the nature of NGS and its lack of necessity of a priori knowledge of sequence. However, NGS for oncology specimens suffers from the same drawbacks as mentioned for congenital disorders, in addition to some that are specific to oncology testing. For example, many oncology specimens are small biopsies or fine needle aspirates that generally yield a small quantity of DNA. Furthermore, these specimens are traditionally fixed in formalin or an alternative preservative, which not only degrade genomic DNA but also may induce chemical modifications; however, NGS protocols for materials such as formalin-fixed, paraffin-embedded specimens are being developed [41]. Also important to keep in mind is that unlike a congenital specimen, which is typically homogenous, oncology specimens can have a great deal of heterogeneity. Therefore, it may be difficult to distinguish low level, relevant oncogenic mutations against a background of normal cells, which are often admixed in these specimens. However, there are many potential ways to enrich for tumor cells in these samples, including laser capture microdissection for solid tumors or cell sorting for hematologic specimens. Furthermore, a great deal of heterogeneity can be present even among the tumor cells themselves, which can also complicate the data analysis. Finally, it is currently common to sequence both tumor and matched normal tissue from the patient in order to filter out germline variants. This would, of course, increase the cost of the test. However, there is important information to be gained from also sequencing germline DNA such as potentially discovering pharmacogenetic alterations that may be important for deciding on the drug or dose with which to treat a given patient.

Infectious disease is another obvious niche in which NGS could have a huge impact on clinical testing. Molecular methods have revolutionized testing in the clinical microbiology laboratory; however, the techniques currently utilized typically require suspicion of a particular pathogen or strain, and the molecular assays are designed to detect, confirm, and/or differentiate between different strains (one pathogen-one test). If a negative result is obtained, additional testing may need to be performed. In addition, some pathogens such as RNA viruses mutate at extremely high rates, which could theoretically make molecular detection difficult. The beauty of next-generation sequencing is that, if a capture method is not used up-front, no a priori knowledge regarding the sequence to be interrogated is necessary. Therefore, if the appropriate specimen is tested by NGS, a complete genome sequence of the pathogen will be acquired and can be blasted against known genomic sequence to identify the culprit; hence, testing is for "any" pathogen. In addition, any potentially important sequence variants (drug-resistance mutations, etc.) would be simultaneously identified; in fact, NGS would be particularly amenable to detection of low-level drug resistant strains. The downfall to this approach is that sequence will be obtained from any DNA present in the sample, including that of the human host and other organisms such as bacteria that may be present yet do not contribute to disease.

Future Uses for NGS

In the near future, when whole genome sequencing is both feasible and cost-effective, one could imagine that every person will have their genome sequenced at some point. This opens up additional uses for this technology, such as newborn screening (NBS). NBS is mandatory in most states; however, the number and types of disorders screened for vary widely (anywhere from 3 to 43), but typically are limited to 29 "core" conditions and, in some cases, a number of additional secondary targets, chosen because they satisfy all or the majority of defined criteria, including the availability of a screening test with appropriate sensitivity and specificity, demonstrated benefits of early detection and available treatment [42]. However, there are a number of disorders that are not screened for at birth because they do not sufficiently satisfy these criteria but would still be beneficial to screen for. An example of this type of disorder is Wilson disease (WD). Wilson disease is an autosomal recessive disorder caused by mutations in *ATP7B*. The phenotype of WD can be severe, including liver disease, neurologic dysfunction, and psychiatric disturbance leading to intellectual deterioration. Unfortunately, the age of onset varies widely (early childhood to adulthood) and the symptoms vary to the point where a diagnosis of WD can be difficult to make. The latter point is important to realize because treatment with copper chelating agents can prevent the development of these hepatic, neurologic, and psychiatric symptoms if started in the asymptomatic period [43]. But, as with many autosomal recessive disorders, there are few clues as to the diagnosis until an affected individual presents with symptoms; hence, treatment is often not started until the phenotype manifests.

Wilson disease is only one example of a disorder that is not included in NBS panels yet would be beneficial to detect before symptoms arise. NGS opens the door to screening for this disorder, and essentially every known single gene disorder, at birth. One could simply collect blood from an infant after delivery and perform whole genome sequencing, either alone or (more likely at first) in tandem with the biochemical assays, which have a faster turnaround time. Since the amount of DNA collected from a newborn is typically very low, methods to increase the amount of DNA such as whole genome amplification may be necessary until NGS technology is amenable to such small sample quantities.

It is likely that by the time NGS is utilized for newborn screening, it will be more cost-effective to perform WGS rather than utilizing a capture method to isolate and analyze only the desired genes. Performing WGS at birth would allow for the detection of a multitude of disorders beyond those currently screened for. However, the tradeoff is that WGS will convey information regarding not only treatable disorders but also everything else-untreatable disorders of childhood, disorders with incomplete penetrance, adult-onset conditions, cancer syndromes, etc. This fact leads into a further consideration regarding the analysis of genomic sequence data—WGS can be performed up front, but one does not have to analyze all of the data up front. In fact, this would be ideal in the case of NBS because the analysis would be much faster if limited only to a subset of disorders suitable for screening at birth. The remaining data is stored, but not analyzed, until it is either necessary or requested. Hence, we may one day adapt a model in which every person has his or her genome sequenced, but the data is analyzed in sections as the clinical need for the data arises. Some of this analysis may occur at birth, with the remainder occurring later in life at specified time points. A pilot exploring a similar model is, in fact, currently underway in the Faroe Islands. The goal is to offer WGS to each of its 50,000 citizens but will begin with a pilot involving 100 adults in order to explore the many challenges of such an undertaking. This data will be linked to each individual's health records, and when a physician is questioning a particular condition, an inquiry will be sent in order to gain access to the relevant genomic information pertaining to the questioned diagnosis. Each individual would also have access to their own data, and the goal is to provide education to each person in order to ensure that they are adequately informed regarding such testing [44].

Physician/GC Considerations

With WGS, as with any genetic test, there is much to consider both pre- and posttest on the part of the physicians and/or genetic counselors. Currently, when a sequencing-based test is ordered, there is a specific question in mind, and the appropriate test is ordered based on that clinical question. With disease-oriented NGS panels, this will likely still be the case; however, the patient will need to be appropriately counseled regarding the greatly increased risk of detecting a VUS. However, exome and whole genome sequencing will require much more consideration both pre- and posttest. The physicians and genetic counselors who ultimately order the test are responsible for explaining to the patients, before ordering the test, the information that can be obtained from such studies. For example, individuals must understand that they will not only receive the information they are seeking, such as carrier status for rare recessive disorders, but also incidental information, such as late-onset neurologic (and often untreatable) conditions. Patients must also be cautioned that, even when a gene in which mutations are known to cause a disorder is found to have a sequence variant, there is a chance that the variant will have unknown significance. Additionally, patients and physicians alike must understand that of the 25,000 known genes in the human genome, many have unknown function or have never been described to harbor pathogenic mutations; hence, reporting any variants identified in these genes might not be medically valuable. Finally, it must be clear that every patient will likely be identified as a carrier for an autosomal recessive disorder. From these conversations, the care provider must be able to determine what information the patient wishes to learn. This will determine what test is ordered and what results are given to the patients.

Once the appropriate information is returned to the care provider from the laboratory, the laborious task of explaining the findings to the patient begins. For every possible sequence finding, the physician or genetic counselor must be able to relate the results not only to the immediate health-related question at hand, but also what, if any, future impact these results have. Finally, the physician needs to be able to understand and relay to the patient what implications these findings have for the patient's family members and potential future offspring.

Informatics

Introduction

The emergence of next generation sequencing instruments described in the previous section is poised to enable the implementation of new and revolutionary clinical tests. However, these opportunities are mirrored by formidable challenges associated with managing, processing, and interpreting the large datasets generated by these instruments. This technical complexity has resulted in the critical need for bioinformatics in any institution implementing NGS-based testing. Extracting useful information from the sea of short sequence reads generated by NGS systems requires multistep workflows designed to efficiently analyze the data. Interpreting the results to identify clinically actionable items presents an even bigger challenge, requiring aggregation and integration of multiple data sources to annotate the resulting variants. Finally, infrastructure requirements to analyze and store the data generated by current sequencing platforms often requires substantial investment in, and retooling of, institutional hardware. This section will provide a high-level overview of the informatics aspects of NGS.

NGS data analysis can be conceptualized as a four-step process, including on-instrument signal processing, sequence-read alignment, variant detection, and results annotation. Through this process, the physical readout of the nucleotide sequence is converted into a digital representation and presented, where possible, with specific context to enable an investigator or clinician to interpret the results. While the details of each step in this process vary with the sequencing instrument selected, test being performed, and selection of analytic tools by the lab, this process is conformed to in most sequencing assays and will be used to template our overview of the analytics in this section.

On-Instrument Signal Processing

With every sequencing instrument there are file conversion and signal processing methods that must be executed to convert the initial instrument readings into specific nucleotides and associated sequence reads. This step in the analysis process is often carried out by software provided with the sequencing instrument and is akin to analysis of a trace chromatogram from Sanger sequencing. For example, the Illumina sequencers measure florescent intensities from the flow cells by taking a series of digital images, which are processed into numeric values, and ultimately converted into single nucleotide base calls [45]. Individual base calls are then appended together to create a short-sequence "read" reflecting the sequence of the target DNA. With each called nucleotide base, there is a corresponding quality score that reflects the confidence in the base call and is instrumental in downstream alignment and variant-base detection. The resulting data is written to a file (standard file format FASTQ) for subsequent reference sequence realignment or de novo assembly [46].

Sequence Read Mapping/Assembly

Every NGS experiment generates millions of short nucleotide sequences, reflecting a highly redundant and overlapping set of reads derived from the original DNA. The process of creating a representation of the target DNA sequence involves mapping the reads back to a reference sequence (remapping) or the de novo assembly of overlapping reads to define larger sequences representative of the target (shot-gun assembly). For reasons of computational efficiency and to minimize the algorithmic complexity, most clinical sequencing applications of NGS rely on reference sequence remapping. Despite the relative computational efficiency, remapping still requires vast computational resources. Consequently, numerous mapping programs have been developed to accurately map the short read sequences (35–100 bases long) back to the reference genome using highly parallelized computer systems [47–51]. Many of the most popular programs used for remapping were first developed in academia and are offered under an open-source license. More recently, commercial offerings have increased, providing users with a number of choices when selecting an alignment program. Most alignment programs now support a standard post-alignment output format, the binary alignment map (BAM) [52]. The BAM file is directly viewable by a variety of visualization programs (i.e., IGV) and is the primary input file for most sequence variant detection programs [53].

Since the initial advent of NGS, significant advances have been made in the programs used to map these short-read sequences back to a reference genome. Most sequencing centers employ a complex series of bioinformatics processes to refine the initial read alignments. These include the use of base-quality scores to optimize read alignments, removal of identical short-reads that likely represent PCR amplification artifact, strategies to maximize the likelihood of properly placing a read that aligns to multiple places in a reference genome, and processes for improving the fidelity of alignments around highly variant regions of the target genome, to name a few. Many of these steps are included in current "best-practice" alignment protocols and analysis pipeline, such as the Broad's GATK alignment toolkit [54, 55].

Variant Detection

Following read alignment to the reference genome, the NGS data is processed by one or more programs designed to identify single nucleotide variants (SNVs) and short insertions and deletions (INDELs). Unlike Sanger sequencing, calling variants using NGS data often involves algorithms that incorporate several characteristics of the aligned data, including position-specific base counts (read-depth), quality values for the individual bases in each read aligned to a putative variant region, and quality values associated with how well the short-read aligned to the reference in the putative variant region. These characteristics are often integrated into either probabilistic-based algorithms or used as hard threshold to filter putative variants [54, 56]. The incorporation of these parameters in variant detection algorithms is used to account for potential sequencing and read-alignment errors. Unlike Sanger sequencing, NGS variant calls are often reported with a numeric estimate of the variant frequency in the aligned reads at a given position. Given the digital nature of this data, low-frequency variants arising from heteroplasmy or complex sample types can be identified. However, this is not a trivial process, as biases in the next-generation sequencing and analysis processes complicate the identification of simple heterozygotic variants, which can comprise between 30 and 65 %, and not exactly 50 %, of the bases at a given position. Therefore, all NGS assays will require substantial bioinformatics support to identify and account for sample- and process-specific biases.

Sequence Variant Annotation and Interpretation

Perhaps the single most challenging aspect of the NGS analysis process is curating variants with sufficient supporting information that will allow them to be rapidly and accurately interpreted by the clinical laboratory director. First pass annotation strategies often involve identifying variants with prior evidence that establishes them as benign polymorphic variants (SNPs) or known pathogenic variants. A variety of public data sources can be leveraged for these annotations, including the NCBI database dbSNP (which contains information on known polymorphisms) [57] and the HAPMAP [58] and the 1,000 genomes [59] projects, which contain information on the frequency of variant occurrence in different populations. Information about known pathogenic variants can be found in the Online Mendelian Inheritance in Man (OMIM) [60], the Human Gene Mutation Database (HGMD) [61], the GeneTests website [62], and other disease-specific resources.

Those variants without an unambiguous assignment, VUSs, are more difficult to curate. One can first easily determine whether the given variant is synonymous, non-synonymous (missense), nonsense, or frameshift. However, unless a variant is an obvious loss of function mutation (nonsense or frameshift), additional tools are necessary in order to gather more information as to the potential pathogenicity of the variant. There are many programs that incorporate species conservation, encoded protein structure, and amino-acid substitution properties to predict the likelihood a non-synonymous variant is disruptive to the encoded protein [63, 64].

Additionally, inferences of disruption of known splice sites and regulatory element binding motifs can also be made using publically and commercially available softwares.

As institutions begin adopting this technology for clinical testing, they must be prepared to add bioinformaticians to the staff involved in the assay development and implementation. These professionals will provide the expertise needed to manage, analyze, and aid in the interpretation of the vast amounts of raw data generated. On a related note, one of the potentially unanticipated impacts of next-generation sequencing is the size and scope of the datasets generated and computational infrastructure needed to analyze it. The rapidly escalating output from NGS platforms (measured in gigabases) has lead to the revamping of most institutional computational centers to accommodate requirements for post-sequencing data processing. The volume of raw and processed data has likewise forced institutions to critically assess data storage capacity and more-often-than-not led to the development of highly structured/limited data retention policies. Data retention policies need to be defined and endorsed by the regulatory community, including definitions of what is the primary data generated by NGS instruments and how long should it be stored by a clinical lab. Beyond this, the scope of the raw information that is presented back to investigators is also driving the development of integrated systems for results filtering and interpretation. Despite these technical challenges, NGS is beginning to revolutionize clinical laboratories and is creating exciting new opportunities for the world of clinical diagnostics.

Regulatory Considerations

The transformational power of NGS in the diagnostic arena has been thoroughly discussed in this chapter. With such potential, one might expect that making a decision to implement a clinical diagnostic NGS laboratory would be trivial. However, even after the necessary chemistry and informatics pipelines are in place, significant effort must be put into understanding how the current regulatory environment could impact clinical NGS testing. This is made even more complicated in the light of changing FDA policies regarding laboratory developed tests (LDTs) [65].

In the past, the FDA has exercised what it calls "enforcement discretion" of LDTs, allowing other regulatory bodies and legislation like the Center for Medicare and Medicaid Services (CMS) and The Clinical Laboratory Improvement Amendments (CLIA) to regulate this type of testing [66]. However, with the recent explosion of high-complexity testing and direct-to-consumer (DTC) genetic tests, the FDA is creating new guidance for the development, validation, and implementation of LDTs. There is currently significant uncertainty about what this guidance will look like and what amount of effort it will take to satisfy the new FDA regulations. This concern is so significant that many clinical laboratories have chosen to postpone the implementation of NGS-based assays until these new regulations are clear [67].

Fortunately, there are a number of organizations moving forward with their own draft guidance regarding NGS test development and implementation to help address some of FDA's concerns. Recently, the American College of Medical Genetics (ACMG) published a brief report on one of the FDA's top LDT concerns, the clinical utility of NGS [68]. In the ACMG document, the college outlines three areas where they feel the clinical utility of NGS is well established. The first scenario recognized in this document is the potential for significant improvements in the diagnosis, prognosis, and treatment decisions made for patients suffering from late stage cancers. In another, they describe the clinical utility of sequencing parents and their affected children in cases where the suspicion of a genetic disorder is high, but standard DNA testing has failed to resolve the case and identify a diagnosis. Finally, the ACMG supports (with caveats) the notion that some individuals will want to perform "exploratory sequencing" of their personal genome to be "screened" for health conditions they may be at a higher risk to develop. In this third class, a very clear note is made regarding the higher bar for reporting variants when there is no specific disease pathway under investigation, stating "the threshold for determining which results should be returned to individuals seeking screening should be set significantly higher than that set for diagnostic testing due to the much lower a priori chance of disease in such individuals."

Validation and Quality Control

It could be said that NGS is one of the most complex laboratory methodologies to be implemented in the clinical diagnostic arena to date. It is true that there are many considerations to take into account regarding sample preparation, sequencing equipment, computer hardware, and software. However, the fact remains that this is a controllable process that is not fundamentally different from any other LDT and can therefore be fully understood by performing a robust test validation. Currently, there are no specific FDA, CLIA, or CAP guidelines regarding the validation of a clinical NGS test. While the ACMG addressed regulatory issues like clinical utility, other groups like the Centers for Disease Control and Prevention (CDC), Division of Laboratory Science and Standards, are now focusing on the analytical performance of diagnostic NGS tests. In a developing document, the CDC workgroup plans to address test Validation, Quality Control, Strategies for Proficiency Testing, and the development of Reference Materials all in support of clinical NGS [69]. Briefly stated, it will be important to create a validation strategy that addresses the performance of the specific NGS platform being utilized. This should include all of the reagents for sequence enrichment, library preparation, sequence generation, and the instrument itself. In addition, the bioinformatics pipeline (hardware and software) should undergo rigorous optimization during this platform validation. Finally, the test proper should be validated. This will include running a number of well-characterized samples to be certain the NGS process is identifying the mutations the test has been developed to detect. This is easily accomplished for relatively small panel type tests, but much more difficult for whole exome and whole genome sequencing. In the latter example, it may have to suffice to validate regions of the targeted design, and then extrapolate that performance to the rest of the exome or genome. In addition, the extremely large number of possible variants coupled with the relatively high false positive variant detection rate will dictate that all "reportable" variants be verified by an existing laboratory gold standard methodology. Finally, there is a need to validate the informatics pipeline for its ability to detect the types of mutations expected in the sample population. Currently, most informatics pipelines are very good at finding single nucleotide variants but struggle with accurately detecting insertions and deletions. One interesting method for pipeline validation that has been discussed is to create known synthetic data sets that represent all imaginable types of alterations through the system. The results of such a test should give you a very good idea of what your system will and will not detect.

The adoption of next-generation sequencing as a standard clinical testing modality will also require substantial advancements in quality control and assurance processes for this technology. As is the case for validation, there are currently no guidelines that specifically address clinical grade quality control of next generation sequencing. Additionally, there is often little to no validation or control of the public datasets routinely used for the annotation and interpretation of sequencing results. Despite the need and opportunity for massive growth in this area, steps can be taken to monitor mapping accuracy and feature detection by implementing routine quality-control testing protocols that leverage the same well-characterized datasets used for validation. Understanding the performance metrics of the entire NGS test process, monitoring these metrics over time, and communicating known limitations to ordering physicians will be critical to the successful clinical implementation of this technology.

Intellectual Property

There is very little debate regarding the value of a patent's ability to protect the intellectual property (IP) of scientists and inventors. That general agreement falls to the wayside when the question revolves around processes and compositions that are considered products of nature. In this light, the individual genes in the human genome have historically been patentable, but with much controversy as many feel they are "natural occurrences" and thus not patentable [70]. This is becoming a very important issue as diagnostic laboratories begin to outfit themselves with the technical capabilities to sequence entire exomes and genomes. Even though it is possible to generate a whole exome or whole genome sequence for a single individual in a diagnostic laboratory, with the current patent laws in place, it is illegal for any single laboratory to issue a comprehensive interpretative genome-wide report. In essence, no diagnostic complete genome is truly complete as individual laboratories do not hold rights to the IP required to report mutations found in every gene. This might not be completely accurate, as most current gene patents refer to an isolation process that techniques like WGS might circumvent. This has not been challenged in court yet.

The issue of gene patents has been challenged by the American Civil Liberties Union (ACLU) in a case they have initiated against the United States Patent and Trademark Office and Myriad Genetics *Association For Molecular Pathology, et al., vs. United States Patent and Trademark Office, et al.* [71]. The case, initiated in 2009, revolves around the ability for a patent to be issued for a "natural occurrence," of which the ACLU posits, genes are. The position taken by the ACLU is that by owning patents for *BRCA1* and *BRCA2*, Myriad can essentially monopolize diagnostic testing for these important breast and ovarian cancer-related genes. Allowing gene patents has led to increased costs for diagnostic testing and virtually no recourse for a second opinion. In March of 2010, the ACLU's position was validated by a federal district court, but the judgment was quickly appealed and partially overturned in July of 2011 [72]. Though the ACLU and Myriad would both like to have the case heard by the US Supreme Court, the justices have recommended that the case be reconsidered using the recent *Prometheus v Mayo Collaborative Services* decision [73, 74]. In this landmark case, the Supreme Court has made it clear that "natural observances" are not patentable subject matter.

The decision of this case will have a profound effect on how genome sequencing will be deployed in the clinical setting. At this time, small, focused panels are desirable due to their relative simplicity. However, as the cost of sequencing decreases and sequencers and informatics pipelines become easier to use, many assume that whole genome sequencing will become the default molecular test. If, however, intellectual property rights exist for individual genes, the task of obtaining the appropriate licenses could become logistically and financially prohibitive, so much so that no single institution could realistically provide a true comprehensive genome interpretation.

Conclusions

In a very brief period of time, NGS technologies have transformed from a billion dollar research project to just a few thousand dollars per genome with real clinical value. While the price is still too high for high volume genomes, focused high-content panels have an immediate, value focused, application in the clinical diagnostic laboratory. These panels will continue to grow in number and utilization for the next 2–3 years. Very quickly however, we will see most clinical DNA sequencing switching from panels to whole genomes. The importance of continued bioinformatics investments cannot be understated. Creating high output sequencing data has become routine. Extracting value, in a timely and cost-effective manner, from that sequencing data is the "secret sauce" of the genomics future. Understanding the "whole genome" will be an endless journey. This further understanding is required to fully extract the value of a whole genome sequence. While NGS is indeed a LDT, the workings of the system are of the most complex used in diagnostic laboratories to date. Important issues regarding the oversight of LDT's by the FDA, CMS, CAP, and others will need further clarification in order to promote the full potential of WGS. Finally, even when all the technical and regulatory issues are settled, there remain the complex issues surrounding IP and gene patents. If a full genome sequence exists, but cannot be interpreted, it is of marginal value.

References

1. Watson JD, Crick FH. Molecular structure of nucleic acids; a structure for deoxyribose nucleic acid. Nature. 1953;171(4356):737–8.
2. Maxam AM, Gilbert W. A new method for sequencing DNA. Proc Natl Acad Sci USA. 1977; 74(2):560–4.
3. Sanger F, Nicklen S, Coulson AR. DNA sequencing with chain-terminating inhibitors. Proc Natl Acad Sci USA. 1977;74(12):5463–7.
4. Smith LM, et al. The synthesis of oligonucleotides containing an aliphatic amino group at the 5' terminus: synthesis of fluorescent DNA primers for use in DNA sequence analysis. Nucleic Acids Res. 1985; 13(7):2399–412.
5. Sanger F, Coulson AR. A rapid method for determining sequences in DNA by primed synthesis with DNA polymerase. J Mol Biol. 1975;94(3):441–8.
6. Tsuda T, et al. Separation of nucleotides by high-voltage capillary electrophoresis. J Appl Biochem. 1983;5(4–5):330–6.
7. Venter JC, et al. The sequence of the human genome. Science. 2001;291(5507):1304–51.
8. Lander ES, et al. Initial sequencing and analysis of the human genome. Nature. 2001;409(6822):860–921.
9. Szybalski W. From the double-helix to novel approaches to the sequencing of large genomes. Gene. 1993;135(1–2):279–90.
10. International Human Genome Sequencing Consortium. Finishing the euchromatic sequence of the human genome. Nature. 2004;431(7011):931–45.
11. Collins FS, Morgan M, Patrinos A. The human genome project: lessons from large-scale biology. Science. 2003;300(5617):286–90.
12. Venter JC. Shotgunning the human genome: a personal view. Encyclopedia of Life Science. 2006.
13. Fink L, Collins FS. The human genome project: view from the national institutes of health. J Am Med Womens Assoc. 1997; 52(1):4–7, 15.
14. Nakano M, et al. Single-molecule reverse transcription polymerase chain reaction using water-in-oil emulsion. J Biosci Bioeng. 2005;99(3):293–5.
15. Williams R, et al. Amplification of complex gene libraries by emulsion PCR. Nat Methods. 2006; 3(7):545–50.
16. Metzker ML. Sequencing technologies – the next generation. Nat Rev Genet. 2010;11(1):31–46.
17. Margulies M, et al. Genome sequencing in microfabricated high-density picolitre reactors. Nature. 2005; 437(7057):376–80.
18. Bentley DR, et al. Accurate whole human genome sequencing using reversible terminator chemistry. Nature. 2008;456(7218):53–9.
19. McKernan KJ, et al. Sequence and structural variation in a human genome uncovered by short-read, massively parallel ligation sequencing using two-base encoding. Genome Res. 2009;19(9):1527–41.
20. Rothberg JM, et al. An integrated semiconductor device enabling non-optical genome sequencing. Nature. 2011;475(7356):348–52.
21. Bowers J, et al. Virtual terminator nucleotides for next-generation DNA sequencing. Nat Methods. 2009; 6(8):593–5.
22. Eid J, et al. Real-time DNA sequencing from single polymerase molecules. Science. 2009;323(5910): 133–8.
23. Flusberg BA, et al. Direct detection of DNA methylation during single-molecule, real-time sequencing. Nat Methods. 2010;7(6):461–5.
24. Maglia G, et al. Analysis of single nucleic acid molecules with protein nanopores. Methods Enzymol. 2010; 475:591–623.
25. Lunshof JE, et al. Personal genomes in progress: from the human genome project to the personal genome project. Dialogues Clin Neurosci. 2010;12(1):47–60.
26. Albert TJ, et al. Direct selection of human genomic loci by microarray hybridization. Nat Methods. 2007;4(11):903–5.
27. Gnirke A, et al. Solution hybrid selection with ultra-long oligonucleotides for massively parallel targeted sequencing. Nat Biotechnol. 2009;27(2):182–9.
28. Tewhey R, et al. Microdroplet-based PCR enrichment for large-scale targeted sequencing. Nat Biotechnol. 2009;27(11):1025–31.
29. MacConaill LE, et al. Clinical implementation of comprehensive strategies to characterize cancer genomes: opportunities and challenges. Cancer Discov. 2011;1(4):297–311.
30. Riordan JR, et al. Identification of the cystic fibrosis gene: cloning and characterization of complementary DNA. Science. 1989;245(4922):1066–73.
31. Smith RJH, Sheffield AM, Van Camp G. Nonsyndromic hearing loss and deafness, DFNA3. 1998 Sep 28, 2012 Apr 19 [cited 2012]. Available from: http://www.ncbi.nlm.nih.gov/books/NBK1536/
32. Schouten JP, et al. Relative quantification of 40 nucleic acid sequences by multiplex ligation-dependent probe amplification. Nucleic Acids Res. 2002;30(12):e57.
33. Ijssel P, Ylstra B. Oligonucleotide array comparative genomic hybridization. Methods Mol Biol. 2007; 396:207–21.
34. Lockwood WW, et al. Recent advances in array comparative genomic hybridization technologies and their applications in human genetics. Eur J Hum Genet. 2006;14(2):139–48.
35. Gross SJ, Pletcher BA, Monaghan KG. Carrier screening in individuals of Ashkenazi Jewish descent. Genet Med. 2008;10(1):54–6.

36. Ku CS, Naidoo N, Pawitan Y. Revisiting Mendelian disorders through exome sequencing. Hum Genet. 2011;129(4):351–70.
37. Chen W, et al. Breakpoint analysis of balanced chromosome rearrangements by next-generation paired-end sequencing. Eur J Hum Genet. 2010;18(5):539–43.
38. Gonzaga-Jauregui C, Lupski JR, Gibbs RA. Human genome sequencing in health and disease. Annu Rev Med. 2012;63:35–61.
39. Berg JS, Khoury MJ, Evans JP. Deploying whole genome sequencing in clinical practice and public health: meeting the challenge one bin at a time. Genet Med. 2011;13(6):499–504.
40. Kaminsky EB, et al. An evidence-based approach to establish the functional and clinical significance of copy number variants in intellectual and developmental disabilities. Genet Med. 2011;13(9):777–84.
41. Wood HM, et al. Using next-generation sequencing for high resolution multiplex analysis of copy number variation from nanogram quantities of DNA from formalin-fixed paraffin-embedded specimens. Nucleic Acids Res. 2010;38(14):e151.
42. Newborn screening: toward a uniform screening panel and system. Genet Med. 2006;8(Suppl 1):1S–252S.
43. Cox DW, Roberts EA. Wilson disease. 1999 Oct 22, 2006 Jan 24 [cited 2012]. Available from: http://www.ncbi.nlm.nih.gov/books/NBK1512/
44. Kupferschmidt K. Danish Archipelago launches mass sequencing plan. ScienceInsider. 2011
45. Ansorge WJ. Next-generation DNA sequencing techniques. New Biotechnol. 2009;25(4):195–203.
46. Cock PJ, et al. The Sanger FASTQ file format for sequences with quality scores, and the Solexa/Illumina FASTQ variants. Nucleic Acids Res. 2010;38(6):1767–71.
47. Langmead B, et al. Ultrafast and memory-efficient alignment of short DNA sequences to the human genome. Genome Biol. 2009;10(3):R25.
48. Li H, Durbin R. Fast and accurate short read alignment with Burrows-Wheeler transform. Bioinformatics. 2009;25(14):1754–60.
49. Li H, Ruan J, Durbin R. Mapping short DNA sequencing reads and calling variants using mapping quality scores. Genome Res. 2008;18(11):1851–8.
50. Li R, et al. SOAP: short oligonucleotide alignment program. Bioinformatics. 2008;24(5):713–4.
51. Li R, et al. SOAP2: an improved ultrafast tool for short read alignment. Bioinformatics. 2009;25(15):1966–7.
52. Li H, et al. The sequence alignment/map format and SAMtools. Bioinformatics. 2009;25(16):2078–9.
53. Robinson JT, et al. Integrative genomics viewer. Nat Biotechnol. 2011;29(1):24–6.
54. DePristo MA, et al. A framework for variation discovery and genotyping using next-generation DNA sequencing data. Nat Genet. 2011;43(5):491–8.
55. McKenna A, et al. The genome analysis toolkit: a MapReduce framework for analyzing next-generation DNA sequencing data. Genome Res. 2010;20(9):1297–303.
56. Goya R, et al. SNVMix: predicting single nucleotide variants from next-generation sequencing of tumors. Bioinformatics. 2010;26(6):730–6.
57. Sherry ST, et al. dbSNP: the NCBI database of genetic variation. Nucleic Acids Res. 2001;29(1):308–11.
58. International HapMap Consortium. The international HapMap project. Nature. 2003;426(6968):789–96.
59. 1000 Genomes Project Consortium, Abecasis GR, Altshuler D, Auton A, Brooks LD, Durbin RM, Gibbs RA, Hurles ME, McVean GA. A map of human genome variation from population-scale sequencing. Nature. 2010;467(7319):1061–73.
60. Online Mendelian Inheritance in Man, OMIM. 2012.
61. Stenson PD, et al. Human Gene Mutation Database (HGMD): 2003 update. Hum Mutat. 2003;21(6):577–81.
62. GeneTests Medical Genetics Information Resource. 2012.
63. Adzhubei IA, et al. A method and server for predicting damaging missense mutations. Nat Methods. 2010;7(4):248–9.
64. Ng PC, Henikoff S. Predicting deleterious amino acid substitutions. Genome Res. 2001;11(5):863–74.
65. Department of Health and Human Services. Oversight of Laboratory Developed Tests; Public Meeting; Request for Comments, Department of Health and Human Services, Editor. 2010. Federal Register http://www.gpo.gov. p. 34463–4.
66. CMS.gov. Clinical Laboratory Improvement Amendments (CLIA). Centers for Medicare and Medicaid Services. Available from: http://www.cms.gov/Regulations-and-Guidance/Legislation/CLIA/index.html
67. Vorhaus D. The FDA and DTC genetic testing: setting the record straight. In: Vorhaus D, editor. Genomics law report. Charlotte, NC: Robinson Bradshaw and Hinson; 2011.
68. American College of Medical Genetics. Points to consider in the clinical application of genomic sequencing [Policy Statement]. 2012. Available from: http://www.acmg.net/StaticContent/PPG/Clinical_Application_of_Genomic_Sequencing.pdf
69. Gargis AS, et al. Next generation sequencing – standardization of clinical testing (Nex-StoCT): approaches to quality assurance and complying with regulatory and professional standards. 2011. Available from: http://www.cdc.gov/osels/lspppo/pdf/2011AMPPoster.pdf
70. United States Patent and Trademark Office Commerce. Utility examination guidelines. Federal Register Online via the Government Printing Office. 2001. http://www.gpo.gov. p. 1092–9.
71. Association For Molecular Pathology. Association for molecular pathology, et al., vs. United States patent and trademark office, et al. 2010. Case 1:09-cv-04515-RWS.
72. United States Court of Appeals for the Federal Circuit. Appeal from the United States District Court for the Southern District of New York in Case No.

09-CV-4515, Senior Judge Robert W. Sweet. United States Court of Appeals for the Federal Circuit. 2011. http://www.cafc.uscourts.gov
73. Supreme Court of the United States. Mayo collaborative services, DBA Mayo Medical Laboratories, et Al. v. Prometheus Laboratories, INC. Supreme Court of the United States. 2011. http://www.supremecourt.gov
74. Supreme Court of the United States. Certiorari – summary despositions. Supreme Court of the United States. 2012. http://www.supremecourt.gov/orders. p. 11–725.

Index

W.E. Highsmith Jr. (ed.), *Molecular Diagnostics: 12 Tests That Changed Everything*, Molecular and Translational Medicine, DOI 10.1007/978-1-4614-8127-0,

I

L

MIX
Papier aus verantwortungsvollen Quellen
Paper from responsible sources
FSC® C105338

If you have any concerns about our products,
you can contact us on
ProductSafety@springernature.com

In case Publisher is established outside the EU,
the EU authorized representative is:
Springer Nature Customer Service Center GmbH
Europaplatz 3, 69115 Heidelberg, Germany

Printed by Libri Plureos GmbH
in Hamburg, Germany